EAR, NOSE, AND THROAT DISORDERS IN CHILDREN

Ear, Nose, and Throat Disorders in Children

John E. Bordley, M.D., F.A.C.S.
Andelot Professor (Emeritus), Laryngology and Otology
Chairman, Department of Laryngology and Otology (Emeritus)
The Johns Hopkins University School of Medicine
Professor, Environmental Medicine (Emeritus)
The Johns Hopkins University School of Hygiene and Public Health
Otolaryngologist in Charge
The Johns Hopkins Hospital (Emeritus)
Baltimore, Maryland

Patrick E. Brookhouser, M.D., F.A.C.S.
Director, Boys Town National Institute for Communication Disorders in Children
Father Edward Flanagan Professor and Chairman
Department of Otolaryngology and Human Communication
Creighton University School of Medicine
Omaha, Nebraska

Gabriel Frederick Tucker, Jr. M.D., F.A.C.S.
Head, Division, Bronchoesophagology–Otolaryngology
Department of Communicative Disorders
Children's Memorial Hospital
Professor of Otolaryngology, Head and Neck Surgery,
Northwestern University, School of Medicine
Chicago, Illinois

Raven Press ■ New York

Raven Press, 1140 Avenue of the Americas, New York, New York 10036

Made in the United States of America

Library of Congress Cataloging-in-Publication Data

Bordley, John E.
  Ear, nose, and throat disorders in children.

  Includes bibliographies and index.
  1. Pediatric otolaryngology.   I. Brookhouser,
Patrick E.   II. Tucker, Gabriel F., 1924–   .
III. Title.   [DNLM: 1. Otorhinolaryngologic Diseases—
in infancy & childhood   WV 100 B729e]
RF47.C4B67   1985   618.92′09751   85-19285
ISBN 0-89004-324-8

Preface

This volume discusses the disorders and diseases of the ears, nose, throat, larynx, and associated structures in children.

Presented in this volume is a description of the embryology and the anatomy and physiology of the particular region under discussion, with directions for the proper clinical examination, followed by a description of the disorders and diseases affecting that region. For each of these disorders and diseases the diagnostic symptoms and physical findings that may be anticipated are presented. The usual clinical course is described, and the pathological changes that can appear during its course are outlined.

Therapy is discussed to the extent that it can be directed from a medical or pediatric point of view. Danger signs are emphasized that may indicate the need for specialist referral. Such specialized consultation, with its own examination techniques and recommendations for more sophisticated therapy and/or surgical intervention, is necessary after failure of time-tried and proved medical treatments. Surgical intervention and surgical reconstruction are discussed in general terms so that the attending doctor can understand the underlying rationale and be better prepared to discuss the surgery with the parents.

At the end of each section is an authoritative bibliography of pertinent articles chosen for the broad coverage of the topics presented in that section. The bibliography should provide the pediatrician, family practitioner, otolaryngologist, house officer, and medical student with a practical, clinical guide.

This volume is designed as a compact reference book that will be useful to pediatricians, general practitioners, resident trainees in otolaryngology, pediatrics, and family practice, and medical students. It will also be useful to the busy practicing otolaryngologist as a ready reference source for pediatric problems.

John E. Bordley, M.D.

Acknowledgments

Credit is gratefully given to the following for their valuable contributions to Chapter 2 of this volume:

David G. Cyr, Ph.D., Coordinator, Vestibular Services, Boys Town National Institute for Communication Disorders in Children; Assistant Professor of Human Communication, Department of Otolaryngology and Human Communication, Creighton University School of Medicine (Section 6: Vestibular Assessment).

Eric Javel, Ph.D., Senior Scientist, Auditory Physiology, Boys Town National Institute for Communication Disorders in Children; Professor of Human Communication, Department of Otolaryngology and Human Communication, Creighton University School of Medicine (Section 1: Anatomy and Physiology).

John T. Lybolt, Ph.D., formerly Coordinator, Speech/Language Services, Boys Town National Institute for Communication Disorders in Children; now in North Brook, Illinois (Section 7: Speech and Language Disorders: A Clinical Perspective).

Betty Jane Philips, Ed.D., Director, Special Clinical Program Development, Boys Town National Institute for Communication Disorders in Children; Professor of Human Communication, Department of Otolaryngology and Human Communication, Creighton University School of Medicine (Section 7: Speech and Language Disorders: A Clinical Perspective).

Shelley D. Smith, Ph.D., Clinical Genetics Research Associate, Boys Town National Institute for Communication Disorders in Children; Assistant Professor of Human Communication, Department of Otolaryngology and Human Communication, Creighton University School of Medicine (Section 4: Childhood Hearing Loss: Medical/Genetic Considerations).

Don W. Worthington, Ph.D., Director, Clinical Communication Sciences, Boys Town National Institute for Communication Disorders in Children; Professor of Human Communication, Department of Otolaryngology and Human Communication, Creighton University School of Medicine (Section 5: Measurement of Hearing).

Many thanks are also due to Judith A. Brookhouser for her artwork of the ear, to Tamara L. Williams for her help as a word processor, and to Gail L. Binderup for her administrative help and editing of Chapter 2.

With regard to Chapter 7, we would like to express our appreciation to Zelda Oser Zelinsky for the excellent line drawings that illustrate this chapter and to the Edward Shedd Wells Foundation for their generous support of the Laryngeal Development Laboratory.

Deep appreciation is extended to Linda Reese (Mrs. Frederic) for typing the original book outline and later for her help in preparation of the remaining chapters of this book. Special thanks are due for her good-humored acceptance of those long Sunday telephone conferences and for her help in the use of the English language.

Last but certainly not least, we wish to thank Dr. Diana Schneider of Raven Press for her unfailing encouragement to undertake and complete this book.

This book is dedicated to our wives with love and apologies for spending so many hours on weekends in its preparation.

Contents

1 Mucous Membranes of the Ear, Nose, Throat, and
    Associated Structures   1

2 The Ear
    Section 1:   Anatomy and Physiology   20
    Section 2:   Ear Examination Techniques and External
                 Ear Disorders   40
    Section 3:   Otitis Media and Mastoid Disease   65
    Section 4:   Childhood Hearing Loss: Medical/Genetic
                 Considerations   98
    Section 5:   Measurement of Hearing   149
    Section 6:   Vestibular Assessment   174
    Section 7:   Speech and Language Disorders:
                 A Clinical Perspective   192

3 Hearing-Impaired Child: The Pediatrician's Role   211

4 Nose and Accessory Nasal Sinuses   228

5 Mouth and Pharynx   317

6 Neck   383

7 Larynx   405

    Subject Index   433

Chapter 1

Mucous Membranes of the Ear, Nose, Throat, and Associated Structures

Histology 1
Functions 2
   Respiration 2
   Olfaction 7
Conditions Causing Injury 8
   Environment 8
   Infections 9
   Man-Made Agents 18
   Trauma 18
Comment 19

HISTOLOGY

Mucous membranes are a modification of the epithelial tissue forming the protective sheet of cells that covers the body as skin and becomes the epithelial lining (mucous membrane) of the primitive digestive tube. The epithelial lining of the respiratory tract originates as an evagination of the digestive tube. The epithelial tissues of the digestive–pulmonary tract arise from the ectoblast or the entoblast.

Mucous membranes are continuous throughout the respiratory and digestive tracts. They are formed by a surface of epithelial cells resting on a thin basement membrane below which lies a network of blood vessels and nerves in loose connective tissue, the tunica propria (Fig. 1-1). Numerous mucous cells (goblet cells) (Fig. 1-2) are distributed along its surface; numerous small mucous and serous glands lie just beneath the surface and empty through small outlets onto that surface. The epithelial surface of mucous membrane varies in composition from ciliated to pavement epithelium according to its function.

1

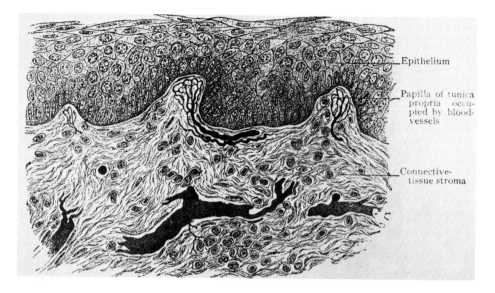

FIG. 1-1. Section of human oral squamous mucous membrane. (×350.) (Piersol Anatomy, 1923.)

Ciliated, columnar epithelium forms the surface of the respiratory mucous membrane found in the respiratory tract except for the nasal vestibule, the lower two-thirds of the nasopharynx, the pharynx, the mouth, the larynx, and the alveoli of the lung (Fig. 1-3). It lines the accessory nasal sinuses, the eustachian tube, and most of the adjacent middle ear. In the upper nasal fossa, from the cribriform plate to the middle of the superior turbinate and extending down the nasal septum to about the same level, the mucous membrane becomes nonciliated and contains olfactory cells. The pharynx, mouth, and tongue are covered with stratified squamous epithelium, whereas the upper two-thirds of the larynx including the vocal cords is lined with nonciliated squamous epithelium that is very tightly bound to the underlying structures. The alveoli of the lung are lined by a single layer of pavement-type epithelium, which forms the respiratory membrane.

FUNCTIONS

Respiration

The mucous membrane in the respiratory tract facilitates preparation of air that passes through the nose, trachea, and bronchi into the alveoli so that oxygen and carbon dioxide exchange can take place. The stratified squamous mucous membranes line the mouth where food particles and the mucous blankets discharged into

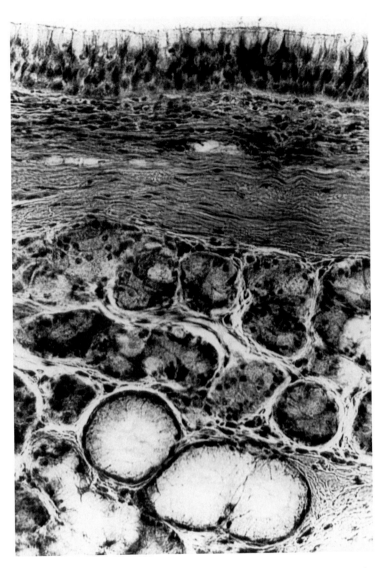

FIG. 1-2. Human ciliated respiratory mucous membrane from near the eustachian tube orifice. Note the ciliated cells, basement membrane, and mucous glands.

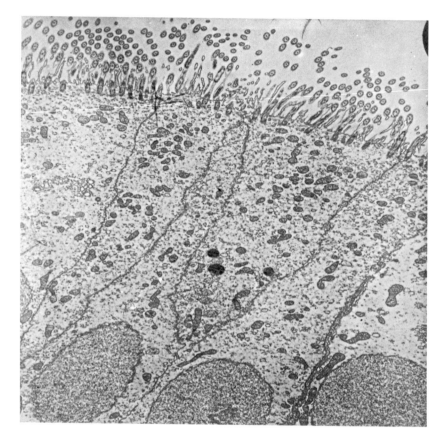

FIG. 1-3. Normal respiratory mucous membrane of a ferret. (From Hotz, G., and Bang, F. B.: Electronmicroscopic study of ferret respiratory cells infected with influenza virus. *Bull. Johns Hopkins Hosp.*, 101:175–208, 1967. With permission.)

the mouth from the nose and bronchi are passed into the digestive tract. Olfactory mucous membranes mediate the sense of smell.

Exchange of oxygen and carbon dioxide in the lung can occur only through a water medium at the membrane barrier in the alveolus. It is therefore necessary that the air be cleaned and heated and reach saturation before entering the alveolus. There, oxygen diffuses from a region containing a higher concentration of gas molecules, the alveolus, to a region of lower molecular concentration, the blood-stream. The same mechanism is responsible for the movement of carbon dioxide into the alveolus from its higher concentration in the blood. Any lack of saturation at the alveolar–pulmonary membrane can interfere with oxygen and carbon dioxide diffusion across that membrane. This mechanism may result from the fact that the respiratory tract in man is the evolution of a system that was originally developed for gaseous exchange in the completely fluid medium of the ocean. It is a system that later had to adapt itself to the gaseous atmosphere found on the surface of the land masses that rose from the sea.

The mucous membranes of the nose are primarily concerned with cleaning and conditioning of inspired air and, secondarily, perform their protective function of olfaction. In conditioning the air, the turbinates covered by erectile tissue play a major role. Under the membranes of these turbinates, arterioles and venules run in an anterior–posterior direction, resembling steam pipes in a boiler. Constriction or dilatation of these vessels through autonomic stimuli controls the hydrostatic pressure in the capillaries of the tissues, thus regulating the pressure of tissue fluids and metering the amount of water delivered to the membrane surface by transudation. Such control of blood flow can also regulate the heat supplied to warm air passing over the mucous membranes on inspiration, so that its temperature can properly be controlled to increase or decrease water content. As inspired air descends into the lungs, its temperature normally increases. As the air warms, more moisture is supplied by the mucous membranes of the nose, trachea, and upper bronchi. Regulation of humidity is controlled in part by the degree of water saturation of the mucous blanket covering the surface of these membranes. According to Starling, some of the water used in this humidification is regained through condensation taking place in the nose on expiration. Inspired air may take up as much as a liter of water a day. Unless the mucosa of the nose supplies most of this fluid, there is dangerous drying of the mucous membrane in the lower respiratory tract, which results in alteration of the moisture content and pH of the mucous blanket and may also interfere with normal streaming of the mucous blanket. Excessively hot inspired air can be low in water content, and the combination of heat and low humidity can cause serious alteration in the normal function of the mucous membrane.

Inspired air is first filtered by the vibrissae of the nose. Smaller foreign particles including microorganisms are entrapped by the mucous blanket covering the surfaces of normal respiratory mucous membranes. This elastic, sticky material is produced by goblet cells and small mucous glands, which extend from the vestibule of the nose to the alveoli of the lungs (Fig. 1-4). Mucus of approximately pH 7 has, according to Fleming, a bacteriostatic effect attributable to lysozymes that dissolve bacteria. Negus stated that mucus also acts as waterproofing for the membrane surface and protects the cilia. By surface attraction under the influence of electrical charges, foreign particles are entrapped in the mucus and are swept with it from the nose into the nasopharynx and from the bronchi and trachea into the larynx, at which point they are discharged into the mouth and swallowed.

Cilia, which were discovered by DeHeide in 1683, play an important role in this cleansing system. In man, nasal cilia measure about 7μm in length and about 0.3μm in diameter and cover the exposed surfaces of ciliated cells. The distance between the cilia approximately equals their diameter, and they are curved in the direction of their beat. Cilia are not activated by any known nerve complex, and individual ciliated cells continue to beat for a long time after total detachment from surrounding mucous membranes. They seem to be genetically coded to beat in a specific direction; when a section of mucous membrane is removed, rotated 180 degrees, and

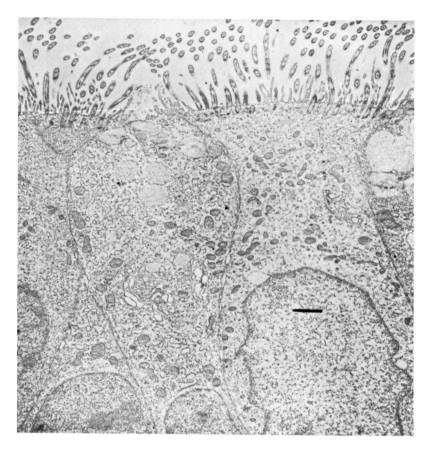

FIG. 1-4. Electron micrograph of normal respiratory mucous membrane from a ferret showing a goblet cell about to discharge into the mucous blanket. (Photo courtesy of F. B. Bangs.)

reimplanted, the cilia beat against the direction of mucous flow. When injured, a ciliated cell (or a mucous cell) in the mucous membrane is extruded into the mucous stream, and neighboring cells close ranks.

Ciliated movement causes streaming of mucus along specific routes. The ciliary beat frequency varies between 8 and 12 Hz; recovery time between beats is approximately five times as long as the stroke. Studies by Hilding and by Proctor have mapped the streaming patterns developed in the nose as well as those found in the bronchial tree and trachea (Fig. 1-5). By damaging areas of the membrane of the trachea and bronchi or by removing islands of ciliated epithelium, Hilding demonstrated an interruption to the normal streaming pattern; he noted that there are deposits of foreign particles upstream to these islands and that the mucus flow is slowed in its passage around them. Streaming is finally reestablished beyond the interrupted areas.

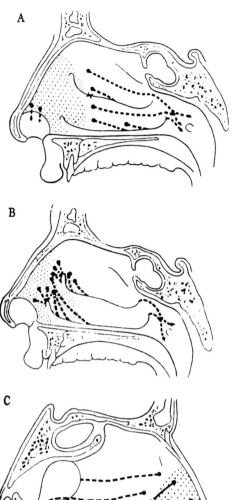

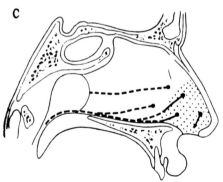

FIG. 1-5. Ciliary streaming of mucous. **A:** Over the active areas of the lateral wall. **B:** Over the inactive areas of the lateral nasal wall. **C:** Over the active areas of the nasal septum. Stippling shows inactive areas of the septum. (From Hilding, A. C.: Phagocytoses, mucous flow and ciliary action. *Arch. Environ. Health,* 6:61–73, 1963. With permission.)

Olfaction

The olfactory mucous membrane is nonciliated, has a yellowish tint, and contains many surface cuboidal cells. It occupies a relatively small area in man (2.5 cm²) in the vault of each nostril. The olfactory receptor fibers pass upward through the cribriform plate of the ethmoid bone, where they enter the olfactory bulb. Olfactory mucosa itself contains two types of cells: sustentacular and receptor cells. Receptor cells are bipolar neurons whose cell bodies lie in the peripheral epithelium, much more exposed than most neural receptors. Each cell has a single axon that clusters with those of other receptors to form a "filia olfactoria"; these are first-order neurons. Olfactory rods of the receptors extend beyond the surface of the epithelium and are highly sensitive. Olfactory mucous membrane is covered with mucus, and in order for a substance to be detected by the receptors, it must be volatile at ordinary temperatures and be lipid soluble. It has been suggested that odor quality depends on the size and shape of the stimulating molecule.

Olfaction may be distorted or completely eliminated by a number of conditions, most frequently by interference with the passage of air over the olfactory mucous membrane as a result of swollen nasal tissues. Masses such as nasal polyps or intranasal tumors can also stop airflow through the nasal vault. Such extradural tumors as neurofibromas or meningiomas can alter or eliminate the sense of smell by pressure on the olfactory nerve along its course to the olfactory bulb; brain tumors that involve the central olfactory pathways, the amygdaloid complex, or the olfactory tubercle also affect the sense of smell. Some cases of unexplained anosmia are thought to be the result of a virus infection that has involved the olfactory mucous membrane.

CONDITIONS CAUSING INJURY

Respiratory mucous membrane is a delicate, highly specialized epithelium, and damage to it can alter its normal physiology and result in serious sequelae, especially in the lower respiratory tract. Factors that can result in physiological derangement of the mucous membrane system may be divided into three broad categories: environmental factors, infections, man-made conditions, and trauma.

Environment

An important environmental factor is climate: air can become too dry and too hot for healthy respiratory exchange. If the necessary cooling and moisture uptake cannot be met by nasal mucous membranes and drying results in the upper trachea, ciliary action may be slowed or inhibited; this predisposes to lower respiratory tract infection (Fig. 1-6). Air also can contain too many particles of foreign matter to be filtered effectively by the body's defenses: anthracosis and silicosis illustrate the consequences of particle deposition at the alveolar level in such quantities as to seriously reduce oxygen and carbon dioxide exchange. Deficiency of calcium may also cause changes in cell permeability, which are reflected in changes in water

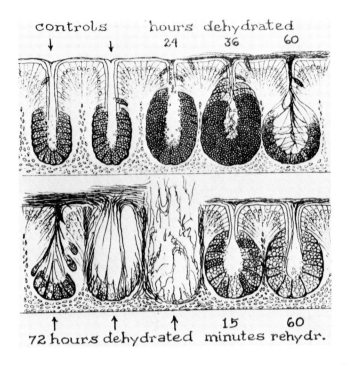

controls   hours dehydrated
        24   36   60

72 hours dehydrated   15   60
                      minutes rehydr.

FIG. 1-6. Dehydration effects on respiratory mucous membrane of the chick. (From Bang, B. G., and Bang, F. B.: Nasal mucociliary systems. In: *Lung Biology in Health and Disease,* Vol. V, Part I, Chap. II, Respiratory Defense Mechanisms. edited by J. D. Brean, et al., p. 407, 1977. Marcel Dekker, New York. With permission.)

output of the membrane surfaces and the viscosity of the mucus. Vitamin A plays an important role and has been shown by Fell and Mellanby to exhibit some control of keratinization of the mucous membrane and to play a part in the actual maintenance of the ciliated form of mucous membrane. Avitaminosis, as well as a lack of calcium in the diet, may result in serious changes in the mucous membrane. Likewise, any autonomic imbalance can result in viscosity changes in the mucus that affect ciliary action and the speed of streaming.

Infections

Very serious damage can be done to the mucous membrane as the result of certain infectious agents. The enteric diseases such as typhoid fever and cholera have long been associated with thrombotic desquamation of the mucous membrane surfaces in the nose and, at times, in the lower respiratory tract. In severe cases, such enteric infections have caused perforation of the nasal septum and destruction of wide areas

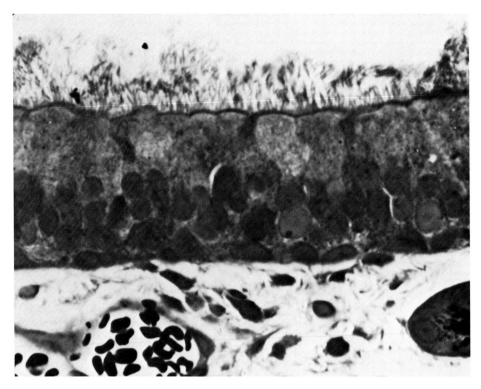

FIG. 1-7. Enlarged view of normal respiratory mucous membrane of a ferret showing the cilia and underlining goblet cells. (Photo courtesy of F. B. Bang.)

of mucous membrane, resulting in severe scarring, crusting, obstruction of proper mucous flow, and exposure of the lower respiratory tract to concurrent infections.

Bang and his associates, employing the Newcastle fowl virus, were able to show a loss of cilia and ciliated cells in the mucous membranes of the fowl's turbinates and trachea. Other work by the same group (Fig. 1-7) using human influenza A virus to infect the ferret (Fig. 1-8) has shown a loss of cilia (Fig. 1-9) followed by gradual replacement after resolution of the infection (Fig. 1-10). Laryngotracheitis virus applied to a chick nasal septum denudes the septum of cilia and greatly reduces the number of acinus glands on the side to which the virus has been applied (Fig. 1-11). Pertussis and influenza have caused the destruction of ciliated membranes in the trachea with resultant difficulty in removing lower respiratory tract discharges. Although many believe that whooping cough is the result of *Bordetella pertussis* infection, postmortem sections have revealed inclusion bodies, and there has been much discussion about the possibility of a viral component in this illness. Certainly, the destruction of ciliated membranes during an attack of whooping cough suggests the possibility of viral infection.

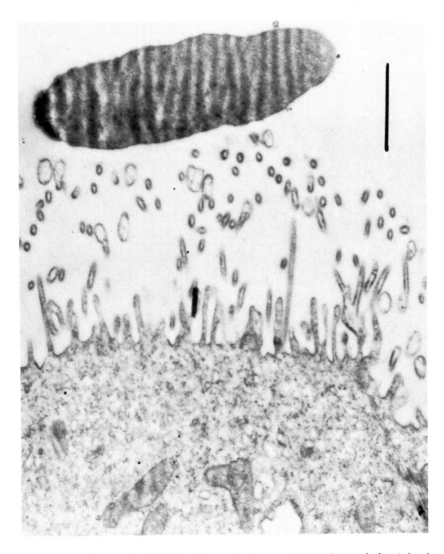

FIG. 1-8. Early influenza virus infection of the respiratory mucous membrane of a ferret showing a red blood cell resting on the cilia. (Photo courtesy of F. B. Bang.)

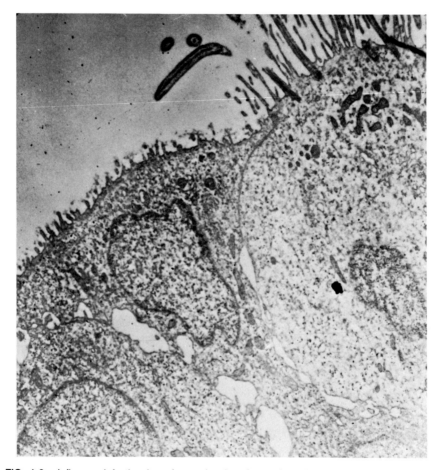

FIG. 1-9. Influenza infection in a ferret showing destruction of cilia with adjacent normal-appearing cilia. (Photo courtesy of F. B. Bang.)

Certain viruses can produce vesicular lesions in mucous membrane. Chickenpox produces a small vesicle surrounded by a red areola and a small macule that is red and raised. When the vesicle is ruptured, it leaves a raw area. Herpes, which characteristically spreads in the mouth along the distribution of the sensory division of a cranial nerve, presents a slightly larger vesicle, which can be quite painful when ruptured. Smallpox, in its milder form, produces practically the same lesions as found in chickenpox and herpes. Scrapings studied from these three infections show multinucleated giant cells typical of varicella and herpes; in smallpox many inclusion bodies are found, and atypical cells known as "Guarnieri's bodies" (Fig. 1-12) can be seen. With measles, Koplik's spots, which appear along the gums

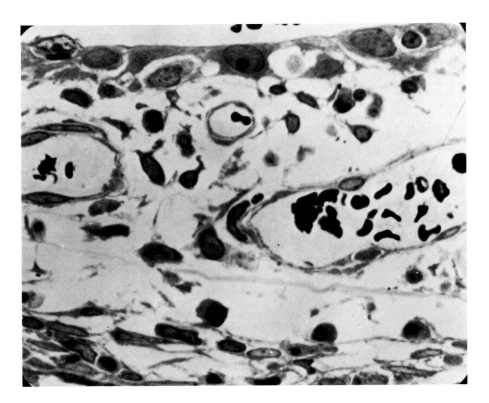

FIG. 1-10. Influenza infection of the mucous membrane in a ferret after 73 hr showing undifferentiated epithelial cells covering the membrane surface at the earliest regeneration. (From Hotz, G., and Bang, F. B.: Electronmicroscopic study of ferret respiratory cells infected with influenza virus. *Bull. Johns Hopkins Hosp.,* 101:176, 1967. With permission.)

and on the buccal surfaces of the mouth and palate, present as small, raised areas and consist of mononuclear infiltration, cytoplasmic and nuclear inclusions, subepithelial round cell infiltration, and multinucleated giant cells (Fig. 1-13). Measles, chickenpox, and smallpox viruses cause a very marked polypoid reaction and wide destruction of the mucous membrane in the middle ear in children (Fig. 1-14).

Pemphigus produces a similar reaction to that seen in chickenpox: the mucous membrane presents a number of thin-walled, bullous-type lesions that ruptures very easily, leaving crater-like erosions. These bullae form just above the basal layer, and healing may result in scarring. Most of these lesions are found on the skin, but a number appear in the mucous membranes.

Characteristic changes in the mucous membrane of the nose, particularly in that of the accessory nasal sinuses, are seen in mucormycosis, a fungal infection closely associated with diabetes (see Chapter 4). The mucous membrane shows evidence of arteritis and thrombotic infarction. Giant cells are seen occasionally. The general

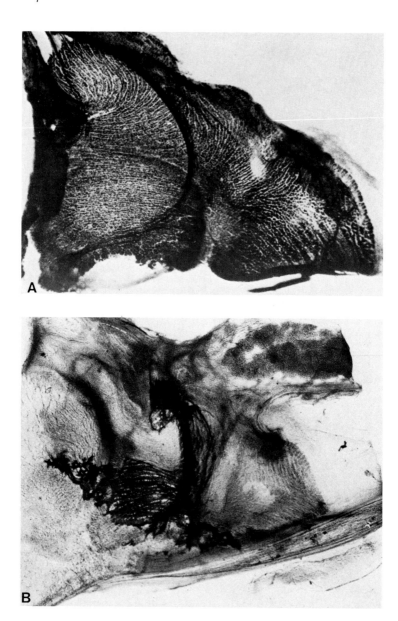

FIG. 1-11.   A: Normal pattern of acini in chick septum after application of india ink in uninfected check. **B:** Acinar pattern on infected chick respiratory mucous membrane after 72 hr showing incomplete clearance due to ciliary damage. (From Bang, B., and Bang, F. B.: Laryngotracheitis virus infection in chickens. *J. Exp. Med.,* 125(3):plates 27A and 27B, 1967. With permission.)

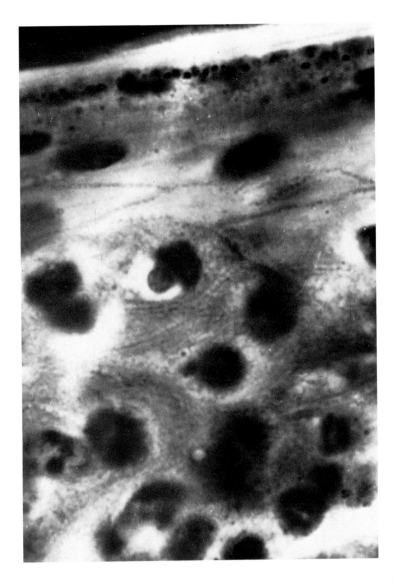

FIG. 1-12. Guarnieri's body in middle ear mucosa seen in a child dying of smallpox. (From Bordley, J. E., and Kapur, Y. P.: Histopathological changes in the temporal bone resulting from acute smallpox and chickenpox infections. *Laryngoscope,* 33(8):1484, 1977. With permission.)

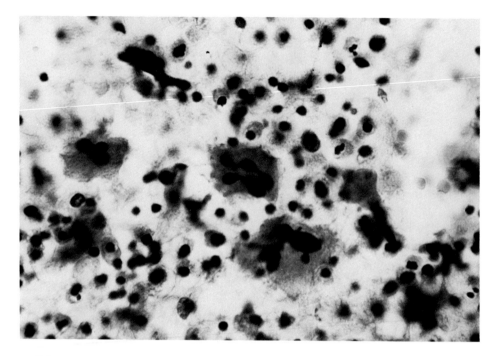

FIG. 1-13. Multinucleated giant cells (Warthin-Finkeldey cell) in middle ear mucosa. They appear in the mucous membranes in the presence of a measles virus infection. (From Bordley, J. E., and Kapur, Y. P.: Histopathological changes in the temporal bone resulting from measles infection, *Arch. Otolaryngol.,* 103:163, March, 1977. With permission.)

picture is one of extensive necrosis and is the result of an invasion of the fungal phycomycete *Mucor* involving the vascular bed of the mucous membrane.

Until the development of drugs effective in the treatment of tuberculosis, this disease was one of the more common causes of mucous membrane destruction in the mouth, pharynx, larynx, trachea, and middle ear. Large areas of destruction could be seen as a complication of severe acute pulmonary tuberculosis. Such lesions were also commonly found as ulcers on the vocal cords and in the posterior commissure region of the larynx. Tubercular lesions consist of tubercles containing epithelioid cells surrounding multinucleated giant cells and infiltrated with round cells. There is marked local edema followed by necrosis and ulceration of the membrane itself. The ulceration is sometimes followed by fibrous tissue infiltration. Large areas of ulceration in the mouth, middle ear, larynx, or trachea should always arouse the suspicion of a possible tuberculous infection.

The mucous membranes of the mouth and respiratory tract can also show the morphologic changes found in the epithelium of other parts of the body as a result of malignancies or so-called premalignant lesions. Such growths are discussed in

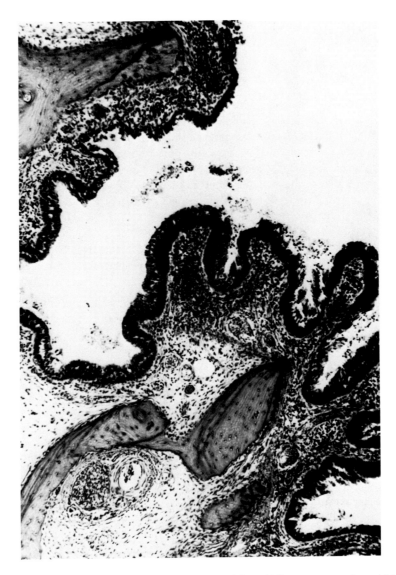

FIG. 1-14. Polypoid changes and marked edema of the middle ear mucosa in a child with smallpox. (From Bordley, J. E., and Kapur, Y. P.: Histopathological changes in the temporal bone resulting from acute smallpox and chickenpox infections. *Laryngoscope,* 33(3):1481, 1972. With permission.)

subsequent chapters as each anatomic division of the ears, nose, throat, and associated structures is presented.

Man-Made Agents

Various man-made agents act on normal ciliated movement, thereby affecting the functions of the mucous membranes. Such agents can cause serious damage to the respiratory tract. The most common vehicle in general use is distilled water, which is used in many solutions applied to the respiratory mucosa. Every effort should be made to buffer such solutions to avoid damage to the cilia. Drugs such as atropine, scopolamine, and morphine are known to slow ciliary activity. Atropine and scopolamine, which act on the parasympathetic nervous system, also impede the function of the goblet cells, causing changes in the viscosity of the mucus with subsequent loss of streaming. Large doses of atropine and scopolomine administered at the time of surgery should be avoided if possible. Other agents that have been known to impede ciliated movement and to be injurious to the goblet cells and ciliated cells are the wetting agents such as triethanolamine. Such agents are used in sprays as a vehicle for various chemical compounds; therefore, great care should always be taken when selecting drug preparations to administer to a patient, particularly a patient who has any upper respiratory infection or pulmonary disorder. In the treatment of sinusitis, it is important to avoid any vehicles for the application of drugs that may impede ciliary action because this is the sinus's best defense in the presence of infection.

Trauma

Local treatment and local operations in the nose, larynx, nasopharynx, and throat that involve sclerosing techniques, which in many instances cause membrane injury, should be avoided. Sclerosing materials that have been commonly used in the nose, trachea, and larynx for many years—silver nitrate and trichloroacetic acid—may, if carelessly handled, cause a great deal of mucous membrane scarring. The use of electric cautery and electric coagulation may also destroy large areas of ciliated membrane so thoroughly that there will be no proper regeneration. Such agents can also do much damage to nature's air-conditioning system if used around the turbinates.

Nasal endotracheal tubes employed for many respiratory problems and routinely employed during anesthesia for operative procedures in children have been the agents of much destruction of the mucous membrane of the nose and lower respiratory tract, in many cases destroying ciliated mucous membrane and cartilage and resulting in prolonged serious danger to the lower respiratory tract and to vital respiratory exchange. Great care should be exercised in employing these tubes.

Finally, surgery, a tool carefully developed by man over the years to help cure or alleviate disorders or disease, may become an agent for his destruction if not carefully planned. Planning must take into consideration the physiological factors relating to the respiratory tract, because surgery carelessly executed along this tract with little thought to tissue damage may result in serious consequences for the patient.

COMMENT

The mucous membranes of the trachea, bronchi, alveoli, middle ear, nose, pharynx, larynx, and mouth are vital to health. They are exposed to many dangers throughout life. Serious damage can result from infections, especially viral, which can destroy large areas of ciliated membrane surface. The environment in which we live may also contribute to damage to such membranes, and many drugs when administered and chemicals when applied to mucous membrane surfaces can cause serious long-lasting damage. Destruction of the normal physiology of the mucous membrane can be accomplished, particularly in the lower respiratory tract, by errors in judgment committed in the upper respiratory tract.

SELECTED READING

Bang, B. G., and Bang, F. B. (1967): Laryngotracheitis virus in chickens. *J. Exp. Med.*, 125(3):409–427.

Bang, F. B., and Bang, B. G. (1966): Responses of upper respiratory mucosa to drugs and viral infections. *Am. Rev. Respir. Dis.*, 93:142–149.

Bang, F. B., and Bang, B. G. (1977): Mucous membrane injury and repair. Respiratory defense mechanisms. *Lung Biology in Health and Disease*, Vol. V, Part I, Chap. 13, edited by J. D. Brain, D. F. Proctor, and L. M. Reid. Marcel Dekker, New York.

Bordley, J. E., and Kapur, Y. P. (1972): Histopathological changes in the temporal bone resulting from acute smallpox and chickenpox infection. *Laryngoscope*, 82:1477–1490.

Fell, H. B., and Mellanby, E. (1953): Metaplasia produced in cultures of chick ectoderm by high vitamin A. *J. Physiol. (Lond.)*, 119:470–488.

Hilding, A. C. (1931): Ciliary activity and course of secretion currents of the nose. *Proc. Mayo Clin.*, 6:285.

Hilding, A. C. (1963): Phagocytosis, mucous flow, and ciliary action. *Arch Environ. Health*, 6:61–73.

Hilding, A. C. (1968): Experimental bronchoscopy: Resultant trauma to tracheobronchial epithelium in calves. *Trans. Am. Acad. Ophthalmol. Otolaryngol.*, 72:604–613.

Mountcastle, V. B. (1968): *Medical Physiology*, ed. 12, Vol. II, Chap. 69. C. V. Mosby, St. Louis.

Proctor, D. F. (1977): State of the art: The upper airways. *Am. Rev. Respir. Dis.*, 115:97–129.

Ressig, M., Bang, B. G., and Bang, F. B. (1978): Ultrastructure of the mucociliary interface in the nasal mucosa of the chicken. *Am. Rev. Respir. Dis.*, 117:327–341.

Chapter 2

The Ear

Section 1: Anatomy and Physiology

Embryology of the Ear 20
Clinical Anatomy and Physiology of the Ear 25
Temporal Bone and Skull 29
Temporal Bone Neuroanatomy 30
Cochlear Morphology 31
Labyrinthine Fluids 32
Coding of Auditory Information 33
Central Auditory Pathways 36
Olivocochlear Bundle 37
Auditory Neurochemistry 38

EMBRYOLOGY OF THE EAR

During the third week of embryonic development, a plate-like thickening of ectoderm (otic placode) appears on either side of the head adjacent to the neural tube and lateral to the acouticofacial ganglion. This plate subsequently invaginates, forming the otic pit, which seals by the fourth week to form the otocyst. By 7 weeks the fluid-filled otocyst has undergone a complex series of folds and elongations resulting in formation of the semicircular canals and the beginning of the cochlea, which by 11 weeks has formed nearly all of its 2.5 turns. These ectodermal derivatives, including the endolymphatic duct, comprise the membranous labyrinth, which eventually contains the primary end-organs of hearing and balance surrounded by endolymph (Fig. 2.1-1).

After the endolymphatic duct is formed, the cartilage-encased membranous labyrinth enlarges, reaching adult size by midterm, at which time ossification of the otic capsule prevents further growth. The space between the membranous labyrinth and its bony encasement is called the periotic labyrinth. The portion of this peri-

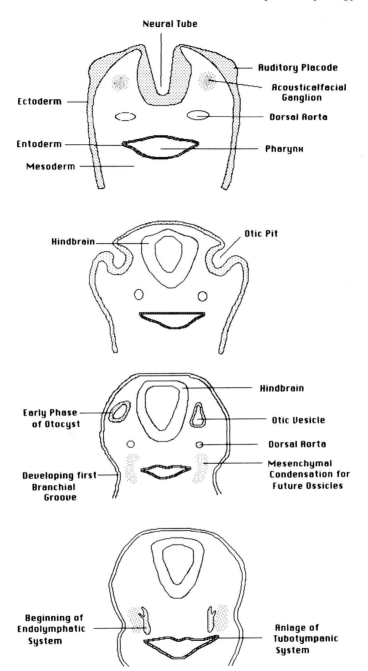

FIG. 2.1-1. Embryologic development of the inner ear. (Redrawn from Goodhill, V.: *Ear Diseases, Deafness and Dizziness.* Harper & Row, Hagerstown, 1979.)

lymph-filled space surrounding the cochlear duct and associated structures is divisible into the scala vestibuli connected via the helicotrema with the scala tympani, which in turn terminates in the round window membrane (Fig. 2.1-2). The perilymphatic duct is a narrow space filled with fluid and arachnoid-type connective tissue extending from the scala tympani near the round window to the subarachnoid space near the emergence of the glossopharyngeal nerve. Cerebrospinal fluid (CSF) is believed to filter slowly via this duct through the helicotrema and scala vestibuli to the remainder of the perilymphatic spaces, thus explaining perilymph's biochemical similarity to CSF. Concurrent with formation of the macrostructure of the membranous labyrinth, the neuroepithelial anlage of the organ of Corti and the vestibular sensory end-organs are taking form.

Whereas the sound perception mechanism takes shape from the ectodermally derived otocyst, the sound conduction elements of the external and middle ear originate from ectodermal, mesodermal, and entodermal components of the branchial arch/groove and pharyngeal pouch structures formed on either side of the embryonic head. In the 4-week human embryo, three branchial arches separated by two grooves appear, following which the third arch and second groove normally disappear. In rare cases, a cleft may persist as a congenital facial cleft anomaly. The first branchial cleft, on the other hand, persists and deepens to give rise to the external auditory meatus. An outpouching from the primitive pharynx, the first pharyngeal pouch, evaginates toward the deepening cleft, which it contacts for a short period. The pharyngeal pouch is the embryonic anlage of the eustachian tube, middle ear cleft, and mastoid air cell system.

Mesoderm soon separates the first cleft and pharyngeal pouch, giving rise to the cartilaginous elements of the first (Reichert's cartilage) and second (Meckel's car-

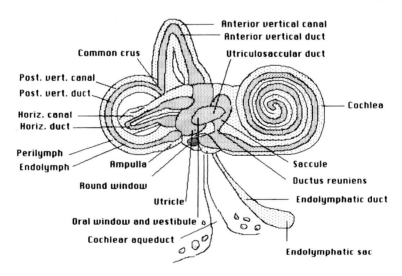

FIG. 2.1-2. Fully developed bony and membranous labyrinth. (Redrawn from Goodhill, V.: *Ear Diseases, Deafness and Dizziness.* Harper & Row, Hagerstown, 1979.)

tilage) branchial arches. The cartilaginous components of the first arch differentiate to form the heads and upper portions of the malleus and incus. The second arch cartilage forms the incus lenticular process, malleus handle, and superstructure of the stapes. The stapes footplate develops from fusion of a lateral cartilaginous plate with a medial plate derived from the otic capsule. By mid-gestation, the ossicles have reached full growth and undergo ossification. Primitive endochondral bone persists throughout life in both the ossicles and labyrinthine bony capsule, neither of which proceeds to the formation of haversian periosteal bone as is characteristic of the remainder of the bony skeleton.

Once the ossicles have formed, the remaining mesenchyme in the primitive middle ear begins to resorb, allowing further inroads of the expanding first pharyngeal pouch into the developing tympanic cavity. The mucosal lining of the middle ear, thus formed, further evaginates into the developing temporal bone to form the epitympanic space, aditus ad antrum, mastoid antrum, and related air cell system. The epitympanum is bounded superiorly by the tegmen tympani, the relatively thin bony plate separating the middle ear from temporal lobe dura in the middle cranial fossa, and the prominence of the lateral semicircular canal forms the medial wall of the aditus. Although cellular development in the mastoid normally proceeds during the early years of life, episodes of otitis during this period can result in a hypocellular mastoid system.

At the same time that middle ear development is proceeding, a solid cord of epithelial cells grows inward from the primitive external meatus toward the advancing pharyngeal pouch epithelium. These two elements are separated by a thin layer of mesoderm, thus giving rise to the three layers of the tympanic membrane: external epithelium, middle connective tissue, and internal mucosa. The connective tissue at the periphery of the developing tympanic membrane (TM) undergoes ossification to form the tympanic sulcus in which the thickened and rolled edge of the tympanic annulus develops. By the middle of the seventh month of gestation, the sound conduction and perception elements of the developing ear have reached nearly complete development. Only then does the solid core of epithelial cells between the primitive external meatus and the tympanic membrane begin to pull away from the TM to form the lumen of the external auditory canal. The progressive cavitation of the canal proceeds from medial to lateral, accounting for the possibility of congenital meatal atresia coexisting with a normally developed tympanic membrane, middle ear, and ossicular chain.

The pinna is formed from six hillocks, arising from the first and second branchial arches by the sixth week of embryonic development, which fuse to form the auricle by the end of the third month (Fig. 2.1-3). Except for the tragus, the remainder of the complex, skin-covered elastic cartilage folds and recesses of the external ear are formed by the hillocks derived from the second arch. Failure to complete the fusion process can result in the fairly common malformation of a preauricular sinus. This small opening near the incisura between the tragus and the anterior superior termination of the helix can extend inward to terminate in a multilocular cyst. Recurrent infection may necessitate surgical removal extensive enough to encompass

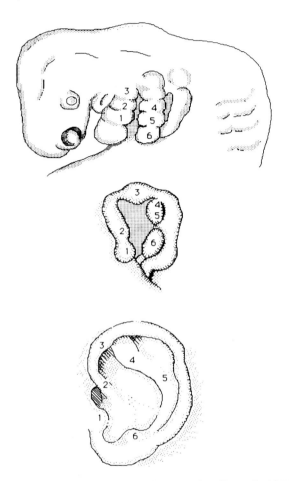

FIG. 2.1-3. Developmental stages of the pinna. (Redrawn from Paparella, M. M., and Shumrick, D. A.: *Otolaryngology, Vol. I: Basic Sciences and Related Disciplines.* Saunders, Philadelphia, 1980.)

the entire cystic mass. The anomaly commonly shows a familial distribution compatible with a dominant inheritance pattern. Very rarely, a first branchial cleft anomaly is reported which presents as a cystic structure anterior to the pinna but which may open into the external auditory canal rather than the preauricular area. Again, safe removal requires surgical familiarity with the anatomy of the parotid, facial nerve, and auricular region. Specific auricular malformations resulting from failure in differentiation of the first and second branchial arches include anotia, microtia, malformations of the cartilaginous structure or folds (e.g., lop ear), as well as malpositioning of the auricles on the side of the head. Congenital atresia of the external auditory canal results from interruption of normal developmental progression of the first branchial cleft.

CLINICAL ANATOMY AND PHYSIOLOGY OF THE EAR

Skin on the posteromedial surface of the pinna is loosely attached and movable over the underlying elastic cartilage, whereas the anterolateral skin is firmly attached to the auricular folds (Fig. 2.1-4). Penetrating vessels from the closely attached anterior covering are important in supplying nutrients to the cartilage, and this blood supply can be compromised by a subcutaneous collection of blood, serum, or pus between the anterior skin and cartilage. Partial resorption of the cartilage may result in a "cauliflower ear," quite common among wrestlers and other athletes prior to the advent of ear protectors.

The S-shaped external auditory canal extends from the concha to the external surface of the tympanic membrane, a distance in the adult of some 2.5 cm but shorter in the newborn. The tragus at the external meatus, together with the narrowed canal lumen at the isthmus, serve as anatomic barriers to the entrance of foreign material which might injure the tympanic membrane or middle ear structures. In addition, cerumen provides a water-repellent coating for the canal skin, minimizing the impact of short periods of exposure to liquid contamination. Cerumen consists of a complex mixture of sebaceous and apocrine glandular secretions combined with exfoliated cornified cells of the stratum corneum which can dissolve during periods of prolonged exposure to water. Parents of small children often attempt to clean all visible cerumen from the child's ear during bathing, thereby removing an important barrier to infection and injury of the external canal skin.

The tympanic membrane, approximately 9 mm in diameter, is positioned obliquely, with the anterior inferior wall of the canal being longer than the posterior superior wall. As the child grows, the tympanic membrane assumes a more upright position. The cartilaginous lateral portion of the canal is directed slightly upward and backward, and the osseous canal slightly downward and forward. Visualization of the

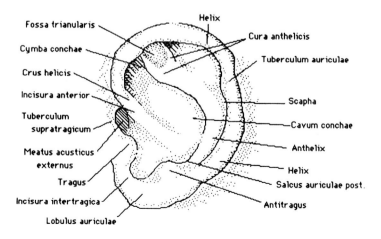

FIG. 2.1-4. Surface anatomy of the pinna.

tympanic membrane is facilitated in the older child by pulling the pinna gently upward, outward, and backward so as to straighten the canal. In infants whose shorter canals are principally cartilaginous, gently pulling outward produces the desired view. Just medial to the junction of the cartilaginous and bony portions is the isthmus, the narrowest portion of the canal.

Lined with keratinizing stratified squamous epithelium which is continuous with the lateral surface of the tympanic membrane, the external auditory canal represents the only skin-lined cul-de-sac in the body, with attendant susceptibility to certain dermatoses (Fig. 2.1-5). Skin lining the cartilaginous canal contains epidermal, dermal, and subcutaneous elements, varying from 0.5 to 1 mm in thickness; the bony canal is lined by a 0.2-mm layer of skin devoid of papillae or subcutaneous tissue with firm attachment to the periosteum of underlying bone. The skin of the bony canal is quite sensitive to trauma, and a painful hematoma readily forms if a shearing force pulls the thin skin layer over the bone, as may occur with vigorous attempts at cerumen or foreign body removal. As might be expected, hair follicles occur almost exclusively in the skin of the cartilaginous canal, and the bony–cartilaginous junction can be visually defined by the examiner who notes the demarcation between hair-bearing and nonhair-bearing skin.

The tympanic membrane is attached both at its circumference and to the manubrium of the malleus, assuming a conical shape, with the bony umbo of the manubrium as the medial apex. The pars tensa comprises the majority of the TM,

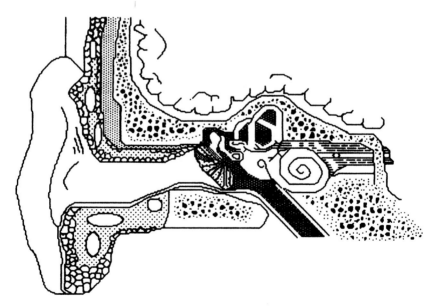

FIG. 2.1-5. External auditory canal. (Redrawn from Goodhill, V.: *Ear Diseases, Deafness and Dizziness.* Harper & Row, Hagerstown, 1979.)

consisting of an outer layer of keratinizing squamous epithelium, a middle layer of fibrous connective tissue, and an inner layer of mucosa continuous with the remainder of the middle ear lining. A small superior portion of the TM, the pars flaccida (Shrapnell's membrane), is superior to the short lateral process of the malleus and is further defined by the anterior and posterior malleal folds. The pars flaccida is devoid of the fibrous tissue layer found in the pars tensa with consequent impairment of elasticity and predilection for medial retraction in the presence of negative middle ear pressure. The lateral short process of the malleus constitutes a diagnostic landmark in otoscopy and appears more prominent as the TM retracts medially.

The pars tensa is normally pearly gray and translucent enough to occasionally permit visualization of the long process of the incus as it descends, turning medially (lenticular process) to meet the capitulum of the stapes in the posterior superior quadrant of the tympanic cavity. The stapes extends medially to the oval window from the incudostapedial joint and therefore is not visible through the drum (Fig. 2.1-6). The partly hollow stapedial crura form the boundaries of the obturator (stapedial) artery, which occupies this space during fetal life and, very rarely, persists as a congenital anomaly. The malleus and incus are stabilized in position by suspensory ligaments arrayed in such a way as to enhance their mobility in response to sound pressure changes against the surface of the tympanic membrane. The tensor tympani muscle, which arises from within a canal parallel to the eustachian tube and is innervated by a branch of the trigeminal nerve, attaches to the malleal manubrium and maintains a variable tension on the tympanic membrane. The stapedius muscle, innervated by a branch of the facial nerve, inserts near the capitulum of the stapes and undergoes bilateral reflexive contraction in response to a loud sound delivered to either ear. This reflex serves to protect the sensitive inner ear structures and provides a useful tool for evaluating the site of a lesion in the auditory system using an impedance bridge.

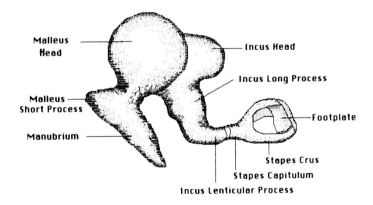

FIG. 2.1-6. Developing ossicular chain.

The tympanic membrane's conical apex near the umbo is the most sensitive region to minimal changes in sound pressure level. As the sound pressure increases, the vibration amplitude increases, and a large portion of the TM participates in the vibratory motion. High-frequency sounds produce a more complex vibrational pattern than those of lower frequency. In an ear with a normally mobile, articulated TM/ossicular complex, frequency vibrations are transmitted through the manubrium of the malleus to the incus and stapes, which in turn transmits airborne acoustic energy to the inner ear fluid system (Fig. 2.1-7).

When airborne sound waves contact an air/liquid interface, e.g., the surface of a swimming pool, 99.1% of the sound energy is reflected back into the air. Such an observation is easily validated by the underwater swimmer who cannot hear his companion's call from above water. By serving to efficiently match the impedance at the air/fluid interface between the external ear and the inner ear fluid, the tympanic membrane and ossicular chain conserve and transmit a much larger fraction of available sound energy. Elementary principles of physics can help explain the amplifier effect of the middle ear; 55 mm^2 of the 85 mm^2 tympanic membrane are tightly attached to the manubrium. If one divides this area by the 3.2 mm^2 area of the stapedial footplate, a mechanical advantage of 17:1 is computed. A further mechanical advantage imparted by the middle ear system derives from the lever arm differential between the malleal manubrium and the incus/stapes combination. The joints between the ossicles normally remain immobile as the chain moves in unison, imparting a piston-like motion to the stapes in the oval window. The favorable ratio between the lengths of the lever arms increases the force at the stapes to 1.3 times that being applied at the manubrium. The overall mechanical advantage imparted through the variable-size piston effect and the lever arm differential approximates 20 to 25 times, which translates into a 30 dB gain in sound

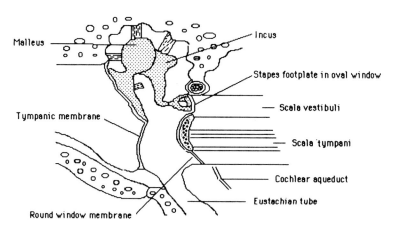

FIG. 2.1-7. Middle ear transformer. (Redrawn from Goodhill, V.: *Ear Diseases, Deafness and Dizziness.* Harper & Row, Hagerstown, 1979.)

intensity. This gain, however, is necessary to overcome the loss of acoustic energy resulting from the transfer of energy from air to the fluids in the inner ear where it produces a traveling wave through the perilymph system of the cochlea. The interaction of the hair cells of the organ of Corti with other cochlear elements, e.g., the tectorial membrane, converts the transmitted sound energy into bioelectric signals to cochlear nuclei and to components of the central auditory nervous system, as explained below.

Depending on their location and size, perforations of the tympanic membrane can produce variable degrees of conductive hearing impairment. Other pathologic conditions, such as atrophy of the tympanic membrane, tympanosclerosis, otosclerosis, and chronic tympanomastoid disease, can result in fixation of the tympanic membrane and/or ossicular chain with a resulting decrease in the efficiency of sound energy transmission. Disarticulation of the TM/ossicular chain complex, resulting from such causes as trauma or infection, can lead to a maximal conductive deficit, particularly if the TM remains imperforate. Necrosis of the lenticular process of the incus, which receives a tenuous vascular supply, is a common cause of ossicular discontinuity following injury or disease. Increasing stiffness in the middle ear structures affects the transmission of low frequencies much more than high frequencies, whereas impedance changes due to an increase in mass are greater as the frequency of sound is higher, thereby affecting high-frequency transmission.

TEMPORAL BONE AND SKULL

The large squamous portion of the temporal bone, forming part of the lateral wall of the middle cranial fossa, articulates with the occipital bone, the parietal bone, and the sphenoid bone. The anteromedial surface of the temporal bone contributes to the floor of the middle cranial fossa contact with temporal lobe dura. Within the mastoid air cell system, the periantral triangle is defined by the posterior fossa and sigmoid sinus plates, in addition to the middle fossa plate and posterior bony canal wall. These relationships are important when considering the potential complications of otomastoiditis, which include epidural abscess, temporal lobe abscess, meningitis, and lateral sinus thrombosis.

Just as the skull of an infant differs from that of an adult, so does the infant temporal bone. The bony external canal rudimentary consists primarily of the bony tympanic sulcus, with the remainder of the canal being cartilaginous. The mastoid air cell system usually contains at least one sizable air cell, the mastoid antrum, a primordium for development of the rest of the mastoid air cell system. Because the remainder of the mastoid air cell system has yet to develop, the facial nerve in the infant exits through a more laterally placed stylomastoid foramen which is not protected by the usual mastoid process. This anatomic feature governs the safe placement of postauricular surgical incisions in the young infant with surgical otomastoiditis or congenital ear deformity.

TEMPORAL BONE NEUROANATOMY

The facial nerve enters the internal auditory meatus with the cochlear and vestibular branches of the eighth nerve. Viewed from the medial aspect, the internal auditory canal may be subdivided into four quadrants. The posterior quadrants contain the superior and inferior branches of the vestibular nerve, and the anterior superior and anterior inferior quadrants contain the facial and cochlear nerves, respectively. The fibers of the cochlear nerve fan out through the bony modiolus of the cochlea to join the cell bodies of the spiral ganglion. The dendritic processes of these cells, by means of which information is sent from the receptor to the central nervous system, become unmyelinated as they leave the cochlear modiolus to terminate in nerve endings in close contact with the hair cells of the organ of Corti (Fig. 2.1-8). The hair cells are the sensory receptors for sound characterized by a distal flat portion that is provided with a bundle of nonmotile cilia protruding from its surface. Also terminating near the base of the hair cells are axons of efferent fibers from the olivocochlear bundle, the apparent function of which is to provide feedback to modify the response of the receptors.

Taking origin from bipolar cells in the vestibular ganglion (Scarpa's ganglion) at the lateral end of the internal auditory meatus, the peripheral vestibular fibers are distributed as follows: superior branch to the macula of the utricle and the cristae of the superior and lateral semicircular canals; inferior branch to the saccular macula; and a small posterior branch through the singular foramen to the posterior semi-

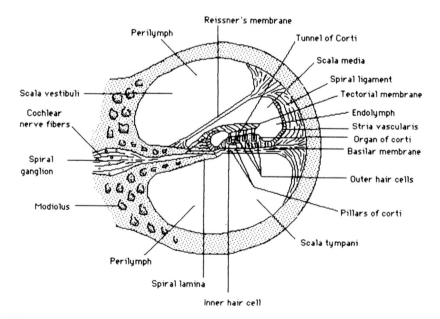

FIG. 2.1-8. Cross section of the cochlea. (Redrawn from Goodhill, V.: *Ear Diseases, Deafness and Dizziness.* Harper & Row, Hagerstown, 1979.)

circular canal. The semicircular canals are arranged in three mutually perpendicular planes of space: horizontal (lateral), anterior vertical (superior), and posterior vertical (inferior). The utricle, semicircular canals, and saccule constitute the membranous vestibular labyrinth containing the receptor organs for sense of motion and position.

The facial nerve leaves the geniculate ganglion in the anterior portion of the middle ear at the anterior genu, coursing backward and downward, and traversing the tympanic cavity as an important surgical landmark, where it forms part of the medial wall above the oval window, usually but not always protected by a bony canal. Just posterior to the oval window, the posterior, or second, genu occurs as the nerve bends downward to pass through the vertical fallopian canal within the mastoid and finally emerges into the upper neck through the stylomastoid foramen. Important branches emerging from the vertical segment include the nerve to the stapedius muscle and the chorda tympani which passes forward across the tympanic cavity between the long processes of the malleus and incus.

COCHLEAR MORPHOLOGY

The organ of Corti contains approximately 13,000 receptor hair cells divided into two rows; the 3,500 cells contained in the inner row are anatomically different from those in the outer row (Fig. 2.1-9). Of the 30,000 neurons whose dendrites

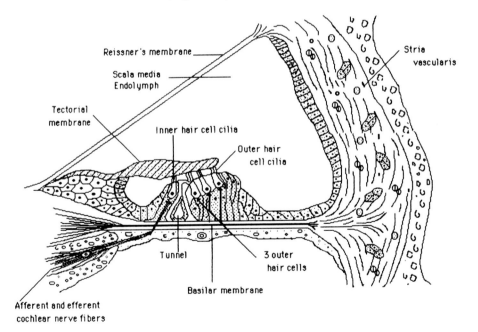

FIG. 2.1-9. Organ of Corti. (Redrawn from Goodhill, V.: *Ear Diseases, Deafness and Dizziness.* Harper & Row, Hagerstown, 1979.)

course along the organ of Corti, 95% innervate the inner hair cells, each neuron branching to only one or a few hair cells. Those innervating the outer hair cells, however, branch to several cells. Efferent nerve fibers, which originate from neurons in the superior olivary complex of the brainstem, are also of two types, one ending directly on outer hair cells and the other on the auditory nerve fibers innervating inner hair cells. A gelatinous tectorial membrane rests over the organ of Corti, supported medially at the wall of the cochlear duct at the limbus and laterally at the outer edge of the organ of Corti. Studies of the tectorial membrane have shown it to be an independent medium with its own ionic composition which is osmotically sensitive to hydration changes. During vibrations of the basilar membrane, the tectorial membrane is subjected to shear displacements in relationship to the motion of the hairs of the sensory cells. Displacement of the hairs relative to the tectorial membrane constitutes the physiological stimulus to the acoustic receptor organ. Stimulation of the dendritic processes of the spiral ganglion cells probably involves a neurochemical transmitter which has not been positively identified.

LABYRINTHINE FLUIDS

The function of the fluids surrounding the various tissues of the membranous labyrinth include: providing nutrients and removing catabolic end products; providing an ionic environment conducive to neurochemical and neuroelectric transmission of acoustic impulses; and conveying a fluid wave from the stapes footplate to interact with the energy-transforming elements of the cochlea. Chemically, perilymph has a sodium/potassium ratio similar to that of CSF, and the high potassium and low sodium concentrations of endolymph are similar to those found intracellularly elsewhere in the body. The concentration of proteins in the endolymph is 127 mg/100 ml; in the perilymph it is approximately 300 mg/100 ml. These figures are different from that of the concentration of protein in CSF, which is about 35 mg/100 ml. Volume approximations in the human include 78.3 mm^3 for perilymph compared with only 2.76 mm^3 for endolymph.

The high potassium concentration in endolymph led to speculation that a third type of fluid, given the name cortilymph, more suitable to neural function must surround the hair cells and unmyelinated fibers of the organ of Corti. Of the three major capillary systems in the cochlea contained in the stria vascularis, the spiral prominence, and the osseus lamina, it appears that the arcade of spiral vessels supplying the capillary loops beneath the basilar membrane and tunnel serves as the source of nutrients for cortilymph. Perilymph, although having many similarities to CSF, is sufficiently different to suggest a more complex derivation than simple filtration through the cochlear aqueduct. Lawrence suggested three possible sources for perilymph, including: ultrafiltration from blood; derivation from endolymph with active maintenance of chemical relationships by endolymphatic membranes; or a slow enough filtration process from CSF to explain chemical differences.

Attempts at measuring pressures within the various membranous spaces of the labyrinth have been fraught with technical difficulties. It has been postulated, however, that one function of the endolymphatic sac and duct is to transmit changes in intracranial pressure to the endolymph so as to maintain a pressure balance with perilymph, thus preventing a shift in position of Reissner's or the basilar membrane with resultant changes in auditory function.

Theories regarding the putative source or sources of endolymph relate to speculation about the nature and direction of flow within the cochlear duct. Some investigators have postulated a longitudinal flow of endolymph from a hypothesized origin in the stria vascularis to a point of absorption in the endolymphatic duct and sac. On the other hand, proponents of radial flow suggest that flow exists from the perilymph through Reissner's membrane to endolymph, with the stria vascularis providing the necessary alterations in chemical composition through selective absorption, utilizing an ion-exchange mechanism similar to that in renal tubules. The selective permeability characteristics of Reissner's membrane, separating endolymph from perilymph, help maintain the differences in potassium/sodium concentrations. After reviewing the evidence, Lawrence concluded that circulation of endolymph is local and radial with specific areas of the organ of Corti being nutritionally independent of adjacent areas. He believed that secretion and absorption of endolymph occur continuously along the entire length of the cochlear duct, with only a very slow longitudinal flow toward the endolymphatic duct. The ionic differences across the cochlear partition give rise to a resting direct-current potential unique in biological systems because endolymph, with a high potassium concentration similar to that in intracellular fluid, has a high positive potential unlike that found in the interior of cells. Measured potentials of $+80$ mV in the endolymph and -80 mV in the organ of Corti have been reported. The exact contribution of these potentials to the energy transformation taking place in the cochlea has yet to be defined, but many theories ascribe an essential role to them.

CODING OF AUDITORY INFORMATION

Frequency and intensity are the two aspects of acoustic signals that are most relevant to the neural coding of auditory information. Frequency or pitch is encoded in two ways. One of these is the "place" mechanism, and the other is the "temporal" mechanism.

Hermann von Helmholtz originally proposed the place mechanism during the 1850s. He theorized that tones of differing frequency possessed different pitches because they stimulate different cochlear regions. In this scheme, high frequencies produce vibrations that are localized to the base of the cochlea, i.e., near the stapes, and low frequencies produce vibrations that are localized to the cochlear apex. During the mid-twentieth century, Georg von Bekesy verified and extended Helmholtz' place principle. He determined that cochlear frequency analysis is a consequence of structural or mechanical factors, the most important of which are a spatial gradation of the mass of the basilar membrane and the degree of coupling between adjacent sections of the membrane. Because of these factors, the pressure differentials that arise across the basilar membrane as a result of stapes motion cause it to vibrate in sections for most frequencies, thereby producing a traveling wave. Von Bekesy found that, depending on frequency, the traveling wave peaks at different places along the cochlear duct in a manner roughly similar to that which Helmholtz had predicted earlier. Von Bekesy also discovered that the buildup to the traveling wave peak is rather gradual, and after the wave peaks it dies out rapidly. Owing to the mechanics of the traveling wave, then, a neuron connected to a given point on the basilar membrane would be expected to respond only to a limited set of frequencies, with the bandwidth of effective frequencies increasing as stimulus intensity increases.

At low intensities, basilar membrane motion is restricted to specific cochlear positions; thus the stimulated cochlear region is highly localized, and encoding of frequency by place is possible. At high intensities, however, the gradual buildup of wave amplitude causes the spatial localization to be lost, more so for low frequencies than for high. To resolve this problem, theorists such as E. Glen Wever proposed that frequency information could be transmitted in the temporal relationships among discharges in auditory nerve fibers. Here basilar membrane vibration, which of course occurs at the stimulus frequency, causes neurotransmitter release from cochlear hair cells only during a half-cycle of the stimulus, with the other half-cycle being inhibitory. Action potentials therefore arise only at times that are related to the stimulus period. Even though a given nerve fiber may not respond with an action potential at every half-cycle, over a group of fibers there are time-locked responses at every period. The brain need only count or time the volleys of action potentials in the active fiber array in order to arrive at an estimate of stimulus frequency.

It has been shown that the receptor potentials of cochlear hair cells are modulated in an alternating manner when basilar membrane vibration occurs, and that auditory nerve fibers indeed respond in a "phase-locked" manner. However, this mode of response, which is very strong at low frequencies, is gradually reduced as frequency increases. Practically speaking, phase-locking persists only up to 3 to 4 kHz. At higher frequencies, frequency information in the time-locked responses of hair cells and the temporal cadences of fiber discharges is lost. Thus neural coding of low frequencies occurs by both place and temporal mechanisms, but coding of high frequencies can occur only by the place mechanism.

Hair cells and auditory nerve fibers are capable of responding to changes in stimulus intensity only over a restricted range. The "dynamic range" of response extends rather linearly from threshold to about 20 dB above it. At higher intensities, the response grows less rapidly and ultimately saturates or reaches a maximum. Above the intensity where the response saturates, further increases in stimulus intensity produce no change in a neuron's response. In general, then, auditory neurons possess a full dynamic range of 30 to 40 dB. A simplistic view of intensity coding holds that low-level intensity information is transmitted in the discharge rates of auditory nerve fibers that are most sensitive to the stimulus frequency, and high-level intensity information is encoded by the number of active fibers. Thus so long as intensity is within 30 to 40 dB of a fiber's response threshold, the fiber is capable of encoding the intensity accurately. Above this, however, responses of the fibers that are most sensitive to the stimulus frequency are saturated, and the brain must rely on the spatial spread of the traveling wave to provide intensity information. In this scheme, the spreading excitation at higher intensities recruits responses of "new" fibers; and although the intensity is within their dynamic range, the newly recruited fibers are capable of encoding changes in intensity. By integrating the spatial extent of activity elicited by a given stimulus along the cochlear duct and hence across the entire fiber array, the brain can arrive at an accurate estimate of stimulus intensity.

Encoding of frequency and intensity in higher auditory centers is more complicated. The point-for-point projection of the cochlea to specific regions in higher nuclei ("tonotopic organization") can account, at least to a first approximation, for frequency coding, but intensity coding and frequency coding based on temporal mechanisms present problems. Phase-locked activity, for example, persists only to 1 kHz or less in higher centers such as the inferior colliculus, and many neurons in higher nuclei respond to increasing stimulus intensity in a nonmonotonic manner; that is, they increase and then decrease their response as intensity increases. At one time, it was thought that intensity was encoded spatially in higher nuclei, such that different neurons responded when intensity changed. This concept, however, has proved to be untenable. Studies involving ablation of brain regions have shown that frequency discrimination does not require the auditory cortex, but intensity discrimination and sound localization do. In sum, the state of knowledge regarding auditory stimulus coding in higher auditory centers is relatively primitive.

The views of frequency and intensity coding presented here are thought to be basically correct, but research on the coding of speech sounds and complex or multifrequency tones has shown that further refinements of the theory will be required if we are to account for all aspects of auditory stimulus processing. For example, it has been shown that at high intensities frequency information is retained only in the phase-locked or synchronized responses of auditory nerve fibers, i.e., that frequency information based on spatial or place mechanisms largely does not exist, and that there is no easy way to account for changes in perceptual loudness at very high stimulus intensities. Moreover, it has been shown that the response of a hair cell or auditory nerve fiber to a multifrequency complex is not a simple sum of the responses to each of the components. Rather, nonlinear interactions occur, the precise nature of which is not fully understood. Until all of the parameters involved in auditory stimulus coding have been thoroughly studied and characterized, expectations for devices such as the cochlear implant prosthesis must remain low.

CENTRAL AUDITORY PATHWAYS

As stated above, the auditory nerve enters the brainstem after passing through the cerebellopontine angle. It terminates in the primary cochlear nuclei, which is subdivided on the basis of its cytoarchitecture into three divisions (Fig. 2.1-10): anteroventral, posteroventral, and dorsal cochlear nuclei. The auditory nerve bifurcates upon entering the nucleus, with the ascending limb innervating cells of the anteroventral cochlear nucleus (AVCN) and the descending limb innervating both the posteroventral cochlear nucleus (PVCN) and the dorsal cochlear nucleus (DCN). Ascending outputs of the cochlear nuclei follow three fiber tracts. The dorsal acoustic stria, which emanates from the DCN, sends the majority of its fibers to the nuclei of the lateral lemniscus (NLL) and inferior colliculus (IC) on the contralateral side, with other projections going to the cerebellum and to the ipsilateral NLL and IC. The intermediate stria projects primarily from PVCN to the contralateral NLL, with offshoots to the ipsilateral superior olivary complex (SOC). The ventral stria or trapezoid body is the largest fiber tract of the three. It projects bilaterally, connecting the AVCN with the superior olivary complex of both sides; and to a lesser extent it projects to the contralateral NLL.

The SOC is a collection of small nuclei, the largest of which are the lateral superior olive or S-segment, the medial superior olive, and the medial nucleus of

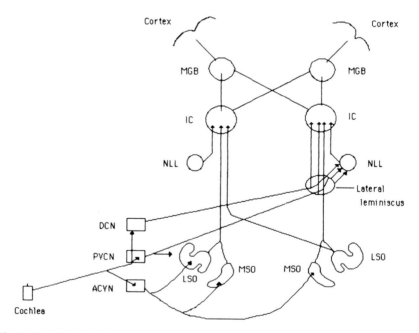

FIG. 2.1-10.   Central auditory pathways. (Adapted from Pickles, J. O.: *An Introduction to the Physiology of Hearing,* p. 170. Academic Press, New York, 1982)

the trapezoid body. The superior olive is the lowest level at which inputs from both ears converge, and its cells are thought to be involved in sound localization. Outputs of the SOC ascend ipsilaterally to the NLL and IC, to the reticular formation, and to the superior colliculi. Other, less numerous outputs travel to the contralateral SOC, to the nuclei of the trigeminal and facial nerve (for the acoustic reflex), and to the cochlear nucleus and cochlea (olivocochlear bundle). Outputs of the NLL project primarily to the IC.

All ascending projections of the auditory system terminate in the IC, which is a structure organized like an onion with a rind. The laminae of the central nucleus, and those for all other central auditory nuclei as well, receive point-for-point projections from the cochlea (tonotopic organization). Although there appears to be a systematic intrinsic organization of the IC with regard to monaurally and binaurally responding cells, the details of that organization have not been worked out in any detail. The outputs of the IC follow the brachium and terminate in the medial geniculate body (MGB) of the thalamus. The MGB consists of two major subdivisions: the pars principalis and the pars magnocellularis. The outputs of the MGB form the acoustic radiations that terminate in an orderly manner on the superior temporal plane of the temporal lobe (Heschl's gyrus). The auditory cortex in humans contains multiple cochlear representations, but only one of these is classified as a primary receiving area, or koniocortex. The primary receiving area, or AI, is surrounded by association cortices, each of which probably possesses a separate cochlear representation. At the superior and caudal extents of the auditory cortex are located cells that respond to somatosensory and visual stimuli, respectively. Outputs of the auditory cortex are not well understood, but it is known that there are numerous orderly connections through the corpus callosum to the contralateral auditory cortex, other connections with the frontal lobe, and numerous descending connections with the MGB and the IC.

OLIVOCOCHLEAR BUNDLE

The organ of Corti is innervated by efferent fibers which originate in the superior olivary complex of the brainstem and reach the cochlea by way of the olivocochlear bundle. Because this innervation is bilateral in origin, the olivocochlear bundle has commonly been subdivided into crossed and uncrossed components. However, more important than this difference in site of origin is the fact that there are two distinct kinds of nerve fiber in the bundle which differ in place of origin and side of termination in the organ of Corti. Olivocochlear neurons located in the *lateral* part of the superior olivary complex project their unmyelinated axons mostly to the cochlea of the same side and terminate on the cochlear nerve fibers innervating the inner hair cells. Olivocochlear neurons located in the *medial* part of the superior olivary complex project their myelinated axons mostly to the cochlea of the opposite side and terminate at the bases of the outer hair cells. Thus there appears to be two separate systems of olivocochlear axons, the lateral system and the medial system, but each contains a different proportion of crossed and uncrossed fibers. The two efferent systems are each associated with only one of the two afferent systems composed of the spiral ganglion cell populations which independently innervate inner and outer hair cells. Although it is still unclear how these afferent and efferent systems work during the process of hearing, it is known that the action of the medial efferent system is to mechanically alter the motion of the basilar membrane, presumably by modulating the motility of the outer hair cell stereocilia which are embedded in the tectorial membrane.

AUDITORY NEUROCHEMISTRY

There are few data available concerning the biochemical characteristics of auditory neurons and how neurochemical events affect the input and integration of auditory information. The field of auditory neurochemistry has lagged well behind those of auditory anatomy and physiology, which have served as models for the study of sensory systems. Advances in methodology and knowledge in the fields of biochemistry and immunology have greatly facilitated our understanding of the brain on a molecular level. These advances have just begun to have an impact on the field of auditory research.

Many putative neurotransmitters are present in auditory neurons. Although some of these may eventually prove to be neurotransmitters, others are found in extremely small quantities and therefore may serve as neuroregulators. In some cases the presence of certain neurochemicals indicate functions not specifically associated with neural transmission. These functions might include an involvement in general processes, e.g., metabolism, or specific processes, e.g., maintenance and formation of synapses.

Some of the neurochemicals present in the auditory nuclei include acetylcholine; the small amino acids glutamate, aspartate, and γ-aminobutyric acid; the catecholamines dopamine and norepinephrine; and the peptide enkephalin. Another neurochemical which may be significant in auditory functioning is the small peptide somatostatin (SS), which was first isolated from mammalian hypothalamus and has been shown to function as an inhibitor of growth hormone release. Its presence in nonhypothalamic areas has led to the suggestion that it might also function as a neurotransmitter. As with most putative neurotransmitters, few data are available concerning the distribution, subcellular localization, or function of SS within the auditory system. Virtually all that is known is that it can be detected with either radioimmunoassay (RIA) or immunocytochemistry tests in several auditory areas of the adult rat. Somatostatin may occur in some nuclei in a higher concentration during the prenatal or early postnatal period of mammals, suggesting a possible role in the formation of synaptic contacts. Additionally, SS has been shown to increase following injury to SS-containing neurons in adult rats, suggesting that such neurons may be involved in synaptic reorganization.

ACKNOWLEDGMENTS

Many of the figures in this chapter have been redrawn from those of Dr. Goodhill in the 1979 work *Ear Diseases, Deafness and Dizziness* (Harper & Row, Hagerstown, Maryland).

SELECTED READING

Anson, B. J., and McVay, C. B. (1971): *Surgical Anatomy,* ed. 5. Saunders, Philadelphia.

Ballenger, J. J. (1985): *Diseases of the Nose, Throat, Ear, Head and Neck.* Lea & Febiger, Philadelphia.

Goodhill, V. (1979): *Ear Diseases, Deafness and Dizziness,* Harper & Row, Hagerstown, Maryland.

Lawrence, M. (1980): Inner ear physiology. In: *Otolaryngology, Vol. I: Basic Sciences and Related Disciplines,* edited by Paparella, M. M., and Shumrick, D. A. pp. 216–240. Saunders, Philadelphia.

Paparella, M. M., and Shumrick, D. A., editors (1980): *Otolaryngology, Vol. I: Basic Sciences and Related Disciplines.* Saunders, Philadelphia.

Pickles, J. O. (1982): *An Introduction to the Physiology of Hearing,* p. 170, Academic Press, New York.

Schuknecht, H. F. (1974): *Pathology of the Ear.* Harvard University Press, Cambridge.

Wolff, D., Bellucci, R. J., and Eggston, A. A. (1971): *Surgical and Microscopic Anatomy of the Temporal Bone,* Hafner, New York.

The Ear

Section 2: Ear Examination Techniques and External Ear Disorders

Clinical Examination of the Ear 40
Assessment of Auditory and Vestibular Function.................. 46
Radiologic Evaluation of the Ear.............................. 47
  Plain Films 47
  Polytomography and Computerized Imaging 47
Disorders of the External Ear 47
Congenital Ear Deformities 48
Trauma, Infections, and Foreign Bodies........................ 53
  Pinna 53
  External Auditory Canal.................................... 55
  Cerumen Impaction 56
  Ear Canal Foreign Bodies 57
  Diffuse External Otitis 59
  Localized External Otitis 62
  Chronic External Otitis.................................... 62
  Eczematous External Otitis 62
  "Malignant" External Otitis 62
  Bullous Myringitis 63
Tumors of the External Ear 63
Acquired External Canal Stenosis 64

CLINICAL EXAMINATION OF THE EAR

Adequate examination of the ears in a child requires patience and planning on the part of the examiner, together with a few instruments for illuminating and cleaning the external canal. Pointers designed to make the encounter atraumatic for both the child and the examiner include:

40

1. Carefully adjusting the maintaining the stability of the child's head position during the course of the examination, often best achieved by placing the young child on an examination table or having a parent help restrain the child on his/her lap; the examiner should be prepared to stand up, lean down, and move about to obtain the desired view.

2. Carefully explaining to the child and his/her parent what you are going to do and reassuring them that you will try to avoid any discomfort. If irrigation or suction are to be used, the examiner might let the child feel the water stream or suction tip against a fingertip to show that it will not hurt before attempting to insert it into the ear canal.

3. Selecting an ear speculum of the appropriate size and shape to achieve an adequate view of the canal and tympanic membrane without pressing against the tender skin of the bony canal.

4. Selecting the appropriate otoscopic head: open (surgical) if instrumentation is to be used; closed (diagnostic) if pneumotoscopy to assess drum mobility is likely to be necessary (Fig. 2.2-1).

5. Keeping in mind that any instrument inserted into the ear canal can inflict serious trauma if the child's head moves unexpectedly; being ready to withdraw the instrument immediately if such movement occurs.

6. Using soft and blunt instruments (e.g., small custom-fashioned, cotton-tipped applicator or blunt-loop curette) rather than sharp instruments (e.g., picks) whenever possible.

7. Opting for the benfits of binocular vision, improved lighting, and magnification afforded by the otosurgical microscope whenever possible.

8. Opting for the improved head stability and resultant safety provided by ear examination under general anesthesia in young and/or particularly uncooperative patients (e.g., mentally retarded or emotionally disturbed).

The first step in examination is to assess the general size and shape of the child's head and face with particular attention to any deformities of the jaws, lip, or palate. The size, shape, and position of the pinnae should be noted together with any evidence of erythema, edema, or discharge. The S-shaped external auditory canal extends from the concha to the external surface of the tympanic membrane, a distance in the adult of some 2.5 cm but less in the young child. The tragus at the external meatus and the narrowed canal lumen at the isthmus serve as anatomic

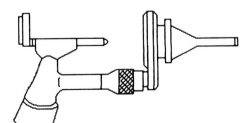

FIG. 2.2-1. Surgical otoscope head.

barriers to the entrance of foreign material which might injure the tympanic membrane or middle ear structures.

In the infant and young child, the tympanic membrane is positioned obliquely, with the anterior inferior wall of the canal being longer than the posterior superior wall. As the child grows, the tympanic membrane assumes a more upright position. The cartilaginous lateral portion of the canal is directed slightly upward and backward, and the osseous canal slightly downward and forward. A prominent anterior bony overhang (the posterior bulge of the temporomandibular joint) may be present in the canal, partially obscuring visualization of a crescent-shaped anterior portion of the tympanic membrane (TM). Visualization of the TM is facilitated in the older child by pulling the pinna gently upward, outward, and backward so as to straighten the canal. In infants, whose shorter canals are principally cartilaginous, gently pulling outward produces the desired view. Standing at the head of the examining table may improve visualization of the TM in the newborn. The examiner should note whether movement of the pinna produces pain (tragal tenderness), as would be compatible with the inflammation of the external ear.

Just medial to the junction of the cartilaginous and bony portions is the isthmus, the narrowest portion of the canal (Fig. 2.2-2). The skin of the bony canal is quite sensitive to trauma, and a painful hematoma readily forms if a shearing force pulls the thin skin layer over the bone, as may occur with vigorous attempts at cerumen or foreign body removal. As might be expected, hair follicles occur almost exclusively in the skin of the cartilaginous canal, and the bony–cartilaginous junction can be visually defined by the examiner who notes the demarcation between hair-bearing and nonhair-bearing skin. The examiner should take note of the general condition of the canal skin and any evidence of inflammation, as well as the presence of cerumen, otorrhea, or foreign bodies.

Next, the condition and position of the TM should be evaluated, keeping in mind

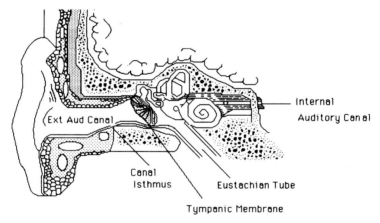

FIG. 2.2-2. External canal landmarks. (Redrawn from Goodhill, V. *Ear Diseases, Deafness and Dizziness,* p. 5. Harper & Row, Hagerstown, 1979.)

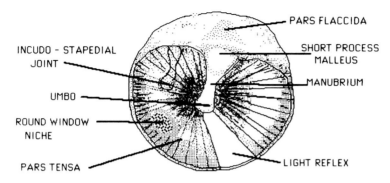

FIG. 2.2-3. Tympanic membrane landmarks.

its normal landmarks (Fig. 2.2-3). The pars tensa is normally pearly gray and translucent enough to occasionally permit visualization of the long process of the incus as it descends, turning medially (lenticular process) to meet the capitulum of the stapes in the posterior superior quadrant of the tympanic cavity. The stapes extends medially to the oval window from the incudostapedial joint and therefore is not visible through the drum. Occasionally the darkish shadow of the round window niche may be visible through the posterior inferior portion of the drum. The pars tensa comprises the majority of the TM consisting of an outer layer of keratinizing squamous epithelium, a middle layer of fibrous connective tissue, and an inner layer of mucosa continuous with the remainder of the middle ear lining. The examiner should determine if the TM is opacified, discolored, inflamed, or scarred, as well as if calcific plaques are present (tympanosclerosis) (Fig. 2.2-4). The extent and location of any pathologic changes should be diagramed for later reference. As hyperemia of the middle ear mucosa occurs with disease, the examiner can observe hypervascularity and pinkish discoloration along the handle of the malleus spreading gradually across the upper portion of the TM. It is important to realize that straining and crying in the young child may be associated with a reddish

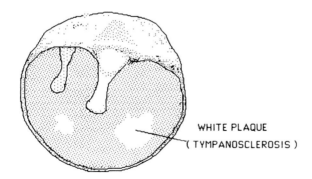

FIG. 2.2-4. Tympanosclerotic plaques in tympanic membrane.

discoloration of the TM leading to mistaken diagnosis of early otitis media. In this case, however, mobility should be unimpaired by either retraction or bulging of the drum.

The TM is attached at its circumference and to the manubrium of the malleus, assuming a conical shape with the bony umbo of the manubrium as the medial apex. If the drum is in normal position, a light reflection (i.e., "light reflex") may be noted in the anterior inferior quadrant of the TM. Special attention should be directed to the small superior portion of the TM, the pars flaccida (Shrapnell's membrane), which is above the short lateral process of the malleus and is further defined by the anterior and posterior malleal folds. The pars flaccida is devoid of the fibrous tissue layer found in the pars tensa with a consequent impairment of elasticity and predilection for medial retraction in the presence of negative middle ear pressure. The lateral short process of the malleus constitutes a diagnostic landmark in otoscopy and appears more prominent as the TM retracts medially (Fig. 2.2-5). Another sign of medial retraction is a foreshortened appearance of the long process (manubrium) of the malleus. Bulging of the drum tends to obliterate rather than enhance the appearance of the TM's bony landmarks (Fig. 2.2-6). Specific attention should be paid to the presence of any retraction pockets often seen in the pars flaccida and the posterior quadrants of the pars tensa.

The mobility of the tympanic membrane may be assessed by means of pneumatic otoscopy (gentle application of positive and negative pressure in an ear canal occluded by a speculum attached to a diagnostic otoscope head). Impedance audiometric techniques to assess mobility of the tympanic membrane/ossicular complex are described in Section 5 of this chapter. Decreased mobility is usually seen with negative middle ear pressure and medial TM retraction, whereas TM atrophy or ossicular discontinuity would be expected to produce hypermobility of the intact drum.

Tympanic membrane findings associated with middle ear disease are discussed in detail in Section 3 of this chapter. Common otoscopic signs of middle ear effusion may include:

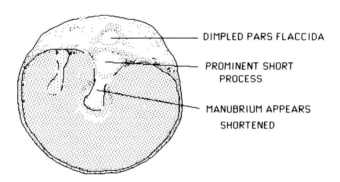

DIMPLED PARS FLACCIDA

PROMINENT SHORT PROCESS

MANUBRIUM APPEARS SHORTENED

FIG. 2.2-5. Retracted tympanic membrane.

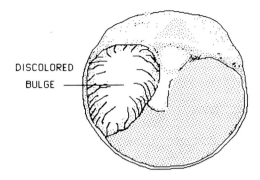

DISCOLORED
BULGE

FIG. 2.2-6. Bulging tympanic membrane.

1. Opaque, amber, or yellowish discoloration of the drumhead with an increase in capillary vascularity and loss of tympanic membrane light reflex. A fluid level or bubbles may also be visible through the drum (Fig. 2.2-7).

2. A blue drumhead, seen in the absence of a history of trauma or middle ear tumor, often associated with long-standing serous otitis media, barotitis/barotrauma, or cholesterol granuloma.

3. Retraction of the tympanic membrane with increased prominence of the short process and apparent shortening of the long process of the malleus.

4. Decreased mobility of the tympanic membrane on pneumootoscopy or Valsalva maneuver.

If pale-colored fluid fills the entire middle ear cavity, it may be difficult to detect otoscopically, but pneumatic compression should reveal a poorly mobile tympanic membrane.

The size, shape, and location of any perforations in the tympanic membrane should be noted, including whether the perforation is surrounded by pars tensa (central perforation) or abuts against the tympanic annulus (marginal perforation) (Fig. 2.2-8). A marginal perforation is more likely to be associated with acquired cholesteatoma formation. The appearance of the underlying middle ear mucosa should also be observed, as well as the nature and amount of any secretions present

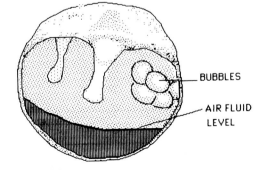

FIG. 2.2-7. Middle ear effusion.

BUBBLES

AIR FLUID LEVEL

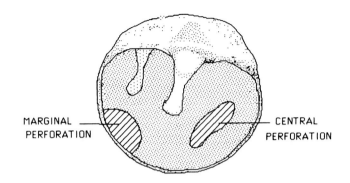

MARGINAL PERFORATION   CENTRAL PERFORATION

FIG. 2.2-8. Tympanic membrane perforations.

in the middle ear. One should be especially wary of an aural polyp which takes origin in the middle ear cleft and may be closely associated with the ossicular chain. Attempts at removing an aural polyp in an uncontrolled situation without adequate magnification and instrumentation can lead to disruption of the ossicular chain and possible destruction of inner ear function.

Depending on their location and size, perforations of the tympanic membrane can produce variable degrees of conductive hearing impairment. Other pathologic conditions such as atrophy of the tympanic membrane, tympanosclerosis, otosclerosis, or chronic tympanomastoid disease can result in fixation of the tympanic membrane and/or ossicular chain with a resulting decrease in the efficiency of sound energy transmission. Disarticulation of the TM/ossicular chain complex, resulting from such causes as trauma or infection, can lead to a maximal conductive deficit, particularly if the TM remains imperforate.

A cholesteatoma may present as a whitish mass behind an intact TM or, more commonly, in the form of a whitish membrane associated with whitish keratin debris and foul-smelling drainage in the canal. An aural polyp is not an unusual finding in association with a cholesteatoma.

A thorough examination of the nose and nasopharynx using anterior rhinoscopy, posterior nasopharyngeal mirror examination, or direct nasopharyngoscopy is essential in determining etiologic factors in cases of middle ear disease.

ASSESSMENT OF AUDITORY AND VESTIBULAR FUNCTION

Although such tuning fork tests as the Rinne, Weber, and Schwabach are still quite useful with adults and older children, they have limited usefulness with the younger child. The tasks of localizing the apparent source of sound delivered through the skull midline (Weber) or comparing the loudness of air-conducted and bone-conducted sound (Rinne) are confusing to many children, and results can be specious. A thorough discussion of pediatric audiologic techniques is contained in Section 5 of this chapter.

Apart from the history of dysequilibrium, the presence of spontaneous nystagmus is the most easily recognizable sign of possible vestibular dysfunction. Vestibular nystagmus should be distinguished from the pendular type characteristic of benign congenital ocular nystagmus. An additional helpful screening test for vestibular and cerebellar disease is the tandem-gait Romberg test (eyes open and eyes closed).

RADIOLOGIC EVALUATION OF THE EAR

Plain Films

In most departments of radiology, a standard series of plain mastoid views has been selected for routine use from among the many possible options. Some of these projections are aimed at assessing the status of the middle-ear cavity and the periantral air cells, likely to be affected in inflammatory conditions. Usually included is a lateral view, most commonly Schüller's view or the Owen's modification of the Mayer view, which approximates the anatomic relationships presented to the surgeon during a standard surgical approach to mastoidectomy. Another common projection is a transorbital oblique view of the mastoid cavity which provides a view of the incus and malleus surrounded by air in the epitympanum. Finally, a view which achieves an overview of the petrous bone as it extends along the base of the skull is included. Stenver's view places the x-ray beam perpendicular to the posterior surface of the petrous bone. This projection provides a view of the mastoid cells around the antrum as well as a useful assessment of the internal auditory meatus, a common site of eighth nerve tumors and occasionally meningiomas.

Polytomography and Computerized Imaging

Assessment of fine structures within the temporal bone, including ossicular structures, the labyrinth, the internal auditory canal (e.g., for acoustic tumors), and the fallopian canal, requires more sophisticated techniques than afforded by plain x-ray films. For a number of years, hypocycloidal polytomography filled this need, but more recently high-resolution computerized tomographic scanning technology has become the evaluative method of choice. It gives enhanced appreciation of cochlear anatomy and results in less radiation exposure than polytomography.

DISORDERS OF THE EXTERNAL EAR

For purposes of this discussion, the external ear consists of the pinna, the cartilaginous and bony external ear canal, and the lateral surface of the tympanic membrane. An extensive discussion of the embryology and clinical anatomy of the ear is included in Section 1 of this chapter, but a brief review is essential to understand congenital ear deformities.

The pinna is formed from six hillocks, arising from the first and second branchial arches by the sixth week of embryonic development, which fuse to form the auricle by the end of the third month. Except for the tragus, the remainder of the complex, skin-covered elastic cartilage folds and recesses of the external ear are formed by the hillocks derived from the second arch. Incomplete fusion can result in the fairly common malformation of a preauricular sinus. This small opening near the incisura between the tragus and the anterior superior insertion of the helix can extend inward to terminate in a multilocular cyst. Recurrent infection may necessitate surgical removal extensive enough to encompass the entire cystic mass to prevent recurrence. The anomaly commonly shows a familial distribution compatible with a dominant inheritance pattern. Rarely reported is a first branchial cleft anomaly which presents as a cystic structure anterior to the pinna but which may open into the eternal auditory canal rather than the preauricular area. Again, safe removal requires surgical familiarity with anatomy of the parotid, facial nerve, and auricular region.

At the same time that middle ear development is proceeding, a solid cord of epithelial cells grows inward from the primitive external meatus toward the advancing pharyngeal pouch epithelium which forms the middle ear cleft. These two elements are separated by a thin layer of mesoderm, thus giving rise to the three layers of the tympanic membrane: external epithelium, middle connective tissue, and internal mucosa. The connective tissue at the periphery of the developing TM undergoes ossification to form the tympanic sulcus in which the thickened and rolled edge of the tympanic annulus develops. By the middle of the seventh month of gestation, the sound conduction and perception elements of the developing ear have reached nearly complete development. Only then does the solid core of epithelial cells between the primitive external meatus and the tympanic membrane begin to pull away from the TM to form the lumen of the external auditory canal. The progressive cavitation of the canal proceeds from medial to lateral, accounting for the possibility of congenital meatal atresia coexisting with a normally developed tympanic membrane, middle ear, and ossicular chain.

CONGENITAL EAR DEFORMITIES

Specific auricular malformations resulting from failure in differentiation of the first and second branchial arches include anotia, microtia, malformations of the cartilaginous structure or folds (e.g., lop ear), and malpositioning of the auricles on the side of the head (Fig. 2.2-9). Congenital atresia of the external auditory canal results from interruption of normal developmental progression of the first branchial cleft.

Congenital malformations limited to the auricle are defects in branchial arch differentiation and are not usually associated with anomalies of the tympanic membrane, middle ear, and ossicles (see Section 1, Anatomy and Physiology, in this chapter). These malformations constitute cosmetic problems unless collapse of the external meatus and canal, resulting in a conductive hearing loss, is an associated

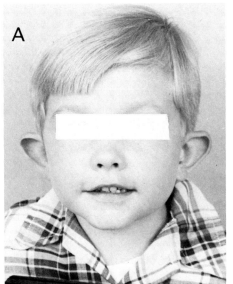 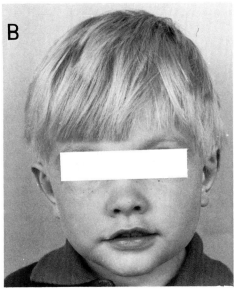

FIG. 2.2-9. **A:** Lop ear deformity pre-operatively. **B.** Post operative bilateral otoplasty.

feature of the anomaly. These anomalies most commonly include auricles which are larger or smaller than normal, as well as those lacking normal architecture, such as "lop" ears in which the absence of the antihelical fold is a common finding. Techniques for surgical correction of these deformities are beyond the scope of this text, but most techniques involve a postauricular approach through which the cartilaginous shape of the auricle can be refashioned into a more cosmetically acceptable form. The usual timing for such cosmetic intervention is during the immediate preschool period when the child is a more cooperative patient and a better anesthetic risk than during infancy.

Moderate and severe forms of congenital aural atresia are encountered in about one of 10,000 to 20,000 individuals, the incidence being equal between males and females. Bilateral atresia is only one-fourth as common as unilateral atresia, which appears to affect the right ear more commonly than the left. Complex ear deformities may include malformations of the external ear and canal, as well as the middle ear in which anotia (absence of external ear structures), microtia, or auricular malpositioning are combined with structural malformations or absence of the external auditory meatus, canal, and middle ear. Aplasia of the auricle may range from partly formed auricles to small cartilaginous or soft-tissue remnants on the side of the head. Placement of the external ear is usually below and anterior to its normal location, so-called "low set" ears. These deformities may be unilateral or bilateral and may occur as isolated anomalies or as one component of a complex syndrome such as Treacher Collins Syndrome (Fig. 2.2-10) (see Section 4 in this chapter).

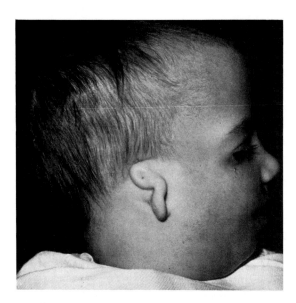

FIG. 2.2-10.   Severe microtia with canal atresia; Treacher Collins syndrome.

In the majority of instances, cochlear function is essentially normal as demonstrated by a careful audiologic evaluation, whereas the hearing loss observed is of the conductive type.

The middle ear cleft and mastoid air cell system can vary in development from being well pneumatized to nearly nonexistent. On surface appearance, the external canal is frequently represented by only a dimple in the skin, underlying which is found in most cases a block of solid bone, the atresia plate, or in rare instances cartilage and soft tissue (Fig. 2.2-11). The only evidence of a tympanic membrane may be a fibrous and mucosal remnant separating the atresia plate from the middle ear cleft. In cases where cartilaginous obstruction of the canal or bony stenosis (as opposed to atresia) is present, a collection of keratin debris derived from the canal skin may become entrapped, giving rise to a canal cholesteatoma or, more properly, keratoma. The range of ossicular chain anomalies found in these patients may include minimal anatomic deformities of the ossicles, fusion of major components such as the malleus and incus, fixation of the stapedial footplate, or nearly total nondifferentiation of the ossicles and oval window.

The approach to correction of these anomalies involves both cosmetic and functional considerations. Correction of the external auricular deformity may involve a multistaged surgical procedure in which the auricular remnants are preserved, rotated into position, and augmented with grafts of cartilage (e.g., costal cartilage) and skin; alternatively, a carefully fashioned prothesis may be utilized to achieve an acceptable cosmetic result. With availability of newer synthetic materials and adhesives, artificial prostheses are gaining wider popularity, even though on initial

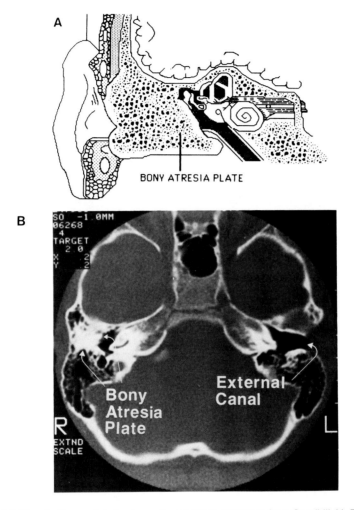

FIG. 2.2-11. **A:** Congenital atresia—external canal. (Redrawn from Goodhill, V. *Ear Diseases, Deafness and Dizziness,* p. 594. Harper & Row, Hagerstown, 1979.) **B:** CT scan showing atresia of the right external auditory canal.

reflection they seem less acceptable to the child. The risk of multiple anesthetics and less than satisfactory results of surgical reconstruction in many instances are factors which must be weighed by parents and physicians as they develop a specific treatment plan for an individual child. Because of their ability to cover the deformed auricle utilizing appropriate hair styles (Fig. 2.2-12), females are less likely to require cosmetic surgical correction of unilateral deformities than males. The need for amelioration of this cosmetic deformity is most urgently felt by parents as the child nears school age, and appropriate referral to a team of specialists including

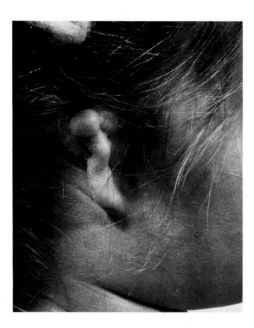

FIG. 2.2-12. Unilateral external ear deformity easily camouflaged by hair style.

otolaryngologists, plastic surgeons, and prosthetists should be undertaken by the primary physician for consultation regarding these complex issues.

The availability of adequate hearing to the developing child with an ear deformity is obviously of paramount importance. Both audiologic and radiologic techniques can be used to assess the nature of the deformity and the status of the inner ear structures. Multidirectional tomography or later-generation computerized axial tomography is useful in assessing the size and location of the middle ear space, mastoid air cell system, ossicular components, and the fallopian canal containing the facial nerve within the temporal bone. Information regarding the general status of inner ear structures can also be gleaned from these radiologic studies.

Auditory habilitation in these cases is usually multifaceted, and the therapeutic plan is greatly influenced by whether the deformity is unilateral or bilateral. In cases of unilateral deformity, with essentially normal hearing in the contralateral ear, no immediate intervention with amplification is necessary, and in the absence of other handicaps the child should be expected to develop normal auditory skills together with age-appropriate speech and language. As with any other unilateral hearing loss, preferential classroom seating that takes advantage of the normal-hearing ear is critical. With regard to surgical reconstruction of the conductive mechanism (i.e., ear canal, tympanic membrane, and ossicles) in these unilateral cases, there is some disagreement among authors reporting large series. The somewhat uncertain benefits to be derived from binaural hearing afforded by tympanoplastic reconstruction in these children must be weighed against the associated risks of anesthesia, damage to the facial nerve or inner ear structures, and suboptimal hearing results achieved in many of these patients. Some patients with unilateral deformities who have undergone reconstructive surgery complain that the contrasting signal provided by subnormal auditory acuity in the reconstructed ear when compared with their normal-hearing ear is more distracting than was the presurgical absence of useful auditory function.

Bilateral involvement poses a more severe developmental problem. Based on audiologic findings, an appropriate bone conduction hearing aid should be fitted on these children as soon as possible and the parents instructed in strategies aimed at developing good auditory listening skills in their child. If these steps are instituted promptly, children with good inner ear function should develop normal communicative skills. The availability of good bone conduction aids has allowed deferral of surgical intervention in these cases until the child's skull growth begins to approach adult proportions. As a general rule, the age-related increased pneumatization of the mastoid air cell system, from which space for the often-deficient tympanic cavity must be "borrowed," makes delay advisable in most cases. Radiologic and audiologic studies are helpful in selecting the ear which presents anatomic features most likely to contribute to a desirable surgical result. Early referral of these cases to a team specializing in congenital deformities is essential because placement of incisions for the tympanoplastic procedure may jeopardize the cosmetic phase of reconstruction and vice versa. Some compromise on the part of all surgeons involved is usually necessary, and the particular psychological needs of the child and family may play a role in rehabilitation planning.

TRAUMA, INFECTIONS, AND FOREIGN BODIES

Pinna

Skin on the posteromedial surface of the pinna is loosely attached and movable over the underlying elastic cartilage, whereas the anterolateral skin is firmly attached to the auricular folds. Penetrating vessels from the closely attached anterior covering are important in supplying nutrients to the cartilage, and this blood supply can be compromised by a subcutaneous collection of blood, serum, or pus between the anterior skin and cartilage (Fig. 2.2-13). Partial resorption of the cartilage may result in the "cauliflower ear" that was quite common among wrestlers and other athletes prior to the advent of ear protectors. Perichondritis of the auricular cartilage may also result following infection, surgery, frostbite, or burns of the external ear. The most commonly identified causative organisms are the gram-negative bacteria *Pseudomonas,* but gram-positive staphylococci may also be present. Local incision and drainage as well as topical drops combined with parenteral antibiotic therapy specific for the causative agent are necessary to prevent cartilage resorption (Fig. 2.2-14). Surgical removal of necrotic cartilage may also be required.

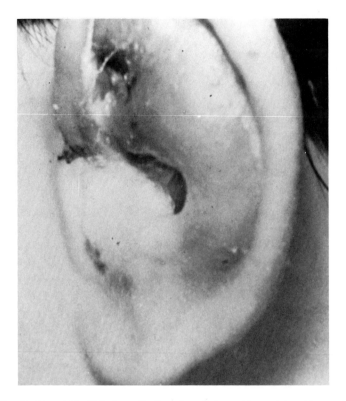

FIG. 2.2-13. Perichondritis. Note the collection of pus between the perichondrium and cartilage.

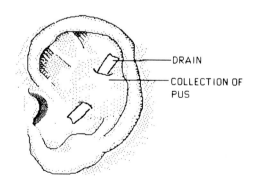

FIG. 2.2-14. Incision and drainage of perichondritis.

External Auditory Canal

The external auditory canal extends from the concha to the external surface of the tympanic membrane; the tragus at the external meatus and the narrowed canal lumen at the isthmus serve as anatomic barriers to the entrance of foreign material which might injure the tympanic membrane or middle ear structures. In addition, cerumen provides a water-repellent coating for the canal skin, minimizing the impact of short periods of exposure to liquid contamination. Cerumen consists of a complex mixture of sebaceous and apocrine glandular secretions combined with exfoliated cornified cells of the stratum corneum which can dissolve during periods of prolonged exposure to water. Parents of small children often attempt to clean all visible cerumen from the child's ear during bathing, thus removing an important barrier to infection and injury of the external canal skin.

Lined with keratinizing stratified squamous epithelium, which is continuous with the lateral surface of the tympanic membrane, the external auditory canal represents the only skin-lined cul-de-sac in the body, with attendant susceptibility to certain dermatoses. Skin lining the cartilaginous canal contains epidermal, dermal, and subcutaneous elements, varying from 0.5 to 1 mm in thickness; the bony canal is lined by a 0.2 mm layer of skin devoid of papillae or subcutaneous tissue with firm attachment to the periosteum of underlying bone (Fig. 2.2-15). A painful hematoma readily forms if manipulation of an instrument such as a cerumen curette is excessively vigorous. As noted previously, the bony–cartilaginous junction can be visually defined by the examiner who notes the demarcation between hair-bearing and nonhair-bearing skin.

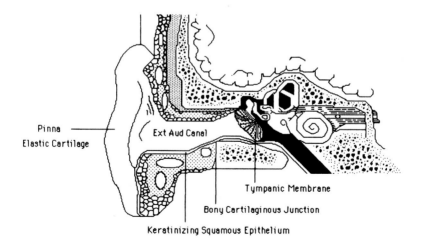

Pinna
Elastic Cartilage
Ext Aud Canal
Tympanic Membrane
Bony Cartilaginous Junction
Keratinizing Squamous Epithelium

FIG. 2.2-15. External ear landmarks. (Redrawn from Goodhill, V.: *Ear Diseases, Deafness and Dizziness,* p. 4. Harper & Row, Hagerstown, 1979.)

Cerumen Impaction

Cerumen impaction is the most commonly treated disorder of the external ear, and predisposing factors may include abnormal external canal shape or size, as well as excessively dry or sticky cerumen. Removal of a cerumen impaction in a young child whose tympanic membrane is intact is best accomplished by gentle irrigation of the ear canal with a solution such as tap water mixed with hydrogen peroxide at body temperature (Fig. 2.2-16). Additional cleaning and drying of the canal with a small cotton-tipped applicator, small cerumen loop curette (Fig. 2.2-17), and/or Baron suction tip (No. 3 or 5) may also be helpful. As during any other instrumentation of the external ear canal in the young child, proper immobilization of the head coupled with careful explanation of the procedure to the older child minimizes the chances for injury to the skin of the canal or the underlying tympanic membrane and middle ear structures. If initial attempts at cerumen removal do not meet with success, several days' delay during which cerumen-softening otic drops (e.g., hydrogen peroxide with oily or glycerine base) are instilled into the canal can facilitate removal and avoid an unpleasant experience for the young child. The examiner should be aware that foreign bodies or bony protuberances (e.g., exostoses or osteomas) can become coated with cerumen, and if careful attempts at removal in the office are unsuccessful, examination and cleaning of the ear under general anesthesia may be the safest alternative.

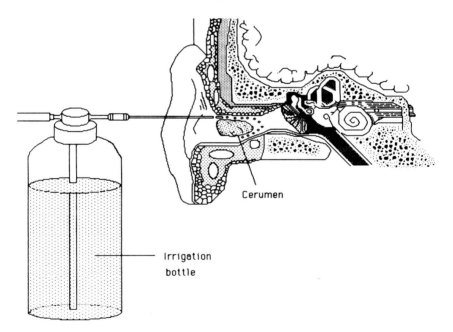

FIG. 2.2-16. Removal of cerumen by canal irrigation. (Redrawn from Goodhill, V. *Ear Diseases, Deafness and Dizziness*, p. 279. Harper & Row, Hagerstown, 1979.)

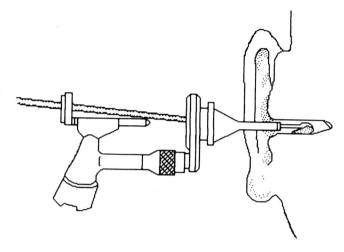

FIG. 2.2-17. Cerumen removal with an ear curette. (Redrawn from Goodhill, V.: *Ear Diseases, Deafness and Dizziness,* p. 277. Harper & Row, Hagerstown, 1979.)

Ear Canal Foreign Bodies

Any small object which finds its way into the hand of a toddler or behaviorly incompetent child (e.g., retarded or emotionally disturbed) is a potential external canal foreign body (Fig. 2.2-18). In the author's experience, this may include vegetable matter, e.g., peas, peanuts, rice, pretzel sticks, and all types of candy, or inert foreign objects ranging from crayons and pencil erasers to styrofoam toy stuffing, beads, extruded tympanostomy tubes, and metal nuts unscrewed from toys. Live insects may even find their way into the warm, dark recesses of the external auditory canal. These foreign objects can be smooth and rounded or jagged and sharp. Although vegetable matter usually provokes a prompt inflammatory response, inert objects may have been present for some time. The child with an external canal foreign body often presents in the emergency room or the primary care physician's office, and it is important to keep in mind a few important management principles:

1. An external canal foreign body seldom represents a true medical emergency.

2. Vegetable-type foreign bodies present a special problem because moisture in the external canal, either naturally occurring or from attempts at irrigation, causes the foreign body to expand.

3. Adequate immobilization of the child's head and proper instrumentation, including good lighting and magnification, are essential to avoid injury to the canal skin, tympanic membrane, or middle ear structures.

4. The use of general anesthesia and the otosurgical microscope, with specially designed microsurgical instruments, should be considered early rather than late in the course of managing external canal foreign bodies, especially in the young or uncooperative child.

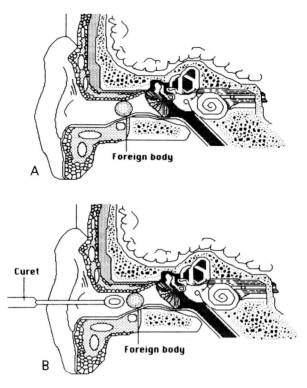

FIG. 2.2-18 A: External canal with a foreign body. **B:** Inappropriate approach to foreign body removal. (Redrawn from Goodhill, V.: *Ear Diseases, Deafness and Dizziness,* p. 281. Harper & Row, Hagerstown, 1979.)

Too often an emergency room physician, lacking proper instrumentation, persists in attempting to remove a difficult foreign body from the ear canal of an unanesthetized child. The child's struggles may lead to a canal laceration with bleeding, a perforated tympanic membrane (Fig. 2.2-19), or, worse, damage to the ossicles and inner ear with resultant risk of infection and hearing loss.

Proper and safe management includes a careful and honest assessment of the child, his/her potential for cooperation, the nature of the foreign body, the instruments available to effect safe removal, and finally the competence of the examiner to deal with potential complications. If the foreign body looks like it would be difficult to remove, given the level of the child's cooperation and available instrumentation, it is appropriate to refer the child to an otolaryngologist. In all but the most favorable cases, the otolaryngologist opts for removal of the foreign object under general anesthesia utilizing the operating microscope and otosurgical instruments. If damage to the tympanic membrane or middle ear structures has occurred, it can be fully assessed and possibly repaired during the same anesthesia.

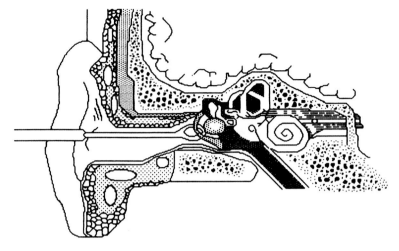

FIG. 2.2-19. Complication of foreign body removal. (Redrawn from Goodhill, V.: *Ear Diseases, Deafness and Dizziness,* p. 282. Harper & Row, Hagerstown, 1979.)

Diffuse External Otitis

Infections constitute the most common diseases of the external ear, with the acute, diffuse form of external otitis (Fig. 2.2-20) most common in hot, humid environments. In addition to high humidity, epidemiologic studies implicate heat, prolonged exposure to water (e.g., swimming) resulting in maceration of the canal skin, trauma secondary to attempts at cleaning or scratching with such implements as cotton swabs and hair pins, and introduction of exogenous bacteria from such sources as lake or pool water. Normal flora of the external auditory canal include *Staphylococcus epidermidis, Corynebacterium,* and micrococci plus, on occasion, *Staphylococcus aureus* and *Streptococcus viridans.* Pathogenic organisms in external otitis can include bacteria, usually gram-negative *Pseudomonas* group, fungi, viruses, spirochetes, and even parasites.

A history of local trauma commonly antedates development of external otitis. This form of trauma frequently occurs on insertion of a foreign object into the ear canal in response to the desire to ease the itching, which is so frequently present in the ear, especially in hot, humid environments.

Diffuse external otitis is characterized by inflammatory edema of the canal lining, pain, itching, a feeling of fullness, drainage, and often some degree of hearing loss due to canal obstruction. The exfoliated keratin debris in the canal constitutes an excellent culture medium, and suppuration generally follows, which may be accompanied by a mild degree of inflammation of the canal perichondrium leading to increasing pain, especially on touching or manipulating the tragus or external meatus, as well as during chewing. The unpleasant-smelling exudate is often green-

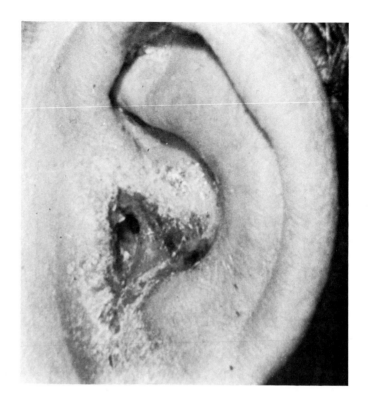

FIG. 2.2-20.   Diffuse external otitis, severe.

ish white and may be accompanied by swelling of the canal lining severe enough to prevent thorough examination and cleaning. In such cases a small wick of gauze or synthetic material may be inserted through the edematous portion of the canal so that drops containing antimicrobials and corticosteroids might be instilled. After several days of such a regimen, edema generally subsides enough to allow a more traditional approach to evaluation and treatment. If resolution does not begin and pain increases, hospitalization with parenteral antibiotics and analgesics may be necessary. In persistent cases, culture of the exudate might be undertaken, but large studies have shown that *Pseudomonas* species are found in one-half to two-thirds of instances; other bacterial pathogens, indicated to a lesser extent, include *Proteus* species, *Escherichia coli*, *S. epidermidis*, *S. aureus*, streptococci, diphtheroids, *Enterobacter aerogenes*, *Klebsiella pneumoniae*, and *Citrobacter*.

Mycotic otitis externa is much less common than generally supposed, constituting about 10% of the otitis externa patients in the United States, although it is more prevalent in tropical climates. Most commonly identified pathogens are *Aspergillus*, which is responsible for about 90% of infections, as well as *Phycomycetes*, *Rhizopus*, *Actinomyces*, *Penicillium*, or yeasts. Patients with immunodeficiency syndromes or who have been receiving immunosuppressive medications or long-term antibiotic therapy are likely candidates for otomycosis. Topical antifungal preparations recommended for use include nystatin, *m*-cresyl acetate, amphotericin B, 1% gentian violet, 1% iodine, or 10% resorcin. Such systemic agents as griseofulvin or amphotericin B are rarely required and of course necessitate hospitalization with careful monitoring for side effects.

Less common forms of diffuse otitis externa include erysipelas and herpes simplex infection, usually limited to the auricle; bullous myringitis with hemorrhagic bullae involving the canal skin and lateral surface of the tympanic membrane, and herpes zoster oticus, which may proceed to involve the seventh and eighth cranial nerves (Ramsey Hunt syndrome).

Senturia et al., in their excellent discussion of external ear disease, defined therapeutic objectives as:

1. Elimination of the microbiologic agents
2. Reduction of inflammation and edema
3. Elimination of discomfort
4. Removal of cerumen and debris from the ear canal; restoration of hearing
5. Restoration of oil and water content of skin
6. Elimination of recurrent itching and scratching

The approaches to treatment of external otitis are those applicable to dermatoses elsewhere on the body surface. The treatment regimen should include thorough cleaning of the ear canal of all secretions and keratin debris to the extent tolerated by the patient. Gentle irrigation with a mixture of sterile water and 35% isopropyl alcohol is often quite effective. As with cerumen removal, a small cotton-tipped applicator and Baron-type ear suction should be available for use by the examiner. Evacuation of the contents of the canal permits direct contact between the medication to be instilled and the diseased skin. In the face of infection, the pH of the ear canal shifts from its normal value of 5 to 7 toward an alkaline level. Effective preparations for treatment of external otitis contain agents such as acetic acid aimed at restoring a slightly more acidic pH (e.g., Domeboro or Vosol drops).

Selection of the appropriate therapeutic agent should be based on consideration of microbiologic, anatomic, and pathologic factors specific to a particular child's ear. In clinical situations, however, it is desirable to employ an agent aimed at inhibiting gram-positive bacteria combined with another aimed at gram-negative organisms. In addition, the incorporation of a corticosteroid to control inflammatory eczematoid reactions is a distinct advantage. Pharmacologic preparations containing one or more antibiotics, with or without a corticosteroid, are available under an array of trade names (e.g., Cortisporin, Pyocidin, Coly-mycin Otic). It should be kept in mind that some of these antibiotics, particularly topical neomycin, have the potential for skin sensitization with a resultant allergic response. In addition to the possibility of resistant organisms, this potential side effect should be suspected if swelling, pain, and drainage persist after a sufficient therapeutic trial.

Localized External Otitis

A furuncle associated with a hair follicle in the external ear canal results in what has been called acute circumscribed otitis externa. Characterized by severe pain, this entity is most commonly caused by *Staphylococcus*. Local heat and systemic antibiotics are most effective in resolving the disorder, with incision and drainage occasionally necessary. As previously described with the acute diffuse form, a wick impregnated with otic drops or ointment yields symptomatic relief and helps get topical medication into contact with all portions of the canal skin.

Chronic External Otitis

Severe and permanent changes in the external canal skin, occasionally seen in adults after prolonged bouts of otitis externa, are rarely observed in children. Most persistent cases in children respond to careful cleaning and drying, coupled with scrupulous avoidance of exposure to water and other contaminants. Resistant organisms, if present, should be identified by culture, and other sources of chronicity, e.g., sensitivity to one or more of the therapeutic agents in use, should be sought. Other rare forms of chronic external otitis include the tubercular form and, less commonly, that associated with lues, yaws, leprosy, or sarcoidosis.

Eczematous External Otitis

Patients may have inflammatory involvement of the external auditory canal in conjunction with an atopic predisposition, seborrheic dermatitis, psoriasis, systemic lupus erythematosus, neurodermatitis, skin sensitivity to topical medications, contact dermatitis, purulent otitis media, and infantile eczema. Itching is the most common presenting complaint, and attempts at scratching with fingernails or sharp instruments can lead to bleeding and secondary infection with bacteria or other pathogens. Constant scratching and picking at the ear by the child with an underlying emotional disturbance may exacerbate the condition. To ameliorate such irritation, antipruritics, antihistamines, analgesics, or tranquilizers may be necessary. Additionally, topical therapy should be initiated with agents such as Burow's solution for active weeping followed by topical corticosteroid preparations to minimize inflammation and prevent recurrence. The child's environment and daily habits must be examined for such commonly offending contact sensitizers as soaps, shampoos, hair sprays, bubble baths, and spray fragrances.

"Malignant" External Otitis

A severe variant of otitis externa is "malignant" external otitis, which characteristically affects the elderly and debilitated, especially diabetics. It is extremely uncommon in children but usually is caused by *Pseudomonas* species which gains access to the deeper tissues surrounding the ear canal including the temporal bone and parotid gland. Vasculitis followed by thrombosis with necrosis of tissue can involve surrounding cartilage, bone, lymph nodes, middle ear structures, the facial nerve, venous sinuses, other cranial nerves, and intracranial structures as well. Examination of the external canal often shows granulation tissue at the junction of the bony and cartilaginous portions of the canal, and the mastoid process may be inflamed and tender. If extensive encroachment on the temporal bone and the base of the skull occurs, widespread central nervous system involvement and death may ensue. Permanent cranial nerve neuropathies, particularly facial paralysis, may result even if the patient recovers.

Treatment of this serious form of external ear infection requires hospitalization, management of predisposing conditions, intensive parenteral, as well as topical, therapy with antimicrobials effective against *Pseudomonas,* and wide débridement of involved tissues which may include extended mastoidectomy, parotid resection, and facial nerve decompression. Careful monitoring for central spread of the infection or impending toxicities of the antibiotic treatment, e.g., renal failure, during the prolonged treatment course (4 to 6 weeks) is essential. Baseline and follow-up auditory and vestibular testing should be accomplished, but caloric irrigation of the affected ear should be avoided. The availability of computerized rotational testing for vestibular dysfunction provides a safe and repeatable way to assess these patients.

Bullous Myringitis

Although bullous myringitis involves the lateral surface of the tympanic membrane, it is technically a disease process that involves the external ear. Most likely of viral origin, this disorder is of limited duration and is characterized by the presence of a number of large blebs, containing blood and/or serous fluid, on the lateral surface of the eardrum. The patient usually complains of pain and may demonstrate some degree of hearing loss. It can be treated with local antibiotic steroid drops, systemic antibiotics to protect against secondary bacterial infection, and surgical opening of the blebs, which is rarely indicated for severe pain.

TUMORS OF THE EXTERNAL EAR

Benign and, very rarely, malignant tumors may affect the external ear in children. An osteoma of the external auditory canal presents as a rounded, hard, skin-covered mass usually encountered along the superior wall of the canal. It may be covered by a thin layer of cerumen, appearing to be a piece of hardened ear wax. Aggressive attempts at removal produce pain and bleeding, and children with such a finding should undergo radiologic examination of the canal. Fibrous dysplasia, either monostotic or polystotic, may also involve the external auditory canal resulting in hearing loss and bony occlusion of the canal with potential cholesteatoma formation. In both types of bony lesion the bone growth must be removed. Ossifying fibromas have also been seen. These also must be surgically removed from the external canal, and the middle ear must be exteriorized.

Rhabdomyosarcoma is the most commonly observed malignant tumor involving the ear, with reticular cell sarcoma less common. A combination of chemotherapy, irradiation, and surgery must be utilized in treating these often fatal lesions.

ACQUIRED EXTERNAL CANAL STENOSIS

More common than congenital canal stenosis, acquired stenosis of the external canal usually results from a combination of surgery, trauma, or infection. It may occur as a complication of chronic external otitis, perichondritis, bullous lesions, chronic otitis media, tubercular lesions, irradiation, and relapsing polychondritis. Recurrent cerumen impactions, conductive hearing loss, persistent external otitis, and canal cholesteatoma are some of the problems encountered in these patients. Surgical correction of the stenosis is the only definitive therapy, and this approach usually involves excision of the offending tissue with possible grafting and long-term stenting to prevent recurrence of cicatricial stenosis. Surgery should usually be delayed until the etiology is determined and until any active infection is under control.

SELECTED READING

Ballenger, J. J. (1985); *Diseases of the Nose, Throat, Ear, Head and Neck*. Lea & Febiger, Philadelphia.
Compere, W. E., and Valvassori, G. E. (1964): *Radiographic Atlas of the Temporal Bone*. H. M. Smyth, St. Paul, Minnesota.
Goodhill, V. (1979): *Ear Diseases, Deafness and Dizziness*. Harper & Row, Hagerstown, Maryland.
Mouney, D. F. (1979): Differential diagnosis of hearing loss in children. *Ear, Nose, Throat J.*, 58:293–296.
Paparella, M. M., and Shumrick, D. A., editors (1980): *The Ear*, Vol. II. Saunders, Philadelphia.
Senturia, B. H., Marcus, M. D., and Lucente, F. E. (1980): *Diseases of the External Ear: An Oto-logic–Dermatologic Manual*. Grune & Stratton, New York.

The Ear

Section 3: Otitis Media and Mastoid Disease

Otitis Media—General Considerations 66
Anatomy and Physiology of the Eustachian Tube and Middle Ear ...68
Etiologic Factors Associated with Impaired Aeration 69
    Anatomic Deformities or Injuries of the Eustachian Tube 69
    Nasopharyngeal Tissue Masses 69
    Inflammatory Disease 70
    Allergy 70
    Cleft Palate 70
    Barotrauma 70
    Metabolic and Neurologic Disorders 70
    Inadequate Antibiotic Therapy of Suppurative Otitis 72
Nature and Source of Effusion 72
Symptoms and Signs of Nonsuppurative Otitis Media 73
    History 73
    Physical Examination 74
    Audiologic Evaluation 74
Signs and Symptoms of Acute Suppurative Otitis Media 75
Radiologic Examination of the Otomastoid System 76
Neonatal Otitis Media 78
Acute Necrotizing Otitis Media 78
Microbiology of Otitis Media 79
Laboratory Studies in Otitis Media 80
Medical Management of Suppurative Otitis Media 81
Management of Nonsuppurative Otitis Media 81
    Medical Management 82
    Surgical Management 83
Complications of Otitis Media and Otomastoiditis 85
    Tympanic Membrane Atrophy and Retraction 86
    Adhesive Otitis 87
    Cholesterol Granuloma 87

Ossicular Discontinuity 87
Tympanic Membrane Perforation 87
Cholesteatoma 88
Tympanosclerosis 89
Acute Petrositis 89
Facial Nerve Palsy 90
Suppurative Labyrinthitis 90
Nonsuppurative Labyrinthitis 90
Thrombophlebitis of the Sigmoid Sinus 91
Extradural Abscess 91
Brain Abscess 91
Meningitis 92
Tympanoplasty and Mastoidectomy 92
Tumors of the Middle Ear and Temporal Bone 95

OTITIS MEDIA—GENERAL CONSIDERATIONS

Otitis media, in the most fundamental sense, refers to an inflammation of the mucosal lining of the middle ear and associated structures. It is usually accompanied, in its acute suppurative form, by "medical mastoiditis" as well as inflammation and/or edema of the eustachian tube lining. Many authors use the term otitis media in a broader sense to include serous otitis media, mucoid otitis media, acute otitis media, subacute otitis media, and chronic suppurative otitis media. Closely related to a discussion of otitis media must be a review of complications related to oto-mastoiditis involving middle ear and inner ear structures, as well as more severe intracranial complications.

In 1869 Politzer first described a secretory and an adhesive form of a condition called otitis media catarrhalis. Since that time a confusing array of terms (e.g., serous otitis media, secretory otitis media, catarrh of the middle ear, allergic otitis media, and mucoid ear) have been applied to disease processes which result in the accumulation of nonpurulent fluid in the middle ear and mastoid air cell system.

Paparella and Dickson, expanding Senturia's work, presented a categorization of middle ear effusions including:

Serous fluid: sterile, pale, yellow fluid with a low viscosity.
Mucoid fluid: cloudy, translucent fluid that may have a rubbery consistency.
Mucopurulent fluid: grossly similar to mucoid but containing microscopically viable bacteria. Both mucoid and mucopurulent fluid may be seen in "glue" ear.
Bloody fluid: present in idiopathic hemotympanum, barotrauma, and some cases of serous otitis, particularly if a cholesterol granuloma is present.

The potential fluctuation between acute suppurative otitis media and nonsuppurative otitis media in an affected individual must be recognized (Fig. 2.3-1). Even

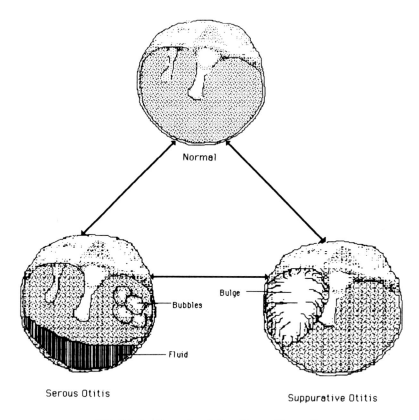

FIG. 2.3-1. Dynamic relationships—otitis media.

as a bout of acute otitis media is controlled with antibiotics, middle ear fluid may persist in the affected ear, providing a culture medium in which bacteria and rarely viruses reintroduced with a subsequent upper respiratory infection may grow, producing a reversion to acute suppurative otitis media. The higher prevalence of persistent middle ear effusions in patients following treatment with antibiotics than was noted during the preantibiotic era has led to speculation that microbial by-products remaining in the middle ear space may play a role in perpetuating the effusion.

The greatest prevalence of otitis media occurs during the first 2 years of life, with 50% of children experiencing at least one episode during the first year and 65 to 75% having had otitis by age two. Approximately 33% of young children experience three or more bouts of otitis during their first 2 years including 15% who are classified as "otitis-prone," suffering six or more episodes by their second birthday. Approximately 50% of children 2 years of age or younger studied by Shurin et al. had effusions that lasted 4 weeks or more after acute otitis media. Significant susceptibility to the disease persists into the early school years, with most studies revealing a rapid decline in incidence after age seven. Early-onset otitis media correlates directly with more severe and persistent episodes during subsequent childhood years. A bout of acute otitis media is a rather infrequent occurrence among the adolescent population.

To help explain the disease's predilection for young children, investigators have implicated factors common to infants and toddlers, such as a higher incidence of respiratory infections, a relatively large mass of adenoid tissue, increased chances for regurgitation of milk and secretions via the eustachian tube during supine feeding, and a highly compliant, less competent eustachian tube.

White children appear to be more likely to suffer from otitis media than Blacks, and Eskimos and American Indians demonstrate a particularly high incidence of the disease. Speculation regarding racial variations in skull base morphology, palatal/eustachian tube relationships, and maturation of defense systems to account for this differential susceptibility await validation. Well-documented longitudinal studies reveal that 60 to 65% of young otitis media patients are males, but a rationale for any sexual predilection for the disease has not been identified. An increased incidence of otitis is also seen among the socioeconomically disadvantaged and those children residing in colder climates. Predictably, otitis occurs with less frequency during warmer weather.

A significant amount of investigative effort has been directed toward describing the chemical components of middle ear effusions, as well as elucidating the pathogenesis of the disease processes which result in these effusions. A point of departure in describing the pathogenesis of otitis media with effusion must be a review of the anatomy and physiology of the tubotympanic system.

ANATOMY AND PHYSIOLOGY OF THE EUSTACHIAN TUBE AND MIDDLE EAR

Development of the eustachian tube, the tympanic cavity, and the mastoid air cell system as derivatives of the first pharyngeal pouch of the embryo results in a system of air-filled cavities that are dependent on intermittent opening of the eustachian tube for pressure equilibration with the surrounding atmosphere. From its pharyngeal orifice, the eustachian tube extends posterior, lateral, and superior to its tympanic orifice in the anterior portion of the middle ear cavity. The length of the tube, which at birth is 17 to 18 mm, is 35 to 36 mm in the adult. The tube is also more horizontal in position in infants than in older children and adults. The lateral one-third of the eustachian tube is bony, and the fibrocartilaginous medial two-thirds is interdigitated between the levator veli palatini and the tensor veli palatini, which courses inferiorly and laterally before rotating about the hamulus, attaching to the posterior margin of the bony palate, and inserting into the anterior margin of the velum. Although the tube is closed most of the time, the pulling of the tensor veli palatini and elevation of the levator veli palatini act to open the fibrocartilaginous portion as part of the process of swallowing. (There is some disagreement in the literature about involvement of the levator in eustachian tube opening.) The junction of the bony and cartilaginous portions of the tube is the narrowest point, or isthmus, which behaves as a one-way valve to open and close the tubal lumen. The isthmus is narrower in children (2.4 × 0.8 mm) than in adults (4.3 × 1.7 mm). The bony portion of the tube does not develop in children until nearly 6 years of age, and the resulting additional compliance of the cartilaginous tube in infants may be a predisposing factor for obstruction at the nasopharyngeal torus. Clinical situations in which middle ear pressure drops significantly below atmospheric pressure, as in rapid descent during air flight, can cause the isthmus to "lock" so that normal physiological maneuvers such as swallowing are unsuccessful in reaerating the middle ear.

In the young child the portion of the tube contiguous with the nasopharynx is lined by a continuation of respiratory-type pseudostratified columnar epithelium which merges into squamous-type epithelium near the aural end of the tube. Sade, as well as Lim and Birck, have described a mucociliary clearance mechanism in the tubotympanic cavity that is compatible with the ciliated epithelium and secretory elements which have been observed in electron microscopic study of the middle ear mucosa.

When the eustachian tube functions properly to equalize intratympanic pressure with ambient pressure, a normally compliant tympanic membrane and ossicles are most efficient in performing the impedance-matching function that is critical to normal auditory acuity. If tubal function is significantly compromised, as Proud and Odoi have demonstrated experimentally, retraction of the mobile tympanic membrane, mucosal edema, and accumulation of middle ear effusion are observed promptly.

ETIOLOGIC FACTORS ASSOCIATED WITH IMPAIRED AERATION

Anatomic Deformities or Injuries of the Eustachian Tube

Eustachian tube deformities or injuries may be seen congenitally, particularly in association with deformities of the base of the skull. They may also be posttraumatic (e.g., skull fractures or surgical trauma to the eustachian tube torus during adenoidectomy or attempted bougienage).

Nasopharyngeal Tissue Masses

Nasopharyngeal tissue masses may be adenoid hypertrophy, congenital lesions (e.g., teratoma), neoplasms (e.g., angiofibromas in child, carcinoma in adult), or, rarely, a vascular deformity (eustachian varices). The mechanism may involve direct closure of the eustachian tube lumen by pressure of the mass or obstruction of eustachian tube lymphatics with resultant middle ear transudate.

Inflammatory Disease

In addition to adenoiditis, mucosal inflammation in association with rhinosinusitis and nasopharyngitis may lead to tubal obstruction as well as to hypersecretion of mucoid fluid by the tympanic cavity epithelium.

Allergy

Allergic edema of the eustachian tube mucosa and/or tympanic mucosal changes associated with allergy are important factors in persistent middle ear effusions. Derlacki reported that the majority of the cases of chronic secretory otitis with either a clear serum or much thicker mucus were due to a definite allergy to house dust or to food.

Cleft Palate

An increase in the incidence of middle ear effusion is seen in children with a cleft palate (Fig. 2.3-2). Tensor and levator palatini muscle dysfunction is believed to be the causative factor. With adolescence, the incidence of middle ear disease drops significantly, reiterating the importance of effective management during the critical early years if hearing is to be conserved.

Barotrauma

Rapid descent from low to high ambient pressure without intermittent equilibration of middle ear pressure via tubal opening results in eustachian tube "lock" secondary to occlusion by suction. Coexisting factors which impede tubal function (e.g., upper respiratory infection or enlarged adenoids) may increase the incidence of barotrauma during air flight. Promotion of repeated swallowing during descent, by gum chewing, for instance, may help children avoid this unpleasant complication of air travel.

Metabolic and Neurologic Disorders

Disorders as diverse as hypothyroidism, collagen diseases causing stiffening of the tubal ligaments and cartilage, paresis of the palate and pharynx, and palatal myoclonus may cause impaired aeration.

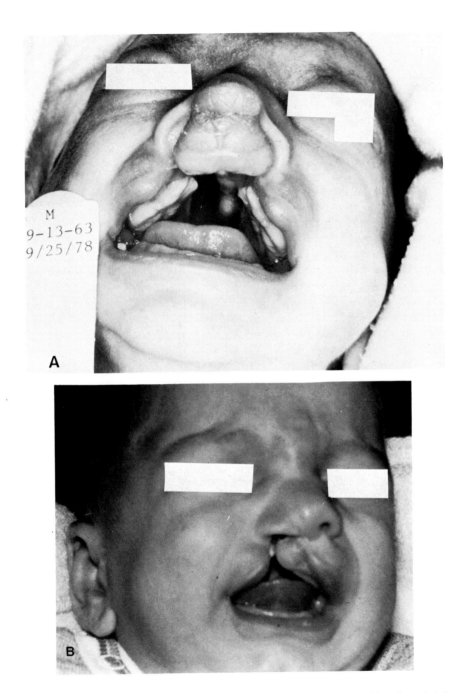

FIG. 2.3-2. **A:** Infant with complete bilateral cleft lip and palate. **B:** Infant with unilateral cleft lip and palate.

Inadequate Antibiotic Therapy of Suppurative Otitis

Early antibiotic therapy is an important tool in the management of suppurative otitis media. Incomplete or ineffective treatment may result in chronic exudative otitis requiring additional therapeutic steps.

NATURE AND SOURCE OF EFFUSION

Although tubal obstruction, with attendant absorption of gases from the closed tympanic cavity and consequent development of negative pressure, has long been implicated in the etiology of middle ear effusions (*ex vacuo* hypothesis), the nature and source of the fluid have been somewhat unclear. Because of the presence of mucociliary activity, the middle ear must be presupposed to contain secretions at all times. The thin, pale, yellow fluid usually associated with mild serous otitis has been described as a transudate derived from lymphatic vessels contained within the edematous mucosal lining of the middle ear. Pulec et al. attributed a significant role in the pathogenesis of middle ear effusions to obstruction of eustachian tube lymphatics which converge on the lateral retropharyngeal nodes. Although obstruction of eustachian tube lymphatics may conceivably result in an effusion in the presence of a patent tube in the same way that negative pressure resulting from tubal obstruction may be present without fluid, both conditions are usually found in clinical situations as evidenced by retraction of the tympanic membrane, negative middle ear pressure, and accumulation of fluid which characterize otitis media with effusion.

Whereas thin serous fluid has been demonstrated to be predominantly a transudate mixed with normal middle ear secretions, thicker mucoid effusions, as seen in "glue" ear, have been shown by the histochemical studies of Palva and Palva, as well as Mogi et al., to have different characteristics. These viscous effusions contain higher concentrations of enzymes than either serum or normal middle ear secretions, together with secretory immunoglobulin A, thus pointing to the presence of enhanced epithelial secretory activity in the middle ear. Disease processes affecting mucosal lining of the tympanic cavity in conjunction with coexisting tubal occlusion may well lead to early evolution of the more difficult to evacuate mucoid effusions with resultant implications for patient management. Research examining the importance of bacterial byproducts often found in middle ear effusions in the absence of signs and symptoms of inflammation appears to relate the presence of these elements with persistence of the effusion. More research is needed to elucidate the specific immunologic competence of normal and diseased middle ear mucosa and the role which localized immunologic dysfunction may play in susceptibility to otitis media.

SYMPTOMS AND SIGNS OF NONSUPPURATIVE OTITIS MEDIA

History

Adults with middle ear effusions are usually acutely aware of a "plugged-up" feeling in the diseased ear or a deep-seated "tickling" sensation, perhaps associated with a popping sound and decreased auditory acuity. Children, apart from a history of ear aches, may be seemingly unaware of a middle ear effusion in one or both ears. The parent may report that the child has persistently been picking at or tugging his ears, which should serve as a clue to underlying disease. In cases of more tenacious middle ear effusions, parents or teachers may observe any of the following abnormal hearing behaviors in the child:

1. Not be able to tell where voices and other sounds are coming from. The child may turn in the wrong direction when you call.
2. Frequently fails to respond when spoken to in a conversational voice, i.e., at a loudness level normally used when talking to a child in a quiet setting. You may find that you must actually tap the child on the shoulder to gain attention.
3. Often responds to what you say with "what?" or "huh?" and you find that you need to repeat what you have said.
4. Has difficulty understanding what is said when other people are talking or when the television, radio, or stereo is playing in the background.
5. Has problems maintaining good attention at story time or when watching television.
6. Tends to sit close to the television set or adjusts the sound so that it is loud.
7. Appears to "tune out," not listen, not pay attention, or ignore you and others around him.
8. Is reluctant to join in group activities and games, preferring to play alone.
9. Not be able to follow several instructions that have been combined in one sentence. The child may hesitate in responding to instructions but then may figure out what to do by watching others.
10. Talks very loudly.
11. Has abnormal speech.

Detection of a hearing loss in the course of a screening program at school is an important means for identifying the school-age child with an unsuspected middle ear effusion.

A history of adenoidectomy or adenotonsillectomy without myringotomy is not uncommon in children with persistent middle ear effusions, indicating the importance of involving a surgeon who has a thorough understanding of the indications and techniques of myringotomy in the management of these patients. Historical clues to underlying etiologic factors, e.g., allergy or rhinosinusitis, may also be present.

Physical Examination

Based on Paparella's categorization of tympanic membrane changes described in patients with middle ear effusions, physical findings on otologic examination may include:

1. Opaque, amber, or yellowish discoloration of the drumhead with an increase in capillary vascularity and loss of tympanic membrane light reflex.
2. A chalky appearing malleus handle.
3. Retraction of the tympanic membrane with increased prominence of the short process and apparent shortening of the long process of the malleus. Retraction of the pars flaccida may produce a small-mouthed retraction pocket, and retraction of the posterior superior drum quadrant may result in draping of the tympanic membrane over the underlying incudostapedial joint.
4. A fluid level or bubbles may be seen indicating some ingress of air via the eustachian tube into a fluid-filled middle ear cavity (Fig. 2.3-3).
5. A blue drumhead, seen in the absence of a history of trauma or middle ear tumor, is often associated with long-standing serous otitis media, barotitis/barotrauma, or cholesterol granuloma.
6. Decreased mobility of the tympanic membrane on pneumo-otoscopy or Valsalva maneuver may also be present. If pale-colored fluid fills the entire middle ear cavity, it may be difficult to detect otoscopically, but pneumatic compression should reveal a poorly mobile tympanic membrane.

A thorough examination of the nose and nasopharynx using anterior rhinoscopy, posterior nasopharyngeal mirror examination, or direct nasopharyngoscopy is essential for determining etiologic factors in cases of chronic middle ear effusion.

Audiologic Evaluation

Pure tone audiometric testing usually reveals a mild to moderate conductive hearing loss (the loss is generally greater with mucoid effusions), confirming a Rinne tuning fork test in which bone conduction is more acute than air conduction in the affected ear. Tympanometry is an increasingly popular audiologic technique in which a pressure/compliance curve relates the compliance of the tympanic membrane–ossicular system to changing pressure artificially produced in the airtight external canal which is occluded by a probe with openings to allow for pressure alteration and transmission/recording of test tones. The measured pressure at which maximal compliance of the middle ear system occurs is directly related to the existing middle ear pressure level. Specific tympanometric patterns are also indicative of the presence of middle ear fluid and have been described (see Section 5, Measurement of Hearing, in this chapter). With the potential of detecting both negative middle ear pressure and/or the presence of a middle ear effusion, tympanometry is fast becoming a mandatory part of the otologic/audiologic evaluation of patients with middle ear disease.

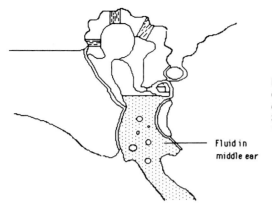

FIG. 2.3-3. Middle ear effusion. (Redrawn from Goodhill, V.: *Ear Diseases, Deafness and Dizziness,* p. 325. Harper & Row, Hagerstown, 1979.)

Fluid in
middle ear

SIGNS AND SYMPTOMS OF ACUTE SUPPURATIVE OTITIS MEDIA

From a theoretical point of view, the tympanomastoid system can become infected from the nasopharynx via the eustachian tube, externally through a perforation or tympanostomy tube connecting the middle ear with the external canal, and finally by hematogenous spread. Most common in infants and children with intact tympanic membranes is the trans-eustachian tube route, and in many cases a preexisting middle ear effusion may act as a ready culture medium.

Regardless of whether the child has a preexisting middle ear effusion, pain in the ear is the most common presenting symptom of acute otitis media. This stage may have been preceded by signs and symptoms of an upper respiratory infection, which in older children is often accompanied by vigorous nose blowing and sniffing, both of which may play a role in regurgitation of nasopharyngeal secretions into the middle ear. As hyperemia of the middle ear mucosa becomes evident, the examiner can observe hypervascularity and pinkish discoloration along the handle of the malleus, spreading gradually across the upper portion of the tympanic membrane. It is important to realize that straining and crying in the young child may be associated with reddish hypervascularity of the tympanic membrane, leading to mistaken diagnosis of early otitis media. In this case, however, mobility should be unimpaired by either retraction or bulging of the drum.

As the disease progresses, the patient experiences increasing pain and fever, often accompanied by systemic complaints such as myalgias, restlessness, and rarely meningismus. The entire tympanic membrane becomes reddened and thickened, eradicating such commonly observable landmarks as the short process of the malleus. Tympanometry at this stage may demonstrate increased middle ear pressure. As suppuration progresses in untreated patients, fever as high as 40°C is not uncommon, pain in the ear becomes more intense, and tinnitus with hearing loss may be described by the older child. In a small but significant number of children vertigo may also be present. As pus fills the tympanic cavity, the tympanic membrane assumes a whitish discoloration reflecting the color of the underlying pus, loses its concavity, begins to bulge outward, and reveals decreased mobility on pneumatic otoscopy. With pressure necrosis, usually of the central portion of the pars tensa, a perforation can occur, often heralded by a sudden flow of purulent material, blood, or in some cases straw-colored fluid from the ear. Following this spontaneous evacuation of the middle ear, pain usually subsides as do signs and symptoms of generalized toxicity.

The tympanic membrane perforation that occurs spontaneously with a bout of acute otitis media is usually of a small central type which heals in 80 to 90% of cases without incident with return of normal auditory acuity. Treatment of a patient in the early stages of acute suppurative otitis media with antibiotics often provides symptomatic relief and prevents further evolution of the disease to the point of tympanic membrane rupture, but such therapy may be associated with persistence of a middle ear effusion following apparent recovery from the infection. Hearing loss and tympanographic abnormalities may be the sole remaining evidence of an effusion, thus reinforcing the need for clinical follow-up of otitis media patients utilizing both visual examination and audiologic evaluation to document resolution of the disease process.

During this era of antibiotic therapy for otitis media, only a small percentage of patients experience persistence of the drainage for longer than 2 weeks or recurrence of pain and copious purulent drainage 7 to 14 days after the initial episode of otorrhea has subsided. Both of these signs suggest mastoiditis, and they may be accompanied by tenderness and edema over the postauricular mastoid process. On examination of the ear, edema and sagging of the posterior superior canal wall may be noted, and the middle ear mucosa visible through the persistent perforation may appear beefy red, suggestive of granulation tissue. A mucosa-covered polyp may protrude through the perforation. Erosion of the mastoid cortex can, in a small number of cases, lead to the classic protruding ear presentation of a postauricular subperiosteal abscess. Other life-threatening complications, e.g., meningitis, lateral sinus thrombophlebitis, suppurative labyrinthitis, or brain abscess (temporal lobe or cerebellar), occur rarely but are more often associated with chronic mastoiditis accompanied by cholesteatoma.

RADIOLOGIC EXAMINATION OF THE OTOMASTOID SYSTEM

On plain films the normal mastoid system has the appearance of an air-containing honeycomb with the delicate boney latticework surrounding black air-containing cells. The extent to which the mastoid air cell system is developed is generally directly related to the age of the patient, together with the frequency and severity of previous attacks of otomastoiditis.

As the mastoid mucoperiosteum becomes infected during a bout of acute oto-mastoiditis, it thickens, reducing the size of the air spaces visible radiographically. As fluid or pus fills the cells, a clouding is apparent on the x-ray film with no air

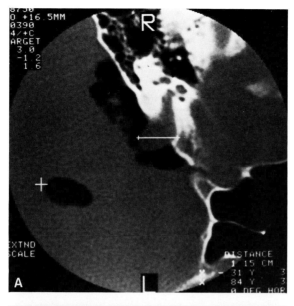

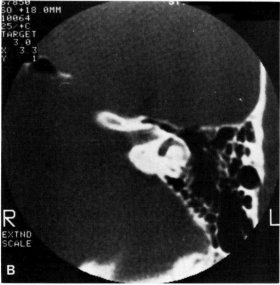

FIG. 2.3-4. **A:** CT scan showing a right acoustic neuroma. **B:** CT scan showing a normal internal auditory canal.

spaces being visible. Coalescent mastoiditis is accompanied by resorption of the bony latticework separating the air cells and consequent loss of normal markings on mastoid films.

The presence of a cholesteatoma may be heralded by a lytic area in the mastoid, particularly in the attic, aditus, and antrum, with the surrounding bone appearing relatively thickened or sclerotic on x-ray films. The availability of polytomographic and computerized imaging technology (CT scan) has added a greater dimension of resolution to radiographic examination of the temporal bone. The integrity of the ossicular chain as well as the relationship of lesions such as cholesteatoma to the underlying labyrinth can be accurately assessed. The size of the internal auditory canal can be accurately measured to aid in the identification of neoplasms involving the eighth nerve and the cerebello-pontine angle region (Fig. 2.3-4).

NEONATAL OTITIS MEDIA

Otitis media in the newborn must be considered as a possible occult cause of septicemia, meningitis, or fever of unknown origin. Otitis-related complications such as labyrinthitis and facial nerve paralysis can also occur early in life. Seen most often in high-risk, low-birth-weight infants, neonatal otitis also appears to be related to such invasive therapeutic techniques as long-term placement of a naso-tracheal or nasogastric tube. Hypoxic stress episodes leading to respiratory efforts by the infant *in utero* have been suggested to explain regurgitation of vernix caseosa, epithelial cells, and amniotic fluid into the middle ear cavity, as has been documented at autopsy. The examiner must take pains to thoroughly clean the neonate's short external auditory canal of vernix and associated debris in order to ensure good visualization of the tympanic membrane. Some clinical studies have suggested a higher incidence of gram-negative pathogens in neonatal otitis, and this evidence must be considered when selecting an appropriate antimicrobial agent.

ACUTE NECROTIZING OTITIS MEDIA

A particularly virulent form of acute otitis media, more prevalent in past decades, can occur in a child severely ill from a systemic infection, generally scarlet fever or measles. This type of otitis has been characterized by the name acute necrotizing otitis media based on the association in these cases of copious foul-smelling drainage with extensive necrosis of the tympanic membrane, ossicular structures, and often middle ear mucosa. The end result can vary from a large central permanent tympanic membrane perforation to ossicular destruction and/or cholesteatoma formation caused by ingrowth of squamous epithelium. Prompt recognition of the disorder, coupled with intensive systemic and topical antibiotic therapy, is indicated to minimize its destructive course. Surgical intervention may be necessary to manage the various sequelae of the disease.

MICROBIOLOGY OF OTITIS MEDIA

Acute suppurative otitis media is most appropriately viewed as a bacterial disease; large clinical studies have demonstrated that pathogenic bacteria may be recovered from middle ear exudates in as many as 75% of cases, the remainder yielding no growth or nonpathogenic organisms. Culture techniques in some studies were not designed to reveal the presence of anaerobes, which may explain some of the remaining 25%. Careful attempts to recover viruses from the middle ear of patients suffering from acute otitis media have yielded only 5% positive results. Although viruses have been postulated to play a role in the early pathogenesis of otitis media in a larger percentage of cases, they were apparently no longer present or were inactivated by host factors at the time the samples were obtained. Attempts to isolate *Mycoplasma* from middle ear exudates have not shown these organisms to play a significant role in the disease.

A number of well-documented bacteriologic studies of acute otitis media have indicated the two most commonly isolated pathogens to be *Streptococcus pneumoniae* and *Hemophilus influenzae*, with the former being the most frequent organism found across all age groups. The common misconception that *H. influenzae* is the most common bacterial agent causing otitis in young infants is not supported by available data. *H. influenzae* is the second most common bacterium cultured from children with otitis up to 8 years of age, with older children being affected much less frequently. Group A β-hemolytic-*Streptococcus, Nisseria catarrhalis,* and *Staphylococcus aureus* are the next most commonly isolated pathogens. Some studies have reported recovery of gram-negative bacilli (*Klebsiella pneumoniae, Pseudomonas aeruginosa,* and various *Proteus* species) from as many as 20% of infants with acute otitis media. These bacteria are much less commonly present in the middle ear exudates of older children. Brooks et al., using careful technique, were successful in isolating anaerobic bacteria from 28% of 62 children with acute otitis media, thus implicating this category of organisms to help explain the sterile cultures obtained from as many as 25% of cases in large studies.

The middle ear fluid obtained from patients who present no symptoms of acute infection (chronic nonsuppurative otitis media) has also been subjected to bacteriologic study. Bacteria were noted to be present on gram stain in approximately 50% of cases with positive cultures for *S. pneumoniae, H. influenza,* or group A *Streptococcus* in 10 to 20% of cultures.

In everyday clinical practice, an attempt to obtain middle ear fluid for culture is not usually necessary. The spectrum of pathogens involved in most cases has been well demonstrated, and they are generally susceptible to a group of antimicrobial agents with minimal associated toxicity. For this reason, myringotomy for acute otitis media is performed infrequently. In certain circumstances, however, positive identification of the infectious agent may be necessary to obtain symptomatic relief or treat complications. These cases may be broadly categorized to include:

1. Otitis with impending sepsis in young infants or immunosuppressed patients
2. Otitis with associated complications such as mastoiditis, meningitis, facial nerve paralysis, labyrinthitis, etc.
3. Otitis which fails to respond to usual antimicrobial therapy, particularly when ampicillin-resistant strains of *H. influenzae* are being reported

Cultures of secretions obtained from the nasopharynx of otitis patients has a reasonably high correlation with cultures of direct aspirates of middle ear fluid, thereby allowing the use of such cultures in epidemiologic studies. In the presence of impending sepsis or otitis-related complications, however, the middle ear fluid should be obtained utilizing more often the invasive techniques of myringotomy or tympanocentesis. It is essential to instill an antiseptic solution, e.g., 70% ethanol or Betadine, in the external ear to remove potential contaminants before the tympanic membrane is penetrated. After removing the antiseptic, entry into the tympanic cavity with a small-gauge tympanocentesis needle or sharp myringotomy knife should be made through the inferior quadrants of the tympanic membrane. Aspiration following myringotomy should be done utilizing a sterile baron-type ear suction cannula with secretions being collected in a sterile trap tube, which can be easily sealed for transmission to the laboratory. Although tympanocentesis and myringotomy can provide useful clinical information, the procedures are not without potential hazard to the structures of the underlying middle and inner ear. It is essential to restrain and/or sedate the patient adequately prior to undertaking the procedure. Magnification is important, and the improved depth perception provided by an otosurgical microscope allows greater precision in placement of the incision.

LABORATORY STUDIES IN OTITIS MEDIA

Appropriate laboratory studies should be completed in children with recurrent bouts of otitis media, including a white blood cell count with differential to rule out neutropenia. Varying degrees of transient hypogammaglobulinemia or agammaglobulinemia, which may be associated with recurrent infection including otitis, may be detected by quantitative immunoglobulin electrophoresis. Increased understanding of the function of various cells types involved in the immunologic response, e.g., T- and B-cells, has made possible detection of specific defects in their activity. Syndromes in which immunodeficiency plays a role should be considered and ruled out in the otitis-prone child.

MEDICAL MANAGEMENT OF SUPPURATIVE OTITIS MEDIA

Paradise, in an excellent review of otitis media, stressed the need for antimicrobial treatment routinely for acute middle ear infections. The high probability of a bacterial etiology, coupled with the widely observed decline in otitis-related complications following the introduction of antibiotics, reinforces the prudence of this therapeutic course. Based on previously cited studies identifying *S. pneumoniae* and *H. influenzae* as the primary pathogens in childhood otitis, the physician may select an appropriate treatment regimen using antimicrobials with known effectiveness against these bacteria. If anaerobic bacteria ultimately prove to be important etiologic agents in childhood otitis, as some studies indicate, these organisms are known to be susceptible to penicillin and its derivatives.

After its introduction, ampicillin gained wide popularity as a safe and effective agent for treatment of otitis. The emergence of ampicillin-resistant strains of *H. influenzae,* however, has prompted the growing use of alternatives such as amoxicillin or combination preparations (phenoxymethyl penicillin plus a sulfonamide or an erythromycin/sulfonamide combination). Later-generation cephalosporins, e.g., cefaclor, have been reported effective in refractory cases of otitis as has the non-antibiotic combination trimethoprim-sulfamethoxazole. Continued emergence of resistant strains of *H. influenzae* coupled with introduction of new antimicrobials make definitive statements regarding the appropriate choice of treatment impossible. The physician should carefully monitor the course of the disease, particularly in neonates, and be ready to obtain cultures and alter the therapeutic regimen as required.

The child with recurrent bouts of acute otitis media which respond to medical therapy presents a therapeutic challenge. Some clinical investigators have reported lower recurrence rates in otitis-prone children with daily oral prophylaxis using less than usual therapeutic doses of antimicrobials, particularly during the high-risk winter months. This approach is still somewhat controversial, and it seems imprudent to utilize long-term antibiotic prophylaxis with any agent having potential toxic side effects greater than those of a bout of otitis media. Additional studies of the effect of long-term prophylaxis on nasopharyngeal flora, as well as the prevalence of complications when a "break through" bout of otitis occurs, are necessary before more definitive recommendations can be made concerning this option.

MANAGEMENT OF NONSUPPURATIVE OTITIS MEDIA

Therapy for persistent middle ear effusions, in the absence of symptoms for acute inflammation, must be directed toward both evacuation of the effusion and alleviation of underlying etiologic factors which may be causing eustachian tube dysfunction. Initially, all middle ear effusions should be treated with medical therapy. Acute serous effusions, as well as barotrauma otitis, may well resolve on a medical regimen, but more viscid effusions, such as those which characterize the "glue" ear, are more likely to be refractory to conservative management.

Medical Management

Antibiotics

Antibiotics are useful in cases of inadequately treated suppurative otitis media and when adenotonsillitis or rhinosinusitis are primary underlying causes of tubal dysfunction. In view of studies in which viable bacteria can be cultured from certain middle ear effusions, a course of antibiotic seems justified in a child not recently treated.

Decongestants

Both topical and systemic decongestants have been reported to be of value, although none has been demonstrated to be clearly superior. Double-blind studies have raised questions about the efficacy of some of the oral agents. One must be careful with topical decongestants to limit their use to a few days in order to avoid the complication of rhinitis medicamentosa.

Antihistamines

Although patients with a true allergic problem might best be managed with antihistamines, the misuse and abuse of antihistamines in the treatment of middle ear effusions in nonallergic patients is widespread. Mucoid or mucopurulent effusions, which are already quite viscid, can scarcely be expected to respond to antihistaminic therapy.

Allergic Hyposensitization

Close cooperation involving the pediatrician, otologist, and allergist will result in the effective management of patients with middle ear effusion who have a family history of allergic disorders. A judicious combination of allergic hyposensitization in clearly allergic patients and surgical treatment often serve to maximize conservation of hearing in the allergic child. Often surgical therapy (i.e., myringotomy with or without insertion of a tympanostomy tube) is employed to achieve immediate resolution of an effusion with associated hearing impairment while waiting for the longer-term results of a regimen of hyposensitization.

Tubal Inflation

Increasing nasopharyngeal pressure to levels sufficient to overcome a tubal "lock" may aid in resolution of otitis media with effusion. Politzerization (i.e., pressure inflation with a Politzer bag via the nose) may be used in cooperative older patients, and careful attempts at Valsalva maneuver by the patient are also helpful. A Valsalva substitute in children who have difficulty in accomplishing this maneuver may be carried out by having the patient inflate a balloon while at the same time occluding his nostrils, thus producing increased naso-oropharyngeal pressure. Care must be taken to treat concurrent infections of the adenoids and paranasal sinuses before tubal inflation is attempted to avoid introduction of microbes into the middle ear effusion. In addition, the physician must be aware of the significant pressures which can be achieved by politzerization with attendant risk of injury to the delicate lamina papyracea and cribriform plate regions of the nasal/sinus cavities.

Surgical Management

Children with persistent (duration longer than 6 to 8 weeks) middle ear effusions accompanied by retraction of the tympanic membrane and significant conductive hearing impairment (greater than 20 dB) who are refractory to adequate medical management should be treated surgically. Surgical procedures should be designed to achieve evacuation of the effusion from the tympanic cavity, allow an adequate period of reaeration to permit return of hypertrophic middle ear mucosa to normal, and promote normal eustachian function.

Myringotomy (Fig. 2.3-5), usually performed by the author in the anterior inferior quadrant of the tympanic membrane, serves not only to immediately equalize intratympanic pressure with ambient levels but also to help evacuate the middle ear effusion. Additionally, rapid restoration of auditory acuity can generally be achieved. Following the work of Armstrong, the insertion of indwelling tympanostomy tubes has become a popular adjunct to myringotomy. An indwelling tube prolongs the period allowed for return of the middle ear to normal and has proved to be of value in cases where the effusion is particularly viscid, mucoid, or mucopurulent and in which severe edema of the middle ear mucosa is present. Silicone rubber (Silastic) tympanostomy tubes have proved quite satisfactory and are easy to introduce. The tube usually extrudes spontaneously within 6 to 18 months (with an average duration of about 9 months) but may remain longer. Only rarely is it necessary to intentionally remove the tube. Reinsertion of a tympanostomy tube may be necessary, particularly in refractory cases such as those seen in children with cleft palate. In the author's experience, approximately 20 to 30% of children whose initial set of typanostomy tubes are inserted prior to age two require at least one additional set. Tubes with a larger-than-standard lumen and phalanges are available for use if indicated. Care must be taken, while the tympanostomy tube is in place, to avoid violation of the

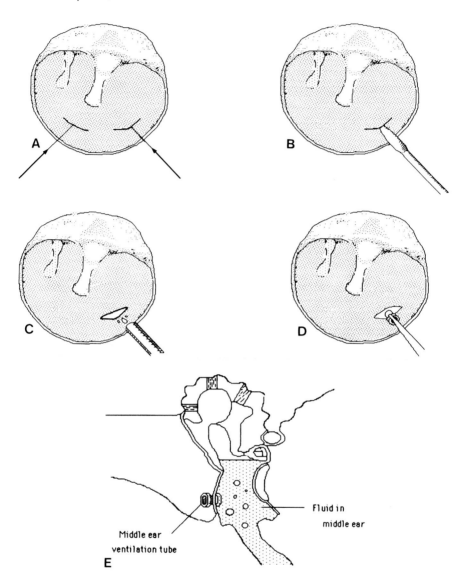

FIG. 2.3-5. **A:** Recommended myringotomy sites. **B:** Myringotomy knife incisions. **C:** Middle ear effusion aspirated. **D:** Tympanostomy tube inserted using forceps. **E:** Placement of ventilation tube. (Redrawn from Goodhill, V.: *Ear Diseases, Deafness and Dizziness,* p. 325. Harper & Row, Hagerstown, 1979.)

middle ear with water or other contaminants. Tubes are not without hazard and should be used only when specific indications are present. Permanent perforations of the tympanic membrane can result, as can tympanosclerosis consisting of calcific deposition in the tympanic membrane and middle ear mucosa. An increased incidence of suppurative otitis media and possibly cholesteatoma has been cited in reviews of large series of patients in whom indwelling tympanostomy tubes have been used.

Chronic otorrhea with attendant foreign body reaction around the tube may necessitate premature surgical removal. While in place, the tube may become nonfunctional when occluded by cerumen or dried secretions. If tympanometry demonstrates normal middle ear function, one may leave the plugged tube in place; but if an effusion recurs, the offending plug must be softened with otic drops and suctioned out in the office, or the tube must be cleaned/replaced surgically.

Surgical measures aimed at restoring eustachian tube function may include adenoidectomy and, less often in children, intranasal or sinus procedures. Adenoidectomy should be done carefully with special attention being paid to removal of adenoidal tissue from the fossa of Rosenmüller and avoidance of trauma to the eustachian tube torus. Cauterization applied to the nasopharynx is unwise as resultant cicatrization can be exceedingly difficult to correct. Children with cleft palate should not, as a rule, have an adenoidectomy performed except in preparation for a pharyngeal flap procedure as the resultant increase in nasal escape of air may be associated with worsening of speech quality. A thorough discussion of the indications for tonsillectomy is not within the scope of this chapter, but tonsillectomy is often performed with adenoidectomy in patients having middle ear effusions if significant evidence of chronic tonsillitis is present. There is no evidence that tonsillectomy has a beneficial effect on eustachian tube function, and the efficacy of adenoidectomy in the absence of associated symptoms of nasal obstruction has been questioned.

A conservative approach would be initially to limit surgical intervention to myringotomy, with or without tympanostomy tube placement, followed by postoperative documentation of eustachian tube function with impedance testing via the patent tube or myringotomy incision. If obstruction of the eustachian tube appears to be a contributory factor and the patient fails to respond to reaeration of the middle ear space, adenoidectomy can be accomplished in conjunction with reinsertion of the tubes, should this step become necessary. The reader may wish to refer to other texts for a more complete discussion of tonsillectomy indications.

COMPLICATIONS OF OTITIS MEDIA AND OTOMASTOIDITIS

Chronic suppurative otitis media (with tympanic membrane perforation) or non-suppurative otitis (without perforation) can give rise to complications.

Tympanic Membrane Atrophy and Retraction

In the face of long-standing negative middle ear pressure, the normally resilient tympanic membrane may atrophy, giving rise to a "chronic retraction." If the retraction involves the pars tensa, particularly the posterior quadrants of the drum, pressure against the underlying ossicles may lead to osteolytic changes. The drum may drape over the incudostapedial joint and reflect into the various recesses of the posterior tympanic cavity, e.g., the facial recess. In such interstices, desquamated keratinizing squamous epithelium may collect giving rise to a cholesteatoma, more precisely called a keratoma, which may result in chronic infection or continual destruction of the surrounding structures.

It is important to know if the retracted drum can be everted with a Valsalva maneuver, negative pneumatic pressure, or, if necessary, direct instrumentation, or if it is permanently adherent to underlying structures. This information is important from both a therapeutic and a prognostic viewpoint as one considers the child's potential for achieving a more normally functional tympanic membrane and middle ear system.

Retraction of the pars flaccida into the area above the tympanic cavity, which is occupied by the heads of the malleus and incus, is referred to as an attic retraction. Because such retractions have a small mouth and are easily occluded by inflammatory edema or polyp formation, it is very important to determine if the deepest extent of the retraction pocket is visible. A cholesteatoma can develop silently (Fig. 2.3-6), hidden by the scutum or lateral wall of the attic, destroying the ossicular heads, spreading into the aditus and mastoid cell system, and threatening to erode the bony covering of the underlying labyrinth and surrounding intracranial structures. The added magnification and binocular vision afforded by an otomicroscope in the ambulatory setting is very helpful in determining the extent of such a retraction pocket and the danger it poses. Prolonged retraction of the squamous epithelium-covered drum segment may necessitate surgical atticotomy or mastoidectomy to

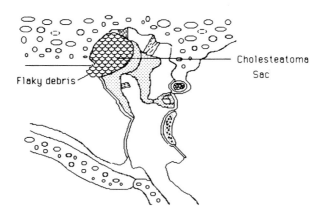

FIG. 2.3-6. Attic retraction cholesteatoma.

eradicate an incipient cholesteatoma if these retraction pockets fail to resolve with more conservative treatment of the middle ear effusion.

Adhesive Otitis

Adhesions may develop between the tympanic membrane and the underlying promontory and ossicles. Although acceptable hearing may be present in cases with adhesions between the drum and the incudostapedial joint, the converse may also be true. The difficulty encountered in surgical management of cases of adhesive otitis speaks eloquently in favor of effective early management of middle ear effusions.

Cholesterol Granuloma

A hemorrhagic effusion into the middle ear and mastoid in conjunction with infection or trauma can give rise to a foreign body-type reaction of fibrosis and phagocytic cell infiltration called a cholesterol granuloma. This lesion, which may be the source of chonic serosanguineous fluid draining through a perforation or tympanostomy tube, requires surgical removal usually by mastoidectomy approach. Although troublesome, cholesterol granuloma is not characterized by the type of irreversible change which typifies cholesteatoma or tympanosclerosis.

Ossicular Discontinuity

A common type of ossicular osteolysis—necrosis of the incus long process, which is supplied by a small end-artery—may produce substantial hearing impairment, requiring tympanoplasty with ossiculoplasty to restore hearing.

Tympanic Membrane Perforation

If a perforation resulting from a bout of suppurative otitis media fails to heal, as occurs in a small percentage of cases, chronic suppurative otitis media may be said to exist. This condition may be either active (with drainage) or inactive (without drainage). The drainage, which is usually purulent and often foul-smelling, may be continuous or occur only after an upper respiratory infection or external contamination of the ear with foreign substances (e.g., water). The drainage is usually accompanied by minimal pain, as is drainage via an indwelling tympanostomy tube. Continuous foul-smelling drainage which is refractory to local and systemic medical treatment is highly suggestive of significant involvement of the mastoid system by granulation tissue or cholesteatoma. Mastoid x-ray films would be expected to show the chronic changes described above. Surgical exenteration of infected mastoid cells may be necessary in cases refractory to medical management.

A perforation is classified as either marginal, i.e., touching the anulus or margin of the tympanic membrane, or central, in which none of the margins touch the anulus. A marginal perforation is viewed as more worrisome by otologists because of a greater potential for squamous epithelial ingrowth into the middle ear cavity from the canal and external surface of the drum giving rise to a cholesteatoma.

Cholesteatoma

The cholesteatoma, more accurately described as a keratoma, is characterized by a sac-like lamellar structure in which a layer of keratinizing squamous epithelium surrounds a collection of desquamated keratin debris within the interstices of the middle ear and temporal bone (Fig. 2.3-7). Although the external auditory canal and lateral surface of the tympanic membrane are stratified squamous keratinizing epithelium, the exfoliated debris is evacuated from the canal naturally under normal conditions. As such epithelium gains ingress into the middle ear and mastoid system, such spontaneous evacuation does not occur and an enlarging sac filled with debris can exert pressure against the bony ossicles and otic capsule, as well as the bony

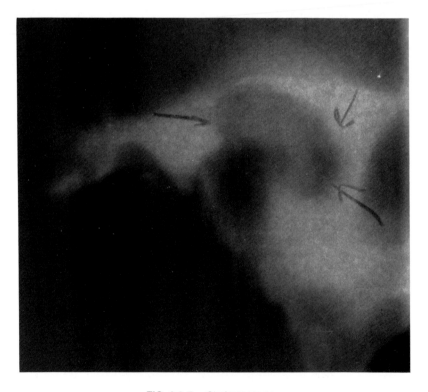

FIG. 2.3-7. Cholesteatoma.

coverings separating the middle and posterior cranial cavities from the mastoid cells. Mechanisms implicated in the formation of cholesteatoma include epithelial migration from the edges of a perforation (usually marginal type), dislocation of squamous epithelium into the middle ear as a result of concussive force (e.g., blast or traumatic perforation), retraction of a squamous covered segment of tympanic membrane into the tympanic or epitympanic cavity secondary to poor aeration, and rarely the presence of an embryonic cellular rest within the air cell system which assumes the histologic pattern of keratinizing squamous epithelium. The latter mechanism can explain the occasional cholesteatoma presenting behind an intact tympanic membrane, usually in children. In addition to osteolysis caused by pressure necrosis, several enzymatic studies suggest chemical components in the matrix which facilitate invasion. The cholesteatoma must be totally removed and/or exteriorized to allow access for cleaning via the external auditory meatus. The various mastoidectomy procedures were designed to accomplish surgical extirpation of these lesions which have a high potential for recurrence.

Tympanosclerosis

Tympanosclerosis, fixing one or more ossicles with conductive hearing loss, is often the result of childhood acute necrotizing otitis media. Tympanosclerosis is characterized initially by hyalinization of the collagen elements in the tympanic membrane and lining of the middle ear and mastoid system followed by deposition of calcium leading to stiffening of the affected tissues. In some cases the tympanosclerotic deposit can be pealed away from the underlying more normal tissue, but all too often the lesion recurs. When limited to the tympanic membrane, the process may coexist with essentially normal middle ear function and hearing. In other instances, a more diffuse involvement of the middle ear structures can lead to ossicular fixation and a significant conductive impairment, this condition is particularly common following childhood acute necritizing otitis media. Surgical removal of these calcium deposits often seems deceptively easy, but maintenance of normal middle ear function and prevention of recurrence during postoperative healing is problematic at best.

Acute Petrositis

The petrous apex of the temporal bone may be aerated to a variable extent, and such air cells may become involved with infection as a result of a bout of otomastoiditis. This complication, more common during the preantibiotic era is usually accompanied by a constellation of signs and symptoms: otitis with otorrhea, pain in the distribution of the trigeminal nerve, and sixth cranial nerve paralysis on the same side as the otitis, called Gradenigo's syndrome. Both intensive antibiotic therapy and surgical drainage of the diseased cells may be necessary to effect resolution of the disease. Polytomography and high-resolution CT scan techniques have added important tools to assist in diagnosis and planning of therapeutic intervention.

Facial Nerve Palsy

Paralysis of the seventh cranial nerve may occur in conjunction with acute otomastoiditis or, more commonly, in cases of chronic mastoiditis with cholesteatoma. It may also follow injury of the nerve during otologic surgery aimed at eradication of disease within the mastoid and middle ear. The bony fallopian canal surrounding the facial nerve has been shown to be dehiscent in certain otherwise normal ears, particularly in the region above the oval window. This condition is usually asymptomatic but symptoms may appear if there is inflammation of the perineural sheath during a bout of otitis media. If facial palsy should develop during an episode of acute otitis, radiologic evaluation of the temporal bone should be carried out followed by immediate myringotomy to drain the suppurative focus in the middle ear. In more chronic cases a mastoidectomy may also be necessary to remove a cholesteatoma and/or chronic granulation tissue as an inciting focus.

Surgical injury of the nerve calls for immediate reexploration of the middle ear and mastoid with careful examination of the course of the nerve within the temporal bone. Decompression of the bony canal and rerouting and reanastomosis of a severed nerve (with or without interposition of a nerve graft) may be necessary to reestablish function.

Suppurative Labyrinthitis

Penetration of the suppurative process in the middle ear and mastoid system into the endolabyrinth may occur via the existing oval or round windows or through a newly formed fistula, most often in the wall of the lateral semicircular canal. Hearing loss, fever, and violent whirling vertigo with accompanying nystagmus may herald the onset of acute suppurative labyrinthitis. Immediate surgical intervention including myringotomy (in acute cases) and mastoidectomy in chronic disease should be carried out in addition to high-dose intravenous antibiotic therapy to prevent intracranial spread of the infection. Severely impaired auditory acuity together with some persistent dysequilibrium may follow this serious complication of otitis media. Histopathologically, the otic labyrinth may be gradually obliterated by new bone formation, thus explaining the term labyrinthitic ossificans, which is often applied to this complication.

Nonsuppurative Labyrinthitis

Nonsuppurative or serous labyrinthitis may accompany a bout of otitis media presenting with a sensorineural hearing loss (usually fluctuating) and varying degrees of dysequilibrium. Symptoms may subside following resolution of the otitis media, although studies by Paparella et al. of large number of patients with long-standing histories of recurrent suppurative otitis media show a higher than expected frequency of persistent sensorineural hearing loss.

Thrombophlebitis of the Sigmoid Sinus

Sigmoid lateral venous sinus thrombophlebitis (rarely of the jugular bulb) may occur in conjunction with both acute and chronic otomastoiditis. The symptoms are sepsis, chills, high swinging fever, generally a positive blood culture, rapid weight loss, and a positive Queckenstedt test, indicating occlusion of the sigmoid sinus on the involved side. Surgical evacuation of the suppurative focus in the temporal bone together with incision and drainage of the thrombosed sinus with evacuation of the thrombus via a transmastoid approach are indicated.

Extradural Abscess

Extradural abscess is usually associated with destruction of the bone adjacent to the dura by cholesteatoma and/or infection. Although an accumulation of pus between the dura and adjacent portion of the temporal bone is occasionally seen, dural granulation tissue observed through a bony defect is a more common finding. Before antibiotics, severe earache, headache in the temporal area, and low-grade fever were observed, although a small, silent abscess may be encountered during mastoidectomy. Otorrhea, if present, is usually pulsatile and characterized by a creamy, often foul-smelling quality. Malaise and anorexia may be present, but no neurologic signs are observed, and CSF findings at lumbar puncture are unremarkable unless coexisting meningitis is present. CT imaging techniques represent a major advance in the detection and localization of an extradural abscess.

Cultures should be taken and appropriate antimicrobial therapy begun, but surgical drainage represents the definitive treatment. A mastoidectomy is performed and enough bone removed to exteriorize the affected dura. Any collection of pus is drained and granulation tissue removed until normal dura is identified. The extent of the mastoidectomy performed should be governed by the therapeutic objective of eradicating the infection and exteriorizing the infected area to the degree necessary to prevent and detect recurrence.

Brain Abscess

Two-thirds of brain abscesses from otitis media are in the temporal lobe of the middle fossa. Symptoms may include vomiting, convulsions, headache, limb weakness, visual hallucinations, visual field defects, nominal aphasia for a left-sided abscess, and motor cortex involvement. One-third of otogenic brain abscesses are cerebellar and generally produce more profound symptoms of increased intracranial pressure, including ataxia, headache, and spontaneous nystagmus that varies in direction and degree. If left untreated, increasing pressure may be exerted upon vital centers in the brainstem, producing Cheyne-Stokes respiration progressing to respiratory arrest and death.

Neurosurgical consultation should be sought immediately if neurologic symptoms are present in conjunction with a bout of otitis media. Neuroradiologic diagnostic procedures including CT scans help to determine the location and extent of intracranial abscesses. Prompt exploration of the affected area with drainage and exteriorization of the abscess may prevent life-threatening progression of the symptoms.

One should not overlook the need to carry out definitive otologic surgery to eradicate the underlying otomastoiditis which initially leads to the complication. If this is not feasible at the time of the neurosurgical intervention, it should be accomplished as soon as the patient's condition permits. Neurologic sequelae such as hemiparesis, hemioanopsia, or seizures may persist following recovery from the acute episode.

Meningitis

Otogenic meningitis is an extremely serious, yet not uncommon, complication of acute and chronic otitis media. As with otitis, *Diplococcus* (*Streptococcus*) *pneumoniae* and *H. influenzae* are the most common pathogenic organisms involved. As stated previously, prompt myringotomy with culture of the middle ear exudate should be carried out in the face of neurologic signs and symptoms accompanying a bout of otitis. High-dose antibiotic therapy has proved effective in controlling the meningitis in most cases, although mastoidectomy may be necessary when chronic otomastoiditis with or without cholesteatoma is present. Sequelae apart from those involving the central nervous system may include severe to profound sensorineural hearing impairment, probably resulting from purulent labyrinthitis. This complication is sufficiently common that all postmeningitic children should have the benefit of audiologic testing as soon as their condition permits. Labyrinthitis and meningitis may be seen with greater frequency in individuals who have sustained traumatic fracture of the temporal bone because the endochondral bone heals only by fibrous union.

TYMPANOPLASTY AND MASTOIDECTOMY

The introduction of antibiotics has greatly reduced the number of patients with coalescent mastoiditis who require life-saving drainage procedures, but the otologist is still confronted by the patient who has a tympanic membrane perforation, possibly a chronic draining ear, and significant hearing impairment of the pure conductive or mixed types. The availability of improved anesthetic techniques, the surgical microscope, and microsurgical instrumentation have contributed to the development of techniques for the restoration of hearing in patients whose major deficit is in the conductive mechanism. Tympanoplasty is the term applied to a category of procedures designed to help restore the integrity of the tympanic membrane together with a functional middle ear. Mastoidectomy, on the other hand, refers to a category of procedures designed to remove diseased bone and soft tissue from the mastoid air cell system and related structures. These procedures may be performed separately or in combination, the latter often called a tympanomastoidectomy. In general, all tympanoplasty procedures (alone or accompanied by mastoidectomy) are aimed at achieving the common goals of a dry ear, an intact tympanic membrane, and the restoration of usable hearing without compromising the patient's chances of avoiding continued infection with possible intracranial complications.

Careful preoperative otologic and audiologic assessments assist the otologist in defining the many variables to be weighed when estimating the chances for success of the various tympanoplasty operations in a particular patient. These considerations include the size and location of the tympanic membrane perforation, the status of the ossicular chain, cochlear function, coexistent allergic or inflammatory disease of the nose and paranasal sinuses influencing eustachian tube function, and finally the presence of processes such as cholesteatoma or tympanosclerosis in the tympanic cavity or mastoid air cells.

A few common principles governing surgical techniques may be distilled from the multitude of tympanoplasty procedures (Figs. 2.3-8 and 2.3-9) which have been described in the literature employing variations in grafting materials and methods for reconstruction of the sound-conducting mechanism of the middle ear. Metabolically inactive tissues such as fascia, perichondrium, and periosteum have proved most successful as grafting material in providing good long-term functional results for closure of tympanic membrane perforations. Homograft tympanic membranes obtained from cadavers have achieved popularity for use as grafts in some centers. The use of these homografts, however, involves substantial effort and expense directed toward their acquisition and storage and is usually reserved for patients in whom total replacement of the tympanic membrane/ossicular chain complex must be undertaken.

Preservation or recreation of a functional middle ear requires careful attention to ossicular chain reconstruction. For best functional results, the tympanoplasty sur-

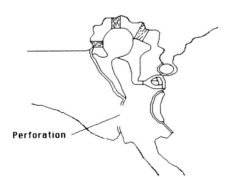

Perforation

FIG. 2.3-8. Tympanic membrane perforation.

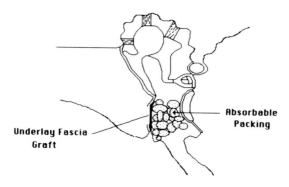

Underlay Fascia Graft

Absorbable Packing

FIG. 2.3-9.   Myringoplasty repair of tympanic membrane perforation.

geon should strive to maintain a mechanical advantage in the mechanism for sound transmission from the tympanic membrane to the oval window, as well as an air pocket overlying the round window to ensure a phase differential in the sound waves reaching the two labyrinthine windows. In cases where ossicular disruption has occurred, various materials have been interposed between the tympanic membrane and whatever ossicular remnant is present. Although many types of artificial protheses (e.g., incus replacement prosthesis, TORPS, PORPS) as well as tissue grafts, ossicular autographs and homografts, and cartilage struts have been employed; the tissue grafts have proved most successful. Homograft and autograft ossicles have demonstrated a capacity to maintain their configuration in the majority of cases and to serve as foci for new bone formation. The use of complete homograft units consisting of a tympanic membrane and attached ossicular chain is being advocated by some otologists, particularly in the reconstruction of the postmastoidectomy ear. Although grafts can be interposed between the eardrum and the footplate of the stapes in an attempt to restore hearing, the presence of a functionally and anatomically intact stapes greatly enhances the chances for a good functional result in these cases.

Exenteration of mastoid air cells with preservation of the bony posterior canal wall is often carried out in conjunction with a tympanoplasty performed in the face of chronic suppurative otomastoiditis without coexisting cholesteatoma. These procedures are variously categorized as simple mastoidectomy or atticoantrostomy. If purulent drainage has persisted until the time of surgery, a staged approach is often taken in which mastoidectomy is performed initially to be followed, after a drainage-free interval, by tympanoplasty.

A cholesteatoma, an epithelial-type inclusion cyst composed of a squamous epithelial lining and a central mass of exfoliated keratin debris, may destroy ossicular structures and erode the bony coverings overlying the endolabyrinth, the dura, and the facial nerve. The demonstrated potential for recurrence of both congenital and acquired cholesteatomas, even after careful removal under magnification, has made otologic surgeons particularly hesitant to compromise traditional surgical techniques for cholesteatoma removal for the sake of preserving more usable hearing. The classic radical mastoidectomy involves removal of the bony wall of the external canal and the tympanic membrane, thereby converting the mastoid system and middle ear into a common cavity accessible through the external meatus. This provides maximum visualization for thorough removal of a cholesteatoma at surgery as well as easy access to the mastoid cavity for early detection of recurrence of the disease. On the other hand, the radical mastoidectomy cavity requires periodic aftercare and leaves the patient with a substantial conductive hearing loss plus a set of anatomic circumstances which offers few opportunities for successful restoration of auditory function without the use of amplification.

Modifications of the radical mastoidectomy, e.g., the Bondy modification, cavity obliteration procedures, and canal wall-preserving procedure (the facial recess approach), strive to provide maximum visualization for removal of the disease process while at the same time avoiding a cavity and preserving hearing. Case selection is the key to successful utilization of these modified procedures while affording maximum safety to the patient during the postoperative period. Most otologists agree that situations including congenital cholesteatoma, intracranial spread of infection, labyrinthine fistula, facial nerve paralysis secondary to infection, and malignant or potentially malignant processes in the mastoid dictate the use of the more conservative classic radical mastoidectomy approach. The test of time must be applied to all of the modified procedures before rendering a final judgment as to their merits, but follow-up studies are showing a higher incidence of recurrent cholesteatoma in the canal wall preserving modifications that require surgical exteriorization of these mastoid systems.

It was supposed by many physicians that widespread antibiotic usage in the treatment of otitis media would definitively eradicate chronic otomastoiditis and related complications. However, although these disease processes have decreased in frequency, they are still a clinical fact of life and must be managed through close cooperation of primary care specialists with otolaryngologists. Methods for the measurement of hearing and middle ear function, even in young children, have greatly improved the physician's diagnostic and prognostic armamentarium.

TUMORS OF THE MIDDLE EAR AND TEMPORAL BONE

As noted in the discussion of external ear disorders, benign and, very rarely, malignant tumors may affect the external ear in children. These lesions include osteomas, fibrous dysplasia, either monostotic or polystotic, and ossifying fibromas. These lesions may involve other portions of the temporal bone, and surgical intervention is indicated if impingement on vital structures is imminent.

Rhabdomyosarcoma is the most commonly observed soft tissue malignancy involving the ear, with reticular cell sarcoma less common. A combination of chemotherapy, irradiation, and surgery must be utilized when treating these often fatal lesions.

Occasionally presenting as lytic lesions of the temporal bone on radiologic examination are the lesions broadly classified as histiocytosis X (i.e., Hand-Schüller-Christian disease, Letterer-Siwe disease, and eosinophilic granuloma). These may present as solitary lesions which are managed with surgical removal and/or radiotherapy.

Another type of radiologically lytic lesion occasionally observed in the temporal bone in the absence of infection is the congenital cholesteatoma, thought to arise from embryonic tissue rests. These lesions may be large and present with signs and symptoms of retrocochlear hearing loss if they are primarily localized in the petrous portion of the temporal bone. Surgical treatment may require a combined otosurgical/neurosurgical approach, and their potential for recurrence dictates a mastoidectomy procedure which permits exteriorization of the affected portion of the temporal bone in the vast majority of cases.

Eighth nerve tumors, which may occur in isolation or in association with neurofibromatosis (von Recklinghausen disease), are discussed in Section 4 of this chapter. These lesions present with hearing loss, tinnitus, dysequilibrium, and audiologic evidence of retrocochlear hearing loss. Facial nerve involvement may also be present with large lesions. Bony erosion of the internal auditory canal may be visible on plain mastoid x-ray films, but the most definitive radiologic study for these lesions is the air contrast CT scan of the cerebellar-pontine angle. Surgical approaches for removal of these tumors are broadly divisible into those procedures designed to spare residual hearing (gaining access to the internal canal via the middle cranial fossa or posterior cranial fossa) and those which sacrifice auditory and vestibular function (e.g., translabyrinthine approach). The neurotologic surgeon, in cooperation with the neurosurgeon, assesses the tumor size together with the degree of residual auditory and vestibular function when selecting the most efficacious surgical procedure to ensure maximal tumor removal with minimal residual deficit.

Meningiomas may involve the petrous portion of the temporal bone in the region of the internal auditory meatus; but rather than presenting as lytic lesions, they may appear radiographically with a halo of bony sclerosis. Again, surgical extirpation, with care to preserve as much auditory, vestibular, and facial nerve function as possible, is the treatment of choice.

SELECTED READING

Armstrong, B. W. (1954): A new treatment for chronic secretory otitis media. *Arch. Otolaryngol.,* 59:653–654.

Ballenger, J. J. (1985): *Diseases of the Nose, Throat, Ear, Head and Neck.* Lea & Febiger, Philadelphia.

Bluestone, C. D., and Stool, S. E., editors (1983): *Pediatric Otolaryngology.* Saunders, Philadelphia.

Brookhouser, P. E., and Bordley, J. E., editors (1980): Childhood communication disorders: Present status and future priorities. *Ann. Otol. Rhinol. Laryngol.,* 89(Suppl. 74):1–184.

Brookhouser, P. E., Hixson, P. K., and Matkin, N. D. (1979): Early childhood language delay: The otolaryngologist's perspective. *Laryngoscope,* 89:1898–1913.

Compere, W. E., and Valvassori, G. E. (1964): *Radiographic Atlas of the Temporal Bone.* H. M. Smyth, St. Paul, Minnesota.

Derlacki, E. L. (1952): Aural manifestations of allergy. *Ann. Otol. Rhinol. Laryngol.,* 61:179–188.

Goodhill, V. (1979): *Ear Diseases, Deafness and Dizziness.* Harper & Row, Hagerstown, Maryland.

Lim, D. J., and Birck, H. (1971): Ultrastructural pathology of the middle ear mucosa in serous otitis media. *Ann. Otol. Rhinol. Laryngol.,* 80:838–853.

Mogi, G., Hanjo, S., Maida, S., Yoshida, T., and Watanabe, N. (1974): Secretory immunoglobulin A (SIgA) in middle ear. *Ann. Otol. Rhinol. Laryngol.,* 83:92–101.

Palva, T., and Palva, A. (1975): Mucosal histochemistry in secretory otitis. *Ann. Otol. Rhinol. Laryngol.,* 84:112–116.

Paparella, M. M., and Shumrick, D. A., editors (1980): *Otolaryngology, Vol. II: The Ear.* Saunders, Philadelphia.

Paradise, J. L. (1981): Otitis media during early life: How hazardous to development? A critical review of the evidence. *Pediatrics,* 68:869–873.

Proud, G. O., and Odoi, H. (1970): Effects of eustachian tube ligation. *Ann. Otol. Rhinol. Laryngol.,* 79:30–32.

Pulec, J. L., Kamio, T., and Graham, M. D. (1975): Eustachian tube lymphatics. *Ann. Otol. Rhinol. Laryngol.,* 84:483–491.

Sade, J. (1966): Pathology and pathogenesis of serous otitis media. *Arch. Otolaryngol.,* 84:79–87.

Shurin, P. A., Pelton, S. I., Donner, A., and Klein, J. O. (1979): Persistence of middle-ear effusion after acute otitis media in children, *N. Engl. J. Med.,* 17:1121–1123.

Smyth, G. D. L. (1980): *Monographs in Clinical Otolaryngology, Vol. 2: Chronic Ear Disease.* Churchill Livingstone, New York.

The Ear

Section 4: Childhood Hearing Loss: Medical/Genetic Considerations

Medical/Genetic Evaluation of the Hearing-Impaired Child 98
  Strategy for Early Identification. 98
  Recommended Evaluation Protocol 100
Etiology of Childhood Hearing Loss 108
  Heredity: History of Familial Deafness and/or Consanguinity 108
  Ear, Nose, and Throat Deformities 122
  Anoxia and Low Apgar Score 122
  Ototoxic Drugs and Chemicals 123
  Viral Infections, Toxoplasmosis, and Syphilis 126
  Other Neonatal Illness, Particularly Sepsis and Jaundice 134
  Growth Retardation: Premature and Full-Term Low Birth Weight . . 134
  Recurrent Otitis Media and Mastoid Disease 135
  Childhood Illnesses: Meningitis and Sudden Hearing Loss 135
  Sound Trauma to the Ear: Acoustic Trauma and Noise 140
  "Knocked-Out": Physical Trauma to Ear and Skull 143

MEDICAL/GENETIC EVALUATION OF THE HEARING-IMPAIRED CHILD

Strategy for Early Identification

Early identification of an educationally significant hearing impairment is an essential public health priority. It is important to be mindful that childhood hearing loss may

1. Occur in either sex and all socioeconomic groups
2. Occur in the prelingual or postlingual age group

98

3. Be congenital or delayed in onset

4. Result from hereditary or environmental etiologies

5. Vary in severity from mild impairment to profound loss

6. Vary in type from a pure conductive or sensorineural loss to a mixed impairment

7. Occur unilaterally or bilaterally, symmetrically or asymmetrically

8. Occur as an isolated disability or as one element in a complex syndrome

9. Exist in a child, without parental awareness, until he/she reaches school age

10. Be relatively stable in severity throughout the child's life, fluctuate as with middle ear effusion, or become progressively worse with age

11. Be confused with mental retardation if the severely impaired child is evaluated with standard tests of mental development

Development of verbal communication skills during the critical preschool years lays the foundation for subsequent learning during the initial grades of elementary school. The severely hearing-impaired child who escapes detection until school age is confronted with the nearly impossible task of trying to catch up with a normal-hearing peer group by telescoping 4 to 5 years of communicative development into a much shorter period.

Given that few types of educationally significant hearing impairment are associated with obvious physical deformities, these disabilities constitute invisible handicaps at birth. Not until the age at which the child is expected to speak does the deficit become manifest. Delayed speech development is often the first indicator to draw parents' attention to their youngster's underlying hearing loss. Diagnosis of hearing impairment by waiting for a demonstrated developmental failure is inefficient and may severely limit the child's achievement potential.

As the physician best acquainted with disorders of hearing, the otolaryngologist must stand ready to help implement a high-risk early identification program for congenital hearing impairment in the community. Pediatricians, particularly neonatologists, and audiologists should be involved in the effort. All participants must become acquainted with those factors that place a neonate in the high-risk category. The authors have found that a list of high-risk factors built around the acronym *HEARING* is easily remembered and used by personnel involved in caring for neonates.

H—heredity: history of familial hearing loss or consanguinity

E—ear, nose, jaw, and throat deformities

A—anoxia and/or low Apgar score

Rx—ototoxic drugs and chemicals, pre- or postnatal

I—infections, prenatal or perinatal

N—neonatal intensive care or complications (jaundice)

G—growth retardation, premature or full-term low birth weight

Once a high-risk infant is identified, appropriate follow-up for definitive evaluation and habilitation planning must be ensured. Any infant admitted to the neonatal intensive care unit is sufficiently at risk to warrant assessment of auditory function at the time of hospital discharge as well as careful follow-up.

A valid and repeatable behavioral audiogram using an appropriate pediatric test battery is the most definitive assessment of an infant's hearing ability, but such a study is not usually feasible until 6 to 9 months of age. Auditory brainstem response (ABR) audiometry can assess the integrity of peripheral and central auditory function as far as the level of the inferior colliculus. It is important to note that an intact ABR does not evaluate a child's ability to utilize auditory input but merely demonstrates, in an objective fashion, whether the auditory system appears to be intact. Maturational changes have been noted in ABR studies of premature infants, and thus serial evaluations may be indicated to distinguish between immaturity and true otoneuropathology. Premature neonates may demonstrate diminished or absent ABRs shortly after birth and develop near-normal behavioral and ABR thresholds with maturation. In addition, it is important to remember that click stimuli used for ABR testing provide information primarily regarding frequencies of 2,000 to 4,000 Hz or greater.

A neonate who demonstrates an ABR compatible with significant hearing impairment should be followed at 3-month intervals through at least the first year of life, during which time repeated electrophysiological and behavioral evaluations of auditory function can be carried out in conjunction with habilitation planning.

Recommended Evaluation Protocol

The medical evaluation of an infant with severe to profound hearing impairment requires familiarity with the various etiologic factors of these disorders. Consideration must be given to whether the loss is hereditary or acquired and if the impairment was present at birth or appeared later in life. It is estimated that 50% of congenital impairment is hereditary, with the remainder representing causative factors, e.g., prenatal viral infections, anoxia, and other perinatal insults. Hearing deficits have been described not only as distinct entities but also in conjunction with abnormalities of nearly every major organ system of the body. A number of relatively exhaustive classification schemes have been developed to help focus clinicians' etiologic search as they confront the hearing-impaired child. A relatively modest example of such a scheme developed by Mouney and the author is contained in Table 2.4-1. For day-to-day clinical utility, a modified version of the high-risk *HEARING* acronym to include four additional childhood risk factors constituting the acronym *RISK* may be used:

R—recurrent otitis and mastoid disease
I—childhood illness, e.g., meningitis and sudden hearing loss
S—sound trauma: acoustic trauma and noise exposure
K—"knocked-out": physical trauma to ear and skull

HEARING RISK has provided an invaluable and easily remembered classification system which is used as an organizing principle for discussing the etiologies of childhood hearing loss in Section 7 of this chapter.

TABLE 2.4-1. *Etiology of deafness in children*

CONDUCTIVE

Nongenetic
  Collapsing external auditory canal
  Stenosis of the external auditory canal
  External otitis or bullous myringitis
  Tympanic membrane perforation with or without ossicular disruption—traumatic or
    postinfection
  Otitis media
    Serous
    Acute
    Chronic
  Tympanosclerosis
  Cholesteatoma
  Neoplastic

Genetic
  Stenosis or atresia of the external auditory canal
  Ossicular fixation with or without associated abnormalities

SENSORINEURAL

Nongenetic, acquired
  Traumatic
  Noise-induced
  Viral
    Mumps
    Measles
    Chickenpox
    Influenza
    Cytomegalic inclusion disease
    Other
  Nonviral infections (syphilis, meningitis, etc.)
  Metabolic disorders
  Neoplastic
  Ototoxic drugs
  Hypoxia

Nongenetic, congenital
  Hypoxia
  Viral (e.g., maternal rubella)
  Rh incompatibility
  Serious maternal metabolic disorder (toxemia, diabetes, etc.)
  Syphilis
  Toxoplasmosis
  Inoculation

Genetic, congenital
  Deafness alone
    Michael's aplasia
    Mondini's aplasia
    Alexander's aplasia
  Deafness with other abnormalities (e.g., Waardenburg's syndrome)

Genetic, delayed onset
  Deafness alone (e.g., otosclerosis)
  Deafness with other abnormalities (e.g., Alport's syndrome, sickle cell anemia)

Evaluation of a child with hearing loss is best carried out by a multidisciplinary team (Table 2.4-2) and should involve detailed examination of the medical history, family history, physical characteristics, laboratory results, and radiologic findings. The medical history includes a complete pregnancy history, with particular questions about possible viral or drug exposures or complications of pregnancy; delivery and neonatal history with review of medical records in questionable cases; and early pediatric history including any serious illnesses, injuries, or hospitalizations, with notation of when hearing loss was first suspected by the parents, how it was documented, and whether there is indication of progression (Fig. 2.4-1).

The physical examination should be done by a pediatrician or medical geneticist trained to look for subtle signs of genetic disorders. This may be especially helpful in the case of an adopted child when little family or early medical history is available.

TABLE 2.4-2. *Pediatric otoneurology team*

Otolaryngologist
  Developmental history
  Otoneurologic testing (vision screening)
  ENG (if appropriate)
  Surgery (if appropriate)

Geneticist
  Family history and pedigree
  Cytogenetics
  Counseling

Audiologist
  Behavioral testing (if possible)
    Behavioral observation audiometry (BOA)
    Visual reinforcement audiometry (VRA)
    Conditional play audiometry (CPA)
    Tangible reinforcement operation conditioning audiometry (TROCA)
  Impedance testing
  Central auditory test battery (if appropriate)
  ABR (if appropriate)

Speech and language pathologist
  Screening examination
  In-depth speech and language evaluation
  Voice evaluation (if indicated)
  Learning disabilities screening

As needed
  Pediatrician
  Ophthalmologist
  Neurologist
  Neuroradiologist
  Early childhood language specialist
  Development psychologist
  Learning disabilities specialist
  Aural habilitation specialist
  Educator of the hearing-impaired

BOYS TOWN INSTITUTE PATIENT QUESTIONNAIRE

Child's Name _____ Date of Birth _____

Date: _____

MEDICAL HISTORY

What are your major concerns about your child? _____

_____

_____

Has your child ever had or presently have:

YES	NO	GENERAL	YES	NO	
☐	☐	Scarlet Fever	☐	☐	Diphtheria
☐	☐	Mumps	☐	☐	Chicken pox
☐	☐	Measles	☐	☐	Rubella
☐	☐	Polio	☐	☐	Rheumatic fever
☐	☐	Tuberculosis	☐	☐	Meningitis
☐	☐	Asthma	☐	☐	Frequent headaches
☐	☐	Anemia	☐	☐	Heart problems
☐	☐	Vision problems	☐	☐	Kidney/bladder problems
☐	☐	Bone or joint deformities	☐	☐	Severe dental problems
☐	☐	Sugar/blood in urine	☐	☐	Fainting problems
☐	☐	Seizures/convulsions	☐	☐	Broken bones
☐	☐	Any serious injuries	☐	☐	Cerebral Palsy
☐	☐	Poor coordination (clumsiness)			
☐	☐	Very high fever (104° or more for longer than 24 hours)			
☐	☐	Frequent Upper Respiratory Infections			
☐	☐	Mental Retardation-if yes, degree _____			
☐	☐	Down Syndrome			
☐	☐	Other syndrome _____			

YES	NO	EAR, NOSE & THROAT	YES	NO	
☐	☐	Constant Cough	☐	☐	Speech problem
☐	☐	Hoarse voice quality	☐	☐	Ear deformity
☐	☐	Larynx deformity (voice box)	☐	☐	Dizziness or balance problems
☐	☐	Difficulty swallowing	☐	☐	"Ringing" in ears
☐	☐	Blood in sputum	☐	☐	Drainage of pus from ear(s)
☐	☐	Tonsillitis or sore throat	☐	☐	Drainage of blood from ear(s)
☐	☐	Mouth breathes/snores	☐	☐	Frequent ear infections
☐	☐	Tongue deformity	☐	☐	Too much wax in ears
☐	☐	Jaw deformity	☐	☐	Hearing problem
☐	☐	Cleft Palate/Cleft lip			

Allergies _____

Previous Hospitalization(s) _____

_____

_____

Present Medication(s) _____

_____

_____

(continues)

Fig. 2.4-1. Patient questionnaire.

DEVELOPMENTAL HISTORY

If appropriate, please complete the following:

At what age did your child sit unsupported? _____

At what age did your child walk? _____

At what age did your child talk? _____

At what age was your child toilet trained? _____

Is your child a bed-wetter? _____

Does your child have learning problems? _____

Has your child ever been in a special classroom in school? _____

Has your child ever attended a School for the Deaf? If so, where and when? _____

FAMILY HISTORY

Has any member of child's family had: GIVE RELATIONSHIP TO CHILD (mother, father, sister, brother, maternal or fraternal aunts, maternal or fraternal uncles, maternal or fraternal grandparents

YES	NO		
☐	☐	Tuberculosis	_____
☐	☐	Syphillis (V.D.)	_____
☐	☐	Diabetes	_____
☐	☐	Kidney trouble	_____
☐	☐	Heart trouble	_____
☐	☐	Asthma, Hay Fever, Hives	_____
☐	☐	Alcoholism	_____
☐	☐	Hemophilia	_____
☐	☐	Taken drugs	_____
☐	☐	Mental retardation	_____
☐	☐	Cleft lip/palate	_____
☐	☐	Speech and/or language problems	_____
☐	☐	Hearing problems	_____
☐	☐	Learning disability	_____

Please list the date of birth and sex of your children (other than the patient):

Date of Birth	Sex
_____	_____
_____	_____
_____	_____
_____	_____
_____	_____

Please list clinics, physicians, agencies, and hospitals where your child has been seen:

Name: _____ _____

Address: _____

Name: _____

Address: _____

Name: _____

Address: _____

PRENATAL/BIRTH HISTORY

MATERNAL ILLNESS DURING PREGNANCY, INCLUDING BLEEDING AND PRE-ECLAMPSIA

Mother's Date of Birth _____

YES   **NO**

☐   ☐   Did you experience any bleeding during pregnancy? If so, what month?
Month   1   2   3   4   5   6   7   8   9 Was it Mild, moderate or severe? _____

☐   ☐   Did you have measles during pregnancy? If so, in what month? Month   1   2   3   4   5   6   7   8   9

☐   ☐   Did you have high blood pressure during pregnancy? If so, in what month(s)?
Month   1   2   3   4   5   6   7   8   9

☐   ☐   Did you experience any labor or leakage of membranes during pregnancy? If so, in what month(s)?
Month   1   2   3   4   5   6   7   8   9

☐   ☐   Did you have any other infections or serious illnesses during pregnancy? If so, name the illness and the month.

Illness/Infection _____ Month   1   2   3   4   5   6   7   8   9

Illness/Infection _____ Month   1   2   3   4   5   6   7   8   9

Illness/Infection _____ Month   1   2   3   4   5   6   7   8   9

YES   **NO**

☐   ☐   Were you hospitalized longer than two days **before** delivery of your child If so, why?

_____

☐   ☐   Did you have any injuries during pregnancy? If so what? _____

RX-OTOTOXIC OR TERATOGENIC DRUGS DURING PREGNANCY
YES   **NO**

☐   ☐   Did you take any medications during pregnancy (exclude vitamins)? If so, what kind(s) of medication(s) and in what month(s)?

Name of Medication _____ Month(s)   1   2   3   4   5   6   7   8   9

Name of Medication _____ Month(s)   1   2   3   4   5   6   7   8   9

Name of Medication _____ Month(s)   1   2   3   4   5   6   7   8   9

Name of Medication _____ Month(s)   1   2   3   4   5   6   7   8   9

Name of Medication _____ Month(s)   1   2   3   4   5   6   7   8   9

STRESS FACTORS IN DELIVERY
YES   **NO**

☐   ☐   Did you have a normal delivery with this child? If you had problems, please explain.

☐   ☐   Was this child a breech delivery?

☐   ☐   Was this child a Caesarean Section delivery?

☐   ☐   Were forceps used in the delivery of this child?

☐   ☐   Was your labor longer than 24 hours? If so, how long? _____

☐   ☐   Was your labor shorter than 3 hours?

(continues)

GROWTH RETARDATION - PREMATURITY OR FULL TERM LOW BIRTH WEIGHT

YES   NO

☐   ☐   How much did your child weigh at birth? _____

☐   ☐   Was your child born prematurely? If so, by how many weeks? _____

☐   ☐   Was your pregnancy greater than 9 months? If so by how many weeks? _____

ANOXIA AT BIRTH OR LOW APGAR SCORE

YES   NO

☐   ☐   Did your child turn blue after birth and require oxygen

☐   ☐   Did your child have a serious problem breathing after birth?

☐   ☐   Did your child have a tube placed in his/her throat to help breathing?

Name of Hospital where your child was born _____

Address _____

City & State _____

Name of Physician who delivered your child _____

NEONATAL INTENSIVE CARE OR PROLONGED HOSPITAL STAY

YES   NO

☐   ☐   Did your child turn yellow after birth? If so did the child have phototherapy (Bililights) and how long? _____

☐   ☐   Did your child require one or more blood transfusions after birth?

☐   ☐   Did your child remain in the hospital more than three days after birth? If so, how long and why? _____

                _____

☐   ☐   Was your child in the Intensive Care Unit or an "incubator" after birth?

**RECURRENT OTITIS MEDIA BEGINNING BEFORE 2 YEARS OF AGE WITH SURGICAL
INTERVENTION AND/OR HEARING LOSS**

YES   NO

☐   ☐   Did your child have ear infections before the age of 3 years? If so, approximately how many? _____

☐   ☐   Has your child had his/her adenoids removed?

☐   ☐   Has your child had tubes placed in his/her ears?

SEIZURES, DIMINISHED SUCKING REFLEX, OR OTHER SIGNS OF C.N.S. DYSFUNCTION

YES   NO

☐   ☐   Has your child a seizure disorder? If so, when diagnosed? Type:

☐   ☐   Is he/she on medication for seizures? If so, name the medication.

☐   ☐   Did your child have problems nursing, feeding problems or sucking a bottle when he/she was a baby?

"KNOCKED OUT" - HEAD TRAUMA WITH LOSS OF CONSCIOUSNESS OR BLOODY OTORRHEA

YES   NO

☐   ☐   Has your child ever fallen or been hit on the head causing him/her to lose consciousness, causing a skull fracture, or concussion? If so, please explain.

☐   ☐   Has your child ever had bloody drainage from his/her ear as a result of a fall or blow to the head? If so, please explain.

_____

Questionnaire completed by:

If the hearing loss appears to be nonsyndromic, selected clinical and laboratory tests may be helpful in delineating certain causes. These include complete blood count; serology for rubella in a child under 1 year and for cytomegalovirus (CMV) in a child under 4 years of age; fluorescent treponemal antibody absorption (FTA) for congenital syphilis; urinalysis to detect Alport's syndrome; thyroid studies for Pendred's syndrome; and an electrocardiogram (ECG) to detect the Jervell and Lange-Nielsen syndrome. An ophthalmologic examination [including an electro-retinogram (ERG) in older children] is mandatory to rule out associated ocular anomalies such as retinitis pigmentosa (Usher syndrome) or viral retinopathy because visual input assumes a dominant role in the child's communicative and learning processes. Imaging of the temporal bone by polytomography or preferably by high-resolution CT scanning can also provide information about the anatomy of the middle ear, inner ear, and internal auditory canal. In addition, audiologic testing of both parents may reveal an unsuspected unilateral loss or other mild expression. Other major and minor anomalies should be noted and a genetic evaluation sought if a heritable syndrome is suspected.

Vestibular evaluation should be routinely completed by age 10 on all children with bilateral severe to profound sensorineural hearing impairment. If significant dysequilibrium exists, it should be carried out at a younger age. Delayed development of motor skills, e.g., standing on one foot and bicycle riding, can be a result of vestibular dysfunction. Parents and physicians should be made aware of this fact.

If a heritable disorder is suspected, the family history should be detailed, with construction of a pedigree at least to the third-degree relatives. Special attention should be paid to findings in other family members which could represent variable manifestations of a syndrome, and the clinician must know the right questions to elicit a complete history. Some manifestations may not be seen as relevant problems by the family, e.g., an ear pit or heterochromia, and may not be volunteered. In some cases it may be necessary for the family to ask their relatives to release their medical records or to submit to examination, and it is often helpful to ask to see family photographs. Consanguinity must be ruled out, particularly in rural areas or ethnic groups where there may not have been much outbreeding.

For most genetic disorders, pedigree analysis for mode of inheritance is fairly uncomplicated. The study of hearing impairment is a notable exception, where complex family histories involving multiple deaf × deaf marriages can make tracing of putative genes very difficult. In addition, families may have assumed various environmental causes for the hearing impairment in their relatives, particularly in previous generations. It may require considerable work and cooperation of other family members to determine the type of hearing loss and mode of inheritance in different branches of the family.

It is difficult to set any firm criteria for ordering a banded karyotype because any part of the genome could be involved and the variability of physical findings is so great that only a few specific syndromes are readily recognizable. The criteria presently followed at Boys Town National Institute are (a) two major malformations,

TABLE 2.4-3. *Examples of minor anomalies and major malformations and disabilities*

MINOR ANOMALIES

High-arched palate	Clinodactyly
Cleft uvula	Hernia
Hypertelorism	Pectus excavatum/carinatum
Abnormal slant of palpebral fissures	Large auricles
Micrognathia	Short neck
Abnormal dermatoglyphics	Synophrys

MAJOR MALFORMATIONS AND DISABILITIES

Growth retardation	Microcephaly
Mental retardation	Cleft lip/palate
Motor delay	Absent or hypoplastic ears
Congenital heart defect	Renal anomalies
Spina bifida	Eye anomalies
Genitourinary malformations	Deafness

or (b) a single major malformation with two or more minor malformations (Table 2.4-3).

Parents, audiologists, and teachers should be made aware also of the need for continued otologic follow-up of the severely to profoundly hearing-impaired child for the diagnosis and treatment of any coexisting middle ear disease which can have a deleterious impact on the child's educational development.

ETIOLOGY OF CHILDHOOD HEARING LOSS

Heredity: History of Familial Deafness and/or Consanguinity

The genes, which are the actual molecular codes for inherited factors, are arranged linearly on long strands of DNA that are packaged into chromosomes. Humans normally have 46 chromosomes in 23 pairs, with one member of each pair contributed by each parent. One of these pairs is composed of the sex chromosomes, two Xs in a female and an X and a Y in a male. Genes on these chromosomes are "sex-linked" and show a distinctive pattern of inheritance, described below. The remaining 22 pairs are termed the autosomes. Each pair of chromosomes carries a distinctive set of gene loci. There may be several alternative codes, or alleles, for a given gene. Thus each genetic trait is controlled by a pair of genes, the genotype, which may have the same code (homozygous) or consist of two different alleles (heterozygous). The physical manifestation of the trait, or phenotype, is determined by which alleles are present and how they interact. A dominant allele is one which is expressed in the phenotype of the individual, whether it is present in the homozygous or heterozygous state, whereas an autosomal recessive allele is expressed in the phenotype only when the individual is homozygous for that allele. An X-linked recessive gene is also expressed in the hemizygous state, i.e., in the male, where the Y chromosome does not carry a complementary allele. The inheritance pattern for a dominant trait, then, is typically one in which the trait goes from generation to generation, with an affected heterozygote having a 50% chance of transmitting the gene to each child. An autosomal recessive trait is generally seen in only one sibship in a family, and the heterozygotic (carrier) parents have a 25% recurrence risk for their children. An X-linked recessive trait is generally not expressed in the heterozygous female, but her sons have a 50% chance of inheriting the gene and showing the full-blown phenotype. The daughters of a carrier woman also have a 50% risk of being carriers themselves. An affected male will not have any affected sons, as they will have inherited his Y chromosome. This leads to the hallmark of X-linked inheritance, the lack of male-to-male transmission. All of the daughters of an affected male will be carriers, however.

Dominant inheritance is not always completely dominant. In some disorders, a dominant gene may show lack of penetrance, that is, not all heterozygotes manifest the disorder. Dominant disorders may also show variable expression of the phenotype, with different family members having different manifestations of the gene. These effects are presumably due to modification of the gene by environmental or other genetic, possibly allelic, influences.

Genetic disorders can also be caused by abnormalities at the chromosomal level, with extra or missing chromosomal material. Because this would involve many genes rather than only one, the phenotypes are generally more severe, with the exception of abnormalities of the sex chromosomes. Chromosomal abnormalities are detected through the construction of a karyotype, in which the chromosomes from a dividing cell are photographed and arranged in their pairs in a standard fashion. In this way, abnormalities in structure or number of chromosomes is readily seen. Before the advent of chromosomal banding techniques, the individual pairs could not be distinguished. The chromosomes were arranged according to size into seven groups, designated A through G. Now, however, each chromosome pair is readily discernible.

Trisomy refers to the presence of an extra chromosome; that is, an individual has three copies of a given chromosome rather than the usual pair. The least severe of the autosomal trisomies is trisomy 21, or Down's syndrome. Trisomy 13 (Patau's syndrome) and trisomy 18 (Edward's syndrome) are also seen but are much more rare and more severe. In the past these disorders were referred to as G, D, or E trisomies, respectively, but with banding it has now been shown that the chromosomes involved in the particular phenotypes are always 21, 13, and 18. Trisomies of the other autosomes are almost always incompatible with a live birth. Autosomal monosomy, or the presence of only one chromosome of a pair, is also almost always lethal.

Parts of chromosomes may be missing (deletions) or extra (duplications). The phenotype and its severity is determined by the amount and chromosomal origin of the material involved. With high-resolution banding, smaller and smaller deletions and duplications can be seen, and the number of chromosomal syndromes described is increasing rapidly.

Genetic Considerations in Hearing Loss

A complete genetic evaluation involves determination and communication of three basic aspects of a disorder: diagnosis, prognosis, and recurrence risk. Precise diagnosis is the most crucial, as it determines both of the other factors. With particular regard to hearing impairment, every effort should be made to determine the etiology. Diagnosis of a particular type of inherited hearing impairment may prompt recognition of other related physical problems, influence the type of treatment, and prevent unnecessary diagnostic procedures. Even if a more precise diagnosis has no effect on presently available treatment options, identification of affected individuals facilitates research on that disorder and allows recontact if advances in treatment occur. Proper diagnostic recognition of a syndrome or family pattern can aid in arriving at a prognosis regarding potential for progression of a hearing loss or the development of other related disorders. Accurate estimation of recurrence risk is also dependent on an accurate diagnosis. It is possible to use empiric risk data if the diagnosis is truly unknown, but a missed diagnosis may prevent early identification of other family members at risk for hearing impairment, thus negating an opportunity for early remedial intervention.

Several population studies have estimated the incidence of childhood hearing impairment due to genetic factors to be approximately 50%. About 20 to 25% of cases are due to identifiable environmental causes, occurring prenatally, during the neonatal period, or later in life; and 25 to 30% are sporadic cases with unknown etiology. These figures vary, however, depending on the population studied. If the cohort born between 1964 and 1966, during the rubella epidemic, is considered, only 15% are expected to have genetically determined hearing loss because of the increased incidence of postrubella hearing impairment; but about 85% of the population of students at Gallaudet College were shown to have a genetic cause for their hearing loss.

Genetic forms of hearing loss may be congenital or of later onset, progressive or nonprogressive, unilateral or bilateral: they may be syndromic (involving other identifiable physical characteristics in other systems) or nonsyndromic, involving only hearing loss. At least 100 genetic syndromes which include hearing loss have been identified, and they are commonly classified according to the other systems involved: craniofacial/cervical, skeletal, integumentary, ocular, neurologic, renal, metabolic, and "other." The nonsyndromic disorders (i.e., hearing loss only) are ususally described by their audiologic characteristics, age of onset, presence or absence of progression, and mode of inheritance. Fraser estimated that 20% of genetic hearing impairment in children in schools for the deaf is due to autosomal dominant genes. However, of the children referred to a university birth defects clinic for hearing loss. Bergström reported that 47% showed autosomal dominant inheritance, which may be a more accurate reflection of a clinician's case load. Fewer than half of these patients had recognizable syndromes, so the genetic mechanism could be identified only through study of the family history.

Inner Ear—Structural Malformations

Those types of hearing loss associated with agenesis or dysgenesis of the inner ear components are common congenital hereditary hearing problems. They are classified clinically and histopathologically by the severity of the loss and the site of developmental failure. The availability of newer imaging techniques, e.g., computerized tomographic (CT) scanning, has made premortem diagnosis of these deformities more precise.

Michel's deformity is characterized by a lack of development of the structures of the inner ear, including in some cases complete agenesis of the petrous portion of the temporal bone. The deformity is transmitted as an autosomal dominant disorder and is usually accompanied by an anatomically normal external and middle ear. The radiologic appearance of the temporal bone is helpful in diagnosing the disorder, although postmortem histopathologic differentiation of this deformity from bony deposition in the labyrinth following labyrinthitis (labyrinthitis ossificans) is necessary for definitive diagnosis. Because the inner ear structures have not differentiated, sensorineural hearing loss is complete in these cases and amplification is not helpful.

Mondini's deformity is characterized by an arrest in cochlear development so that only the basal coil can be differentiated instead of the usually 2.5 turns. The upper coils are seen histopathologically to lack an interscalar septum and assume a cloacal form. This set of anatomic findings, including the tubular shape of the membranous labyrinth, most closely parallels cochlear development at about the sixth week of gestation, and a developmental arrest at this stage seems likely. The underdeveloped vestibular labyrinth observed in most cases reinforces this impression (Fig. 2.4-2). The deformity is transmitted as an autosomal dominant trait and may not be bilateral. Neurosensory structures are present in most of these cases, and therefore the fitting of appropriate amplification based on audiologic testing would be useful in habilitation.

Scheibe's aplasia involves a normally differentiated bony labyrinth, as well as the superior portion of the membranous labyrinth, the semicircular canals and utricle. The saccule and cochlear duct, however, reveal significant abnormalities including lack of differentiation of the organ of Corti, collapse of the scala media and Reissner's membrane, and significant malformation of the tectorial membrane. The commonest form of inherited inner ear aplasia, Scheibe's aplasia demonstrates an autosomal recessive inheritance pattern. As with Mondini's deafness, the presence of some neurosensory elements would warrant the use of selected amplification in the habilitation of these children.

Alexander's malformation includes aplasia of the cochlear duct, specifically affecting the organ of Corti and ganglion cells of the basal turn of the cochlea. Audiometrically, this disorder is characterized by high-frequency hearing impairment, and these patients should be able to use appropriate amplification, taking advantage of residual low-frequency hearing.

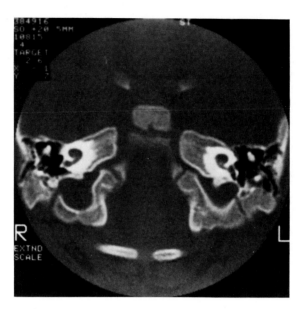

Fig. 2.4-2. CT scan showing Mondini's deformity.

Autosomal Dominant Disorders

Autosomal dominant syndromes appear to be the easiest to recognize, as one should have both a positive family history following the classic dominant pattern and a recognizable phenotype. Unfortunately, this is not always the case. Dominant genes are notoriously susceptible to variations in expressivity, meaning that different characteristics may be present in different family members, and they may have decreased penetrance, such that a gene carrier may not have detectable expression of the gene. Because only one gene is involved in the manifestation of the phenotype, a new mutation may also occur, producing a dominant disorder in an individual with a totally negative family history.

Waardenburg's syndrome is the most commonly cited example of a syndrome with variable expressivity and may account for about 3% of hearing impairment in children. The characteristics include pigmentary anomalies (white forelock, heterochromia irides, premature graying, and vitiligo), craniofacial features such as dystopia canthorum, broad root of the nose, and synophrys, along with unilateral or bilateral sensorineural hearing impairment (Fig. 2.4-3). Only about 20% of patients, however, manifest the white forelock, and it may appear at any time in an individual's life. The other features are equally variable. In addition, only 20% of patients have hearing loss. Questions have been raised concerning the existence of two types of Waardenburg's syndrome based on the presence or absence of dystopia canthorum, with a higher frequency of hearing loss in type II (without dystopia). On the other hand, this observation may reflect a bias of as-

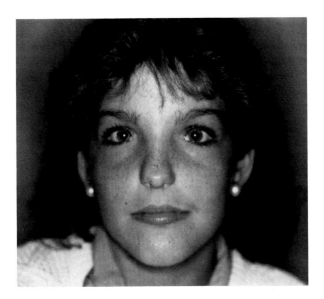

Fig. 2.4-3. Waardenburg's syndrome.

certainment, dystopia and hearing impairment often being the major diagnostic criteria, and the genetic distinctness of the two types remains to be demonstrated. Thus diagnosis of Waardenburg's syndrome may be very difficult if only one or two of the characteristics are observed, and the full-blown syndrome is not seen in the immediate family. In such cases, a complete family history, with attention to the diverse characteristics of the syndrome, is required to make the diagnosis. Audiologic testing to detect previously unsuspected unilateral hearing loss may be particularly informative.

Another variable autosomal dominant disorder which may be relatively common, particularly in the Midwest, is *Stickler's syndrome*. Characteristics include a small jaw, which may produce a cleft palate (Robin's anomaly), severe myopia with risk of retinal detachment or cataracts, joint enlargement and hypermobility with arthritis in early adulthood, and some spondyloepiphyseal dysplasia. About 15% of individuals with this syndrome have sensorineural or mixed hearing loss. Because of the variability in this syndrome, the diagnosis may require careful examination of many family members; however, the severity of two of the findings—hearing loss and retinal detachment—warrants every effort at diagnosis.

The *branchio-oto-renal,* or *Melnick-Fraser, syndrome* is an additional example of a dominant syndrome that can have serious consequences in some gene carriers. Branchial characteristics include ear pits (possibly tags) or cervical fistulas, and the renal findings range from minor asymptomatic dysplasia, seen only on ultrasound or intravenous pyelogram (IVP), to agenesis and renal failure. The hearing loss may be sensorineural, conductive, or mixed. A survey of profoundly deaf school-children revealed that 2% had this syndrome, thus making it an important contributor to hearing loss at all levels. This report further emphasized the need for any child with a hearing loss and ear pit, or branchial cleft anomaly, to have a renal evaluation.

Alport's syndrome also includes renal problems and may account for 1% of genetic hearing impairment. In this syndrome, hearing impairment is sensorineural and progressive: it may not be noted until the second decade, thus paralleling the nephritis, which may be seen as hematuria during infancy, but then remain asymptomatic for several years before onset of renal insufficiency. The renal component is especially severe in males, often resulting in death from uremia before age 30. Konigsmark and Gorlin stressed the importance of early diagnosis of this syndrome to facilitate management of the renal disease and noted that renal transplant was associated with improved hearing in one case. This syndrome is apparently genetically heterogeneous. It has been described as an autosomal dominant trait with decreased expression in females, but there is a dearth of male-to-male transmission, so many cases may actually be X-linked.

Treacher Collins syndrome (mandibulofacial dysostosis) is a craniofacial disorder which includes microtia, meatal atresia, and conductive hearing impairment in about one-third of cases; sensorineural loss and vestibular abnormality may also be present. Although the conductive hearing loss is often due to ossicular malformation, the proportion of patients who can benefit from reconstructive surgery is not clear. The other characteristic facial features are hypoplasia of the malar area and zygomatic arch which produces downward slanting palpebral fissures, coloboma of the lower eyelids, and a hypoplastic mandible. The bilateral symmetry and eyelid coloboma serve to distinguish it from Goldenhar's syndrome and the related oculoauricular vertebral syndromes, which sometimes have similar microtia and craniofacial abnormalities. Treacher Collins syndrome is an autosomal dominant disorder with high penetrance, whereas the oculoauriculovertebral spectrum is probably multifactorial and is usually sporadic (see below). Because the Treacher Collins syndrome is due to a new mutation in as many as 60% of cases, it becomes important to distinguish between the two possibilities in cases with a negative family history. The syndrome can be quite variable in the severity of expression, but the degree of severity tends to be consistent within a family, suggesting that there may be genetic heterogeneity.

Neurofibromatosis exhibits café au lait spots (light brown pigmented spots of varying size) and numerous fibromatous tumors. Cutaneous tumors are most characteristic, but other tumors of the central nervous system, peripheral nerves, and viscera are also common. The phenotype is quite variable, ranging from a few café au lait spots to multiple disfiguring tumors, as in the "elephant man." In some cases tumors of the central nervous system can produce mental retardation, blindness, or hearing impairment. This is also a genetically heterogeneous disorder, and at least two forms are clearly distinct. Classic neurofibromatosis (von Recklinghausen's disease) has a very high frequency of café au lait spots and cutaneous neurofibromas, but the occurrence of acoustic neuromas is infrequent, perhaps around 5%. These are typically unilateral. However, hearing impairment can apparently occur in neurofibromatosis without demonstrable acoustic neuromas, so audiologic follow-up of children with, or at risk for, the disorder is recommended. Central neurofibromatosis is a genetically separate disorder diagnosed primarily by the presence of bilateral acoustic neuromas. These are generally slow-growing and usually are asymptomatic until young adulthood. The first signs may be vestibular dysfunction during adolescence. Café au lait spots and cutaneous neurofibromas may be present but are in much lower frequency than in von Recklinghausen's disease. Some of the other tumors seen in the classic form, e.g., optic glioma, have not been seen in central neurofibromatosis. The distinction between these two disorders is relatively new, and it is likely that cases of von Recklinghausen's disease described in the past with bilateral acoustic neuroma were actually central neurofibromatosis. Both disorders are autosomal dominant with variable expressivity but high penetrance and appear to have very high mutation rates (or further genetic heterogeneity). There is some evidence that they involve different abnormalities of nerve growth factor.

Otosclerosis may represent an autosomal dominant syndrome of conductive or mixed hearing impairment with delayed onset and decreased penetrance. Although the hearing loss generally occurs during adulthood, it may begin in childhood. Penetrance of the gene is estimated at 40%, meaning that only 40% of gene carriers actually demonstrate otosclerosis. Thus the family history may deviate from the expected pattern. In adolescents and adults, stapedectomy, together with insertion of a stapes replacement prosthesis, may be helpful in alleviating a significant portion of the conductive hearing impairment, but a progressive sensorineural component, related to "cochlear otosclerosis," may become apparent with the passage of time. Stapedectomy in infants and children is not generally advisable because of an increased risk of otitis media and associated damage to labyrinthine structures. In cases of bilateral stapes fixation, unilateral mobilization of the stapes can be attempted in children if use of appropriate amplification is not satisfactory. Potential complications include sensorineural hearing loss, vestibular dysfunction, facial nerve paresis, taste change (related to trauma to the chorda tympani), and refixation of the stapes footplate with resultant recurrence of the conductive hearing impairment.

There are several types of *nonsyndromic autosomal dominant hearing loss* which have been described best by Konigsmark and Gorlin. Congenital, severe nonprogressive hearing impairment may actually constitute several disorders, but lack of detailed study of associated temporal bone pathology or changes in vestibular function have made distinguishing the subtypes difficult. *Early-onset, progressive deafness* begins with a high-frequency hearing loss during childhood or early adulthood, gradually progressing to include the middle and finally the low frequencies, with severe hearing loss typical after age 45. Another reported type of high-frequency progressive hearing loss has an earlier onset, but this variant may not truly represent a separate entity. A *low-frequency progressive* type begins with congenital or early onset of a 20- to 60-dB low-frequency loss progressing to include the high frequencies by the third or fourth decade and lastly the middle frequencies. In contrast, mid-frequency progressive hearing loss may be first seen as about an 80-dB loss in childhood in the 1,000- to 2,000-Hz range ("cookie-bite"), which gradually progresses in both the high and low frequencies. Finally, unilateral congenital hearing impairment can be inherited in a dominant fashion, and the family history may contain individuals with bilateral loss.

Autosomal Recessive Disorders

Autosomal recessive inheritance is generally considered to account for about 80% of genetically produced childhood hearing impairment, and about half of these cases represent recognizable syndromes. There is less variability in recessive than in dominant disorders, and penetrance is not decreased, so that diagnosis of a syndrome is not complicated by these factors. On the other hand, carriers of a recessive gene are asymptomatic, and the recurrence risk for a recessive disorder is only 25%, so that most affected families contain only one affected child with an otherwise negative family history. Not until one reaches a sibship size of six is there greater than a 50% chance of having more than one affected child. If the disorder in question is nonsyndromic, it is very difficult to determine that a singleton case actually represents recessive inheritance rather than a nongenetic cause. It follows that a sizable proportion of cases in the "unknown" category can be expected to be undetected autosomal recessive disorders. Empiric risk figures indicate that at least half of the unknown cases have a genetic basis, and one small study has demonstrated, through segregation analysis, that a recessive model could explain both their recessive and unknown etiology families. Because nongenetic causes of hearing loss can be expected to decrease with medical progress, and our ability to detect them should increase, the "unknown" category will contain a larger proportion of singleton cases in the future.

Many recessive syndromes which include hearing impairment as one of the manifestations will be made apparent to the clinician by their other characteristics. The following discussion reviews the more common recessive disorders having hearing impairment as the presenting complaint but requiring specific testing to establish the diagnosis. These tests may be the only way to recognize the genetic component in singleton cases, thereby permitting accurate genetic counseling.

Usher's syndrome may account for as much as 5% of congenital hearing impairment. Because it involves the gradual development of retinitis pigmentosa with eventual visual impairment, early diagnosis is important for educational and career planning. Diagnosis may be made by ophthalmologic examination, including electroretinography (ERG), during childhood before the symptoms of night blindness and tunnel vision become evident. Any child with sensorineural hearing loss should be screened by an ophthalmologist. The age for such screening has been disputed, with some suggesting that it should not be done before high school because earlier detection would only cause extra years of anxiety. However, early detection could be of importance to the parents with respect to future family planning. Some parents may be willing to assume a 25% risk of an isolated hearing loss in future offspring but may see Usher's syndrome as too great a burden. It has been pointed out that early visual deficits, perhaps present before high school age, may represent a danger to children. After the diagnosis has been made, counseling for the child which is age-appropriate must be provided, allowing teachers and parents freedom to help the youngster gradually accept the condition and make realistic educational/vocational plans.

There exist at least four types of Usher's syndrome. Type I, accounting for about 90% of cases, is characterized by congenital profound hearing impairment with onset of retinitis pigmentosa (RP) at about age 10. Type II also has congenital hearing impairment but in the moderate to severe range, and the RP may not present until the early twenties. It accounts for almost 10% of Usher's syndrome patients, with types III and IV being very rare. Type III shows progressive hearing loss, with onset of RP in the early to mid teens, and type IV is phenotypically similar to type II but shows X-linked inheritance. There is some suggestion of further heterogeneity or carrier expression in view of the fact that Usher's syndrome shows a higher frequency in families with isolated retinitis pigmentosa, which in itself is heterogeneous and may be inherited as a dominant, recessive, or X-linked condition.

Pendred's syndrome probably accounts for about 2% of childhood hearing impairment, although a figure as high as 10% has been reported. It is caused by a defect in thyroid hormone organification and is characterized by the development of a euthyroid goiter usually by 8 years of age. Typically, the affected patient presents no other problems, although a few cases of mental retardation have been reported. The diagnosis is made by finding decreased binding of iodine on a perchlorate discharge test; however, the test is not often utilized because it is nonspecific and requires the use of radioactively labeled iodine. Some degree of genetic heterogeneity is probable in that patients with somewhat different defects of thyroid function have been found. Treatment of the goiter is best done by medication, as it generally regenerates following surgical extirpation. Treatment of the thyroid condition has not been shown to affect the hearing loss.

Jervell and Lange-Nielsen syndrome consists of profound congenital hearing impairment and an electrocardial conduction defect, specifically prolongation of the QT interval. It may account for 1% of congenital hearing impairment, and its diagnosis is particularly important because the conduction defect can lead to syncope and even sudden death. In fact, approximately one-half of reported patients died suddenly before age 20. The cardiac defect is effectively treated with β-adrenergic blockers such as propranolol. An ECG is a simple test, and the advantages of diagnosis should make this part of the routine screening provided to any newly identified deaf child.

Nonsyndromic recessive hearing loss has been divided into three types by Konigsmark and Gorlin: congenital severe sensorineural, congenital moderate sensorineural, and early-onset sensorineural. The latter is quite rapidly progressive, with onset as early as 1.5 years of age, and generally the hearing loss is profound by age six. The most common form is the congenital severe sensorineural type, and evidence from matings of individuals who both have this type of hearing impairment but who have normal-hearing children indicates that there are six to 10 different genetic loci which produce indistinguishable disorders.

Sex-Linked Disorders

Sex linkage is rarely observed in childhood hearing impairment, accounting for only about 1% of cases; however, Fraser estimated that it explained about 6% of nonsyndromic profound hearing impairment in boys. As in autosomal recessive disorders, singleton cases are quite possible, which may represent new mutations, so that X-linked recessive disorders often go undetected. X-linked disorders which include hearing impairment are Norrie's disease, the otopalatodigital syndrome, and Wildervanck's syndrome.

Norrie's disease demonstrates congenital or rapidly progressive blindness with development of pseudoglioma, progressive opacification, and degeneration of the eyes leading to microphthalmia. Intellectual functioning also tends to deteriorate, and sensorineural hearing loss, which occurs in about one-third of cases, is progressive with onset usually during the second or third decade.

The *otopalatodigital syndrome* shows characteristic craniofacial malformation with a prominent brow, hypertelorism, flat mid-face and small nose, and cleft palate. There are also skeletal abnormalities, generally with short stature. The fingers and toes are broad and irregular in length, with a wide space between the first and second toes. Conductive hearing loss is probably due to ossicular malformation and may be treatable surgically. Female carriers usually show milder facial features.

Wildervank's syndrome is actually a triad of the Klippel-Feil malformation of fused cervical vertebrae, abducens paralysis producing retraction of the eye when gazing laterally (also called Duane's retraction syndrome), and sensorineural or mixed hearing impairment. It may be inherited as an X-linked dominant with lethality in males; it is almost exclusively observed in females, although one severely affected male apparently representing a new mutation has been reported, and we have seen such a case. Alternatively, the syndrome may be part of a multifactorial continuum. The Klippel-Feil sequence, which is rarely familial, includes hearing impairment in about 30% of cases, and hearing loss is found in about 10% of cases with isolated Duane's syndrome.

Nonsyndromic congenital severe sensorineural hearing loss has been described, and the observation of mental retardation in some cases suggests that there may be more than one type on the X chromosome. Clinical reports also detail a rapidly progressive early-onset type and a moderate, more slowly progressive type, as well as a conductive type with fixation of the stapedial footplate. The latter variant is important surgically, as attempts at stapedectomy usually result in a gush of perilymphatic fluid into the middle ear.

Multifactorial Genetic Disorders

Multifactorial inheritance, which is a combination of multiple genetic factors (possibly including major genes with decreased penetrance) along with unspecified environmental influences, is responsible for some syndromes with associated hearing loss, e.g., clefting syndromes with conductive hearing loss, or the *microtial hemifacial microsomia/Goldenhar spectrum* (Fig. 2.4-4). This spectrum of findings, which are usually unilateral, appear to be part of the same developmental continuum. The family history is positive in about 6% of cases, with different aspects of the spectrum seen within the same family. Preauricular tags or pits are also found and may be the mildest manifestation. Vertebral abnormalities are associated; these are usually hypoplastic or hemivertebrae in the cervical region, but lower vertebrae may also be involved. Eye abnormalities, when present, include epibulbar dermoids and coloboma of the *upper* lid. The most severe manifestation, Goldenhar's syndrome or oculoauriculovertebral dysplasia, has occasionally been described in families with an apparent autosomal dominant inheritance pattern. This may be fortuitous clustering of the multifactorial disorder or may be evidence of genetic heterogeneity.

Increased susceptibility to hearing impairment with diabetes and hyperlipidemia, and perhaps even a genetic susceptibility to the embryopathic effects of the rubella virus, also represent examples of this type of inheritance. It is conceivable that

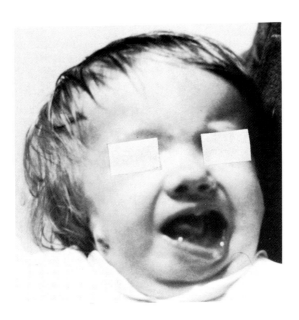

Fig. 2.4-4. Young child with Goldenhar's syndrome.

certain structural characteristics of the temporal bone may make some individuals more susceptible to meningitis and subsequent hearing impairment.

Autosomal Chromosomal Syndromes

Autosomal chromosomal syndromes are generally associated with developmental delays which may obscure the signs and symptoms of an associated hearing loss. All such children should have the benefit of an early comprehensive audiologic evaluation before educational program planning is completed. Children with *Down's syndrome* (trisomy 21) are especially susceptible to middle ear problems and should be checked routinely after about 6 months of age using behavioral, audiologic, and acoustic impedance measures. *Turner's syndrome* is caused by monosomy for all or part of an X chromosome, so that there is only one normal X. The phenotype is that of a female with gonadal dysgenesis and short stature, and occasionally a webbed neck and shield chest. It is often first detected when the girl is evaluated for delayed puberty. This syndrome includes an increased risk of sensorineural, conductive, or mixed hearing loss, and in a young girl between the ages of 3 and 10 there may be no other physical problems to give a clue to the diagnosis. The diagnosis may be suspected in a girl with a history of neonatal lymphedema, particularly is she is short.

Genetic Counseling—A Practical Approach

Genetic counseling involves synthesis of all of the above information in an attempt to reach a diagnosis and communication of the results to the family in terms they can comprehend. The implications of the diagnosis (or lack of one) are discussed, and recurrence risks are given. Genetic counseling, properly done, is nondirective. Many people still fear that the purpose of genetic counseling is to tell them whether to have children, and it is important to defuse this feeling from the beginning. Genetic counseling in regard to hearing impairment is particularly sensitive. When counseling hearing parents of a deaf child, the frequent inability to provide a precise diagnosis can be very frustrating, especially for parents who see this as a high-burden disorder. On the other hand, counseling of deaf parents can be complicated by serious communication problems. The counselor must also be aware that deaf parents may or may not see hearing impairment as a burden in their children. Boughman et al. have developed specific signs for genetic terminology for use with the deaf.

The recurrence risks for an autosomal dominant disorder are straightforward if the disorder is fully penetrant; any child of an affected individual has a 50% risk of inheriting the disorder, whereas the child of an unaffected family member will not be at risk. In disorders with decreased penetrance, allowance must be made for the fact that a child might inherit the gene but may not have a hearing loss; for example, the child of a person with Waardenburg's syndrome may have a 50% risk of inheriting the gene but only a 10% risk of hearing impairment. Allowance must also be made for the possibility of nonpenetrance in some disorders, so an apparently unaffected sibling, for example, may still run a risk of having an affected child.

For an autosomal recessive disorder, the parents have a 25% recurrence risk. They and their affected children are often surprised to learn that the recurrence risk for the affected child is small, depending totally on whom the child marries. If the spouse happens to have exactly the same type of hearing impairment, the recurrence risk would be 100%, but these genes are rare and such an outcome would be exceedingly unlikely. Survey of a school for the deaf revealed that deaf teenagers usually assumed that their risk was 50%, when in fact this was rarely so. Siblings of affected individuals also have very low recurrence risks, on the order of 1 in 100, depending on the frequency of the gene in the general population. Risks would be increased, of course, if either the deaf person or the sibling were to marry a relative.

In families where the mother is a carrier of an X-linked recessive disorder, there is a 50% risk for each son to have the disorders and a 50% chance that each daughter is a carrier. Bayesian calculations can be performed to determine the chance that a given female relative is a carrier by taking into account the degree of relationship, number of unaffected children, etc. A discussion of these calculations can be found in Thompson and Thompson. If the father has an X-linked form of hearing impairment, none of his sons will be affected but all of his daughters will be carriers.

With multifactorial disorders, empiric recurrence risks particular to the disorder in question, are used. Generally, these are quite low for sporadic cases, on the order of a few percent. The recurrence risk for chromosomal disorders is low assuming that both parents have normal karyotypes.

The unique challenge in genetic couseling for hearing impairment is the sporadic case. Because of the multitude of phenocopies, such an individual may have a genetic or nongenetic etiology for his hearing loss, and the recurrence risks for unaffected parents will either be 25% (autosomal recessive or X-linked, if the sex is unknown) or negligible (new dominant mutation, multifactorial, or nongenetic). In such cases, empiric recurrence risks must be used, which give an "averaged" risk over the various possibilities. When such figures are used, it must be stressed that these are averages, and the overall range should also be cited. Recurrence risks cited for the situation of a family with an only child with unexplained hearing impairment have ranged from 10 to 16%. Bieber and Nance have developed a very useful table which specifies the recurrence risk based on the number of affected and unaffected children in the family; for example, the risk for the case described above would be about 10%. If the same family should have a hearing child next, it suggests that the hearing impairment in the first child may not be genetic, and the estimate of their risk would decrease to about 8%. A family with one deaf child and two hearing children would have a 6 to 7% recurrence risk. However, as soon as a second deaf child is born to the family, the assumption of an autosomal recessive (or rarely an X-linked) disorder is made, and a 25% recurrence risk is given. Again, the family should be aware that the recurrence risks given are merely estimates, and that they should recontact the geneticist after any change in their family. Bieber and Nance also found that any history of hearing loss in more distant relatives served to increase estimates of the recurrence risk, presumably due to carrier manifestations in recessives, multifactorial influences, unrecognized dominance, or X-linkage. For example, if there were a positive family history, the recurrence risk for the family with one affected child would be 20% instead of 10%.

The recurrence risk for a couple in which one member has a hearing loss of unknown cause and the other has normal hearing will either be as high as 50% if the affected individual carries a fully penetrant dominant gene or negligible if the hearing impairment is recessive or nongenetic. Again, averaged empiric risks are available. Harper estimated this at 5%. Bieber and Nance gave a similar estimate of 6% and showed that this risk decreases as the number of unaffected children increases. With the birth of an affected child, their recurrence risk becomes 40.8% for each subsequent pregnancy, the discrepancy from 50% presumably due to nonpenetrance.

When both members of the couple have hearing impairment of unknown etiology, the recurrence risk would range from 100% if they have the same recessive type, to 50% if one carries a dominant gene, to negligible. Most observations have shown that the *a priori* risk for such a couple to have a deaf child is about 10%. Again, Bieber and Nance showed that this drops rapidly as they have hearing children, but if their first child is deaf it rises to 62%. Subsequent deaf children would indicate that the couple might have the same recessive disorder, and after five deaf children their risk is virtually 100%. If they should have at least one deaf and one hearing child, their risk is 32.5%, presumably reflecting the averaged effects of dominant genes, some with reduced penetrance, and multifactorial influences.

Genetic evaluation in cases of hearing loss is complex, but the high frequency of genetic causes of hearing impairment indicates that every child with hearing loss should have a thorough evaluation to determine etiology. In particular, genetic evaluation and counseling should be offered in any case where an environmental cause cannot be documented.

Ear, Nose, and Throat Deformities

In addition to deformities of the external and middle ear (see Section 2 in this chapter), and hereditary deformities of the internal ear discussed above, deformities of the jaw, nose, and palate should be looked for by the examiner. The section on middle ear disease discusses the high incidence of eustachian tube dysfunction and middle ear disease among children with skull base and palatal deformities.

Anoxia and Low Apgar Score

Anoxia is the perinatal insult showing the strongest correlation with the subsequent appearance of sensorineural hearing impairment in the young infant. Histopathologic evidence suggests that the anoxic damage occurs not in the cochlea but in the brainstem cochlear nuclei, which show decreased cell numbers and volume in direct proportion to the length and severity of the anoxic episode.

Ototoxic Drugs and Chemicals

The potential toxicity of a number of drugs and chemicals has become increasingly evident as stricter reporting of toxic side effects has become mandatory. The thalidomide tragedy pointed out the danger posed to the developing fetus by otherwise inocuous medications taken during pregnancy. Severe otologic deformities in these infants correlated with consumption of the drug during the gestational period characterized by development of the otologic structures.

In postnatal cases of ototoxicity, tinnitus, hearing loss, and vertigo may all be useful indicators of impending or actual damage to inner ear structures. The young child, however, constitutes a particular challenge to the clinician who vigilantly observes the patient's reaction to therapy and documents inner ear function, using objective techniques in many cases, to avoid potentially irreversible damage to these important neurosensory structures. A partial listing of drugs and chemicals implicated in ototoxicity, taken from Quick, follows:

Drugs

Antibiotics
  Streptomycin
  Neomycin
  Gentamicin
  Viomycin
  Pharmacetin
  Chloramphenicol
  Dihydrostreptomycin
  Kanamycin
  Vancomycin
  Ristocetin

Diuretics
  Ethacrynic acid
  Furosemide

Other drugs
  Salicylates
  Polybrene
  Quinine
  Nitrogen mustard
  Thalidomide

Chemicals

Carbon monoxide
Mercury
Oil of chenopodium
Tobacco
Gold

Lead
Arsenic
Analine dyes
Alcohol

Aminoglycosides

Aminoglycosides in current clinical use for parenteral therapy include streptomycin, kanamycin, gentamicin, tobramycin, and amikacin. Neomycin's nephrotoxicity limits its use to topical application, oral treatment of hepatic coma, and

presurgical bowel preparation. The aminoglycosides must be administered paren-
terally to achieve adequate serum levels; they have a half-life of about 2 hr in the
presence of normal renal functon. They are rapidly excreted by glomerular filtration,
and urine concentration may approximate 100 times the serum levels if kidney
function is unimpaired. Aminoglycosides are removed by hemodialysis and partially
removed by peritoneal dialysis, necessitating close monitoring of serum concentrations in dialysis patients if therapeutic levels are to be maintained and toxic levels
avoided. Streptomycin, gentamicin, and tobramycin have been primarily implicated
in vestibular toxicity, and kanamycin and amikacin are primarily cochleotoxic.
Advanced age and concurrent use of "loop" diuretics potentiate the toxic effects of
the aminoglycosides. Because the margin between effective therapeutic levels and
those which are potentially toxic is small, careful monitoring of peak serum levels
(30 min after intravenous administration) and trough levels (immediately before
administration of the next dose) must be carried out. In patients with renal impairment, drug dosage is adjusted to compensate for the deficiency in elimination.
If levels are carefully maintained, studies have shown that aminoglycoside-induced
auditory toxicity and nephrotoxicity occur independently of each other. In addition
to decreased renal function, factors which may predispose to ototoxicity include
preexisting hearing loss, a history of noise exposure, coexisting otologic infection,
age, duration of therapy, prior use of aminoglycosides, and concomitant use of
other ototoxic drugs (including other aminoglycosides and loop diuretics, e.g.,
ethacrynic acid or furosemide). In an excellent prospective study of the comparative
otoxicity of gentamicin and tobramycin, Fee found that gentamicin was more toxic
than tobramycin, demonstrating significantly more vestibulotoxicity. Other significant associations with tobramycin toxicity were high body temperature, total dose,
and low hematocrit. On the other hand, gentamicin toxic effects appeared to be
potentiated by high hematocrit, high creatinine clearance, criticalness of illness,
and duration of therapy beyond 10 days. Despite their well-known potential for
toxicity, the aminoglycosides are often the drugs of choice in treating serious
infections caused by aerobic gram-negative bacilli.

Although the precise mechanism of aminoglycoside ototoxicity is unclear, it is
known that cochlear damage usually proceeds from the basilar turn toward the apical
coil. Also characteristic is initial destruction of the inner row of outer hair cells
with gradual progression to involve the outer two rows, inner hair cells being spared
except in cases of overwhelming toxicity. Additionally, Fee noted that histopathologic evidence of injury has been noted in the stria vascularis, suprastrial spiral
ligament, pericapillary tissues in the spiral prominence, the outet sulcus, and
Reissner's membrane. He further noted that any pathophysiological explanation
of the ototoxic effects of the aminoglycosides must account for recovery from
ototoxic hearing impairment which has been noted in some patients. The vestibulotoxic effects of the aminoglycosides are less well understood, although type
I hair cells of the crista ampullaris are more sensitive to damage by streptomycin,
kanamycin, and gentamicin than the type II cells.

Aminoglycosides are not uncommonly used during the neonatal period for treatment of sepsis, and it has been generally thought that the neonate is less vulnerable to the toxic effects of these drugs based on the absence of statistically significant hearing test abnormalities and, in some studies, the presence of normal postrotatory vestibular responses. The presence of normal renal function in most neonates together with the absence of other coexistent factors known to potentiate aminoglycoside ototoxicity have been invoked as explanations for this phenomenon. Eviatar and Eviatar, however, have conducted a controlled prospective study of infants treated with aminoglycosides for neonatal sepsis testing the infants and controls (premature infants) for acquisition of head control and vestibular nystagmus induced by position change, prerotatory stimulation via torsion swing, and caloric irrigation of the external ear canals. Nearly 10% of treated infants had multiple vestibular abnormalities and delay in acquiring head control, suggesting some degree of vestibulotoxicity. The most significant delays occurred in the gentamicin-treated group rather than those treated with kanamycin. Treated children were also noted to be at greater risk for static encephalopathy later in life. The study reconfirmed the impression that a combination of ototoxic drugs may have a greater vestibulotoxic effect than when used alone and that prolonged use (25 to 45 days) increases the risk.

Quinine and Chloroquine Ototoxicity

In conjunction with the widespread use of quinine as an antimalarial agent, observations were made regarding its ototoxic potential. Although the ototoxic effects appear to be temporary in all but a few extremely sensitive adults, the developing embryo was noted to be extremely vulnerable. In countries with endemic malaria, mothers receiving quinine during pregnancy gave birth to infants with varying degrees of severe to profound hearing impairment. Animal studies of the ototoxic effects of quinine revealed degenerative changes in the organ of Corti, cochlear neurons, and stria vascularis.

Chloroquine, a synthetic antimalarial agent, has been used as an alternative to quinine. Unfortunately, both retinopathy and ototoxicity have been noted when pregnant mothers have taken the drug in doses above recommended levels or over prolonged periods.

Salicylate Ototoxicity

Salicyclates, most often ingested in the form of aspirin (acetylsalicylic acid), has been noted to produce hearing loss, tinnitus, and occasionally vertigo when taken in high therapeutic doses. The reversibility of these effects has caused tinnitus, in particular, to be used as a useful biologic indicator of dosage levels in patients such as rheumatics who require prolonged therapy. Clinical studies have shown tinnitus and hearing loss to occur as salicyclate concentration in plasma approached 35 mg%, and the audiometric patterns are cochlear as opposed to retrocochlear in configuration. The apparent association of aspirin ingestion in young febrile children with the occurrence of Reye's syndrome has decreased the use of this over-the-counter drug in the absence of strict indications.

"Loop" Diuretics

The introduction of powerful diuretics, e.g., ethacrynic acid, which promote the rapid excretion of large amounts of iso-osmotic urine, led to initial clinical observations of their transient ototoxic effects. Clinical reports have pointed out the potential permanent ototoxic effects of these drugs, particularly when used in association with apparently safe levels of aminoglycoside antibiotics. Animal studies have confirmed the ototoxic potential of these diuretic agents, with histopathologic studies revealing changes in the stria vascularis and significant hair cell loss. Care should be taken when using these drugs in conjunction with aminoglycosides in the presence of compromised renal function so that dosage levels of both these valuable therapeutic agents are adjusted downward appropriately.

When using potentially ototoxic drugs, serial audiograms and, if possible, determinations of vestibular function should be employed during the therapeutic course to achieve early detection of deleterious effects.

Viral Infections, Toxoplasmosis, and Syphilis

A number of viruses have been implicated as causative agents for hearing loss, both congenital and acquired. Although only cytomegalovirus has been isolated from the human labyrinth, seroconversion studies and virus isolation from urine and nasopharyngeal secretions have led to an association of labyrinthitis with rubella, rubeola, mumps influenza, varicella-zoster, Epstein-Barr, poliomyelitis variola, adeno- and parainfluenza viruses. Mumps was traditionally the most common etiology of acquired profound unilateral sensorineural hearing loss during childhood. The advent of effective vaccines for rubella, rubeola, and mumps will hopefully decrease their importance in the etiology of childhood hearing loss, but an understanding of the pathophysiology of these infections in the temporal bone may help in understanding the response of this complex neurosensory organ to infection and insult.

Temporal bone histopathologic studies of labyrinthine disease resulting from prenatal rubella, mumps, rubeola, and cytomegalovirus (CMV) have revealed evidence of an endolymphatic labyrinthitis with pathologic changes limited to the cochlear duct, saccule, and utricle. This would be consistent with a blood-borne spread of infection most likely via vessels of the stria vascularis. On the other hand, measles, mumps, and CMV may also present with a meningoencephalitis permitting direct spread along meningeal and neural structures into the perilymphatic spaces of the labyrinth. Inflammatory changes in the perilymphatic space noted in histopathologic study of these temporal bones may give way to later fibrosis. Bordley and Kapur, studying temporal bones of patients in India who suffered acute small-pox, varicella (chicken pox), or measles, found the most severe pathologic changes in the middle ears, although two cases with measles showed histopathologic evidence of endolabyrinthitis similar to that found in cases of congenital rubella deafness. More detailed discussions of prenatal labyrinthine infections follow.

Additional animal studies are needed to augment the elegant studies carried out by Davis and Johnson which demonstrated selective vulnerability of inner ear structures to specific viruses. Working with newborn hamsters, they demonstrated that influenza virus infected mesenchymal cells in the perilymphatic system, and mumps virus infected principally endolymphatic structures. Rubeola and vaccinia viruses were found to infect both perilymphatic and endolymphatic cells, whereas herpes simplex involvement was essentially limited to the sensory cells of the labyrinth.

Congenital CMV Infection

Congenital CMV infection, diagnosed by isolating the virus from neonates, is the most common cause of intrauterine infection in man, occurring in approximately 1% of all live births. An additional 4 to 10% of infants apparently acquire the infection during and after birth through such sources as cervical virus shedding, virus in breast milk, and blood transfusions. It is estimated that during pregnancy 1.5 to 6% of women have subclinical CMV infections; lower socioeconomic groups, particularly in developing countries, experience the highest prevalence rates. Of the affected infants, 5% demonstrate typical cytomegalic inclusion disease (another 5% demonstrate atypical clinical involvement) characterized by involvement of the central nervous system and reticuloendothelial system, with hepatosplenomegaly, petechiae, and jaundice being common presenting complaints. Microcephaly, in-trauterine growth retardation and prematurity also characterize the population, which may experience a mortality rate as high as 30%. As many as 90% of children with true cytomegalic inclusion disease will develop severe mental and perceptual deficits by 2 years of age, including severe to profound sensorineural hearing impairment and such ocular abnormalities as chorioretinitis and optic atrophy in 25 to 30% of cases.

The remaining 90% of infants infected with CMV demonstrate subclinical in-fection which may become apparent months to years after birth. Although their prognosis for life with normal neurologic development is better, approximately 10 to 17% will develop significant sensorineural hearing loss, ranging from mild to profound. Overall, about 3,000 infants will become severely handicapped annually with typical or atypical forms of cytomegalic inclusion disease, and another 3,000 subclinically infected infants will suffer from significant hearing and mental deficits. Sensorineural hearing loss is the most common irreversible sequela of congenital CMV infection, with an estimated 30% incidence in symptomatic cases and 13% in asymptomatic infants with congenital infection. With the decrease in cases of congenital rubella infection attendant to the widespread use of the vaccine, congenital CMV infection may constitute the major cause of nonhereditary congenital sensorineural deafness. Whereas rubella occurs in epidemic cycles, CMV infection extracts an annually recurring toll on the newborn population.

Congenital CMV infection differs from rubella and toxoplasmosis in that the virus can be transmitted *in utero* in the course of both primary maternal infection and infection resulting from reactivation of the latent virus in immune women. The chance that her baby will have a harmful congenital CMV infection is decreased in the mother with recurrent infection, being approximately one-ninth as great as after primary infection. Stagno found that 52% of babies born after a primary infection during gestation demonstrated congenital infection, whereas this was true of only 6% of babies born after recurrent maternal infections. Hardy found that the gestational age of the fetus is the most important factor determining the extent and long-range consequences of congenital viral infections, but the time of greatest susceptibility for CMV is not known. Regardless of the nature of the infection, CMV is usually found in the affected infant's nasopharyngeal secretions and urine from which it may be isolated for months after birth. Viral culture is the most reliable method for documenting CMV infection, although less expensive serologic methods have been used in some longitudinal studies where seroconversion could be demonstrated.

Histopathologic study of temporal bones of infants dying of cytomegalic inclusion disease revealed characteristic cells with inclusion bodies in the superficial cells of the stria vascularis, Reissner's membrane, the limbus spiralis, saccule, utricle, and semicircular canals. Although no inclusion-bearing cells were present in the organ of Corti, cristae, or ganglia, endolymphatic hydrops was noted to be present in at least a portion of each cochlear duct.

Congenital Rubella

Although rubella, as a disease entity, was first reported in the literature as early as 1752 by de Bergen, the teratogenic effects of the virus following maternal prenatal rubella infection were not recognized until Gregg's report on the Australian epidemic of 1941. Swan and co-workers amplified Gregg's description of the Australian epidemic and were the first to report deafness as a component of the rubella syndrome. Clinical reports prior to 1963, emanating from around the world, showed wide divergence in the estimates of the incidence of fetal damage following first-trimester maternal rubella ranging from 15.9 to 59%. This wide variation is best explained by the inability of the investigators, without laboratory confirmation of disease, to include in their studies the subclinical case of rubella in the mother and the minimally affected rubella child who did not demonstrate the classic clinical triad of congenital cataracts, deafness, and congenital heart defects. Isolation of the rubella myxovirus in 1962 and the subsequent development of serologic techniques for confirmation of rubella infection in both mother and fetus provided the investigators studying the 1963–1965 epidemic with the tools to achieve a new magnitude of specificity in their multidisciplinary investigation of the prenatal rubella victims and their offspring. The availability of the vaccine has led to widespread vaccination of children in the United States with a marked diminution of the usual cyclic epidemics of the disease. Many women of childbearing age are still susceptible, however, and the potential for prenatal rubella in this population persists.

The availability of virologic and serologic documentation of rubella infection in expectant mothers and later in infants has caused investigators to describe rubella-related disorders in addition to the classic triad. Included in the *expanded rubella syndrome* are:

Deafness	Thrombocytopenia
Eye defects	Radiolucencies in long bones
Congenital heart defects	Interstitial pneumonitis
Microcephaly	Encephalitis
Mental and/or motor retardation	Low birth weight
Hepatosplenomegaly during newborn period	

By using paired sera samples taken from mothers in concurrent perinatal research projects during the 1963–1965 epidemic, researchers were able to carry out a prospective study of prenatal rubella which took all cases—clinical and subclinical—into account. In a series of 165 laboratory-documented cases of prenatal rubella studied at Johns Hopkins, 81 (49%) presented typical clinical findings and 84 (51%) were of a subclinical type. The importance of second- and even third-trimester infection in the mother became evident, with offspring of mothers with documented second-trimester rubella manifesting cataracts, deafness, microcephaly, and mental–motor retardation. Infants with only one or two components of the classic rubella triad were clearly demonstrated to be victims of congenital rubella infection, a particularly imporant finding in cases where deafness or retardation occurred as isolated defects. The systematic use of laboratory studies in rubella infants revealed that prolonged virus shedding was most often observed in infants who failed to thrive. The majority of viral excreters were progeny of mothers who experienced first-trimester rubella.

Rubella infants revealed a consistent pattern of low birth weight and a general miniaturization of the fetal organs at autopsy. These organs were noted to be hypocellular, a finding thought to result from the cytopathic action of the virus coupled with a tendency for mitotic inhibition and an increased rate of chromosomal breaks leading to subsequent death of affected daughter cells. Even in the presence of intracellular virus, morphologic differentiation of certain cells appears to proceed unaffected. Whether the physiological integrity of a particular infected cell is maintained during and after differentiation remains unclear. Certain highly specialized cells such as the fiber cells in the lens of the eye appear to become more susceptible to the effects of the intracellular virus as the cells become more specialized, and thus a gradual progression in cataract formation has been noted during the postnatal period. The application of much of the knowledge which has been gained concerning the action of the rubella virus at the cellular level to an understanding of the pathogenesis of congenital rubella deafness must await more widespread application of the techniques of cellular biology in the study of the cells of the scala media.

Of 165 laboratory-proved congenital rubella cases in the Johns Hopkins series reported by Brookhouser and Bordley, those from whom excreted virus was cultured demonstrated a 56.6% incidence of hearing impairment, whereas the group in whom only serologic confirmation of the infection was obtained showed a slightly lower failure rate of 41.5%. Although all major reports confirmed the first trimester as the period during which maternal rubella takes the highest toll of the infant's hearing, 8 of 20 infants in the Johns Hopkins report who were offspring of mothers with second-trimester rubella revealed abnormal hearing tests results (Table 2.4-4). The importance of viral and serologic studies in confirming the diagnosis of rubella was reiterated by a 30% hearing test failure rate in infants with no associated maternal history of clinical rubella but with positive laboratory results indicating a subclinical infection. Hearing loss as the only defect was present in 36 infants with positive laboratory studies, but the usual picture combined hearing loss with one or more additional features of the expanded rubella syndrome. Hearing loss was the single most commonly found deficit in the congenital rubella population.

Brookhouser and Bordley also reported that the pattern of hearing loss found in the Johns Hopkins and Baylor rubella study populations may be summarized as follows:

1. The hearing loss was sensorineural in character with mild conductive component in a few cases.

2. The severity of hearing loss varied greatly from patient to patient and to a lesser degree between the ears of the same patient.

3. Some patients showed no response at any frequency in either ear.

4. Other patients responded to most frequencies but with a distinct asymmetry in performance between ears.

TABLE 2.4-4. *Maternal history: Hearing test results*

Rubella history	Viral positive		Serology positive	
	Passed	Failed	Passed	Failed
First-trimester rubella	3	14	14	22
Second-trimester rubella	2	1	10	7
Third-trimester rubella			4	4
No history of clinical rubella	8	2	51	23

5. Audiograms most frequently associated with rubella showed a "belly-type" or "cookie-bite" curve with greatest loss in the middle frequencies between 500 and 2,000 Hz.

6. Serial audiograms of rubella infants demonstrated nearly a 25% incidence of progressive decrease in auditory acuity.

The histopathologic changes observed in temporal bones taken from patients with documented congenital rubella included cochleosaccular changes of the Scheibe type. No changes were noted in the utricle, semicircular canals, or spiral ganglia. A fairly uniform finding was partial collapse of Reissner's membrane with adherence of the membrane to the stria vascularis and organ of Corti (Fig. 2.4-5). The tectorial membrane was found to be rolled up and lying in the internal sulcus in a number of sections. Collapse of the saccule was observed in the majority of the bones studied, and in some sections the membrane was found to be collapsed and adherent to the macula sacculi, suggestive of a recent acute inflammatory process. Although few changes were noted in the organ of Corti per se, the stria vascularis was found to be smaller than normal, lacking the usual number of capillaries, and in some cases containing significant areas of cystic dilatation at the junction of Reissner's membrane and the spiral ligament associated with a pulling away of the stria and Reissner's membrane from their attachments (Fig. 2.4-6).

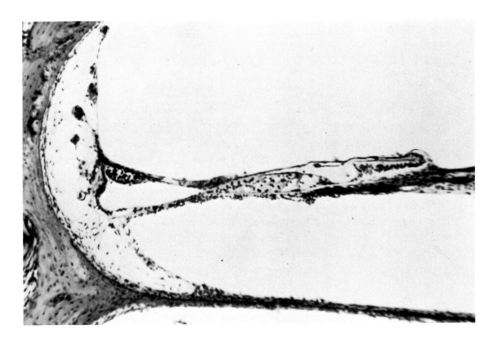

Fig. 2.4-5.   Collapse of cochlear duct in congenital rubella deafness. (Adapted from Bordley, J. E., (Editor): *Arch. Otol.*, 98:217–276, 1973.)

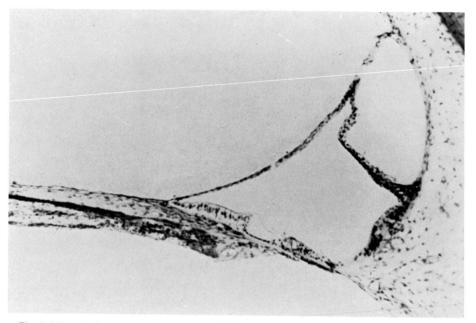

Fig. 2.4-6. Cystic changes in the stria vascularis in congenital rubella deafness. (Adapted from Bordley, J. E., (Editor): *Arch. Otol.*, 98:217–276, 1973.)

Toxoplasmosis

Toxoplasma gondii, a protozoan parasite for which cats are the only natural hosts, represents the third major agent capable of producing intrauterine infection of the fetus leading to congenital hearing loss. The incidence of congenital toxoplasmosis is approximately 1 per 1,000 to 3,000 live births in the United States with the most likely routes of infection of the mother being exposure to infected kittens or consumption of meat containing otocysts taken from infected secondary hosts. As with rubella, only primary infection of the mother poses a threat to the fetus, as maternal immunity protects against intrauterine spread, and the most injurious effects to the fetus occur following first- or second-trimester maternal infection. Ninety percent of cases of congenital toxoplasmosis are subclinical, and the two recognized forms of the disease are the more common neurologically dominant type and a disseminated variant with multiple organ system involvement. If the disease is clinically evident at birth, involving such problems as chorioretinitis, hydrocephalus, and generalized intracranial calcifications, prognosis for normal development is poor. Because of the similarity of presenting signs and symptoms, toxoplasmosis must be differentiated from congenital CMV infection by laboratory means. Subclinical toxoplasmosis carries a much worse prognosis than congenital CMV infection with a high potential for decreasing visual acuity, central nervous system disease with deteriorating intellectual function, deafness, and precocious puberty.

Congenital Syphilis

Congenital syphilis results from transplacental transmission of *Treponema pallidum* to the fetus. In some cases, stigmata and symptoms (e.g., deafness, interstitial keratitis, Hutchinson's teeth, and nasal septal perforation) may be present early in life, but approximately 50% of cases first manifest between 25 and 35 years of age. To promote early case finding, many states require serologic tests for syphilis on cord blood at the time of delivery. The most definitive laboratory determination for patients whose first symptoms appear later in life is the fluorescent *Treponema* antibody absorption test (FTA-ABS), with less than 5% false-negative results. The slightly more specific *Treponema pallidum* immobilization (TPI) test may be used to confirm questionable cases. Sensorineural hearing loss, often a flat audiometric curve, is found in nearly 30 to 40% of cases of congenital syphilis. Speech discrimination is usually worse than one would expect from the pure tone audiometric configuration. If middle ear structures are involved by the disease, a conductive component may also be present. Physical examination of the ear may be normal, but positive results of a fistula test (i.e., brief application of positive and negative pressure in a closed external canal resulting in vertigo and often nystagmus in the presence of a labyrinthine fistula) may be observed (Hennebert's sign). Beginning suddenly in the young child, syphilitic deafness is usually severe to profound, with bilaterally symmetrical involvement being the rule. In contrast to deafness following other types of labyrinthitis or meningitis, accompanying vestibular dysfunction may be minimal to absent. Syphilitic sensorineural hearing loss in adults is usually abrupt in onset but tends to be less severe, more asymmetrical, and more likely to be accompanied by vestibular complaints than is true in the pediatric population.

Temporal bone histopathology in these cases reveals an obliterative endarteritis and ostetitis of the otic capsule giving rise to a secondary labyrinthitis. Degeneration of the cochlear and vestibular end-organs coexisting with endolymphatic hydrops is usually observed.

The mainstay of treatment is, of course, high doses of parenteral penicillin (erythromycin or tetracycline in penicillin-allergic patients). The most recent recommendations regarding minimum dosage and treatment schedules should be in the literature (e.g., publications of the Communicable Disease Center) because some disagreement has arisen regarding the time period during which therapy should be continued. The discovery that treponemes may lie in a semidormant state (multiplying only once in 60 to 90 days) suggests the need for longer-term treatment schedules than previously recommended. In addition to adequate antimicrobial treatment, systemically administered steroids have demonstrated effectiveness in stablizing and/or improving hearing in about 50% of patients with syphilitic deafness. Discrimination scores for speech generally show more improvement than pure tone thresholds, and a maintenence dose of steroids sufficiently low to avoid adverse side effects is achievable in most responsive cases.

Other Neonatal Illness, Particularly Sepsis and Jaundice

The very fact that an infant is at sufficiently high risk to be hospitalized in a neonatal intensive care unit (NICU) puts him/her at risk for hearing impairment. Systematic evaluation of NICU graduates by such objective measures as auditory brainstem response (ABR) testing has revealed an increased incidence of deafness and dysmaturity of the auditory system when compared with results obtained from normal newborns (see Section 5 in this chapter). These infants have a higher incidence of neonatal otitis media and sepsis, often requiring therapy with potentially ototoxic drugs, than a similar population of normal newborns. They are also more likely to be premature, to have sustained neonatal stress, anoxia, and low Apgar scores, and finally to have such complicating problems as jaundice secondary to maternal/infant blood group incompatibility.

A relationship between neonatal kernicterus and sensorineural hearing loss has been appreciated for some decades. Improved perinatal care has decreased the incidence of problems owing to Rh factor incompatibility, but kernicterus resulting from incompatibilities involving the ABO and other groups is still observed. At present, about 0.5 to 1.5% of a population of children with sensorineural hearing loss might be expected to have a history of kernicterus. Most of these children would be expected to have a high frequency loss with poor to moderately impaired discrimination for speech. The coexistence of kernicterus and anoxia in a high-risk neonatal population presents a challenge in sorting out which of the two factors plays the principal etiologic role as far as hearing loss is concerned. As with anoxia, histopathologic study of the brains and temporal bones of deaf children with kernicterus shows the middle and inner ears to be normal, with lesions limited to the central nervous system. Higher levels of the central auditory pathway may show some degree of involvement, but the ventrocochlear nucleus generally reveals the greatest amount of cellular injury.

Growth Retardation: Premature and Full-Term Low Birth Weight

Although such factors as birth stress, sepsis, and kernicterus are often associated with prematurity and dysmaturity, low birth weight of and by itself should be ascertained when searching for the etiology of deafness in the young child. Children with a history of prematurity may represent 10% to as many as 23% of the total population of deaf children. Premature infants are 20 times more likely to be deaf than children of normal birth weight and gestation, with as many as 2% of all infants with birth weight less than 3 pounds manifesting significant degrees of sensorineural hearing loss. In addition to varying degrees of sensorineural impairment, premature infants are far more likely to suffer from additional handicaps with consequent implications for their aural habilitation.

Recurrent Otitis Media and Mastoid Disease

Recurrent otitis media and mastoid disease, which most often result in conductive hearing impairment, are discussed at length in Section 3 of this chapter. Studies by Paparella and others, however, indicate that patients with a history of chronic and/or recurrent otitis media were significantly more likely to have a coexisting sensorineural hearing impairment than would be expected based on general incidence figures. Whether this association results from penetration of the labyrinthine windows (particularly the round window membrane) by infectious elements or toxins, topical medications with ototoxic potential, or a combination thereof is unclear at this time.

Childhood Illnesses: Meningitis and Sudden Hearing Loss

Meningitis

Documented association of childhood hearing loss with prenatal infections and such viral disorders as measles and mumps was discussed above. Another increasingly important cause of hearing impairment in young children is meningitis.

Meningitis, as an etiology of postnatally acquired sensorineural hearing impairment, accounts for approximately 5 to 7% of childhood cases observed in clinical practice. Epidemiologic studies have shown an increasing number of cases, at least partially accounted for by the emergence of resistant strains of *Hemophilus influenzae*. As many as 3% of children with the disease demonstrate bilateral sensorineural hearing loss as a sequela, with an additional 8% suffering from unilateral impairment. The loss may be progressive, and some reports suggest that it may not manifest until some weeks after the acute meningitic episode has resolved. Reports of cases in which postmeningitic hearing levels appeared to improve over time have not been sufficiently well designed to eliminate the potentially confounding variable posed by a coexisting middle ear effusion, perhaps related to the onset of the meningitis. In general, false hope for improvement of a postmeningitic sensorineural impairment should not be fostered in parents by the physician, for often this only delays their acceptance of the child's disability.

Several large studies have examined clinical histories of childhood meningitis victims searching for predictors of hearing loss among such factors as etiologic agent, pretreatment course, type of antimicrobial administered, cerebrospinal fluid (CSF) findings, and coexisting neurologic sequelae. The author and co-workers performed auditory brainstem evoked response testing on 101 children under 2 years of age following an episode of bacterial meningitis:

Hearing	No. of patients
Normal	42
Abnormal	
Conductive	19
Sensorineural	15
Mixed	9
Retrocochlear	16

These results support the assertion that a significant percentage of children who have recovered from bacterial meningitis demonstrate peripheral hearing loss (conductive and/or sensorineural). Although 16% presented patterns consistent with neural maturational delays, suggesting more central involvement, the implications of this finding are uncertain. Among clinical parameters examined, e.g., CSF findings (glucose, proteins, type of organism, cell count, and differential), CSF glucose was found to be significantly lower for children with abnormal ABRs. As the magnitude of hearing loss increased, CSF glucose tended to decrease. Children with bilateral hearing loss had lower CSF glucose than children with either unilateral losses or normal hearing bilaterally. Postmeningitic deafness is usually accompanied by a marked decrease in vestibular function. Unable to orient himself/herself under water, the child with a hypoactive vestibular system may be at greater risk for drowning, and so preventive measures should be taken.

Histopathologic studies of temporal bones from patients with postmeningitic hearing loss confirm multiple pathways (nerves, vessels, and ductal connections between the inner ear and CSF) through which organisms can invade the inner ear. The resulting labyrinthitic infection results in massive destruction of the cochlea and related structures, leading to replacement by fibrous tissue and often by ossification. Postmeningitic ossification of the labyrinth can lead to a radiographic picture similar to that of Michel's deformity (i.e., agenesis of the inner ear).

Sudden Hearing Loss

Sudden onset of hearing loss is a common complaint and may reflect etiologies as simple as impacted cerumen in the ear canal and middle ear effusion or as complex as an acoustic neurinoma. Acoustic trauma and exposure to ototoxic drugs and chemicals are commonly identified precedents to a sudden sensorineural hearing loss. As a specific entity described in the otolaryngologic literature, however, sudden sensorineural hearing loss most commonly refers to a sudden decrease in hearing sensitivity in a patient's ear which has been previously free of otologic disease. Spontaneous sudden cochlear hearing loss (usually unilateral) may be mild, moderate, or severe in degree and may be associated with complaints of tinnitus and/or vertigo. The patient, particularly a young child, may not be consciously aware of a hearing loss but may complain of an "echo" or hollow sound in the ear or a buzzing sensation. Older children and adults may describe hearing loss, tinnitus, and vertigo more specifically, or they may be bothered by a numb sensation in the ear often accompanied by itching or a mildly painful sensation in the ear.

Because sudden hearing loss is not a life-threatening complication, few temporal bones of affected patients have been available for study in the period immediately following onset of the symptom. Speculation as to etiology has ranged the gamut from viral infection, vascular spasm or obstruction, endocrine disease, allergy, and lipid metabolism disorders to, more recently, rupture of labyrinthine membranes within the labyrinth and at the interface with the middle ear (i.e., oval and round windows).

Fistulas of the round window membrane and the oval window ligament around the stapes footplate have been documented at surgery, most often in cases with a history of barotrauma or physical exertion (e.g., scuba diving or snorkeling, weight lifting, excessive straining with coughing, or other physiological maneuvers accompanied by Valsalva maneuver). Hydrodynamic forces in the carotid arterial system and the intracranial venous sinuses directly influence CSF pressure gradient fluctuations within the subarachnoid space (Fig. 2.4-7). Explanations for the propensity of some individuals to suffer labyrinthine membrane rupture during maneuvers safely accomplished by others have invoked increased size and patency of the cochlear aqueduct connecting the perilymph with the CSF. Infant cochlear aqueducts are half as long and relatively wider than those seen in adult temporal bones; Goodhill has postulated that this infantile anatomy may persist in certain adolescents and adults, increasing their vulnerability to damage from sudden CSF pressure changes. This pathway would permit transmission of an explosive force from the CSF to the labyrinth, leading in some cases to rupture of the round window, stapes ligament, or intralabyrinthine membranes.

It is quite possible that the observed association of sudden sensorineural hearing loss with upper respiratory infections, accompanied by sneezing, coughing, and/or nose blowing, may involve spontaneous labyrinthine membrane ruptures in certain cases. Goodhill further pointed out that the implosive route, from sudden Valsalva forces, involves a sudden increase in tubotympanic pressure, with rupture of the round window membrane and/or oval window ligament as sequelae. There may be a reverse chain reaction with disruption of internal labyrinthine membranes (basilar and Reissner's), resulting in hearing loss, vertigo, and tinnitus. Patients with a suspected fistula should be scheduled for a prompt surgical exploration of the middle ear, and reinforcing tissue grafts (e.g., fat or perichondrium) should be available for placement as a seal over the fistula.

If the patient's history is not suggestive of a labyrinthine membrane rupture, other etiologies must be considered. The mumps virus has long been etiologically implicated in cases of sudden unilateral severe cochlear hearing loss which occurs in a small percentage of children and in some adults with epidemic parotitis. As outlined in the section on viral hearing loss, histopathologic findings suggest a mechanism of viremia with the cochlear stria vascularis as the portal of entry. In

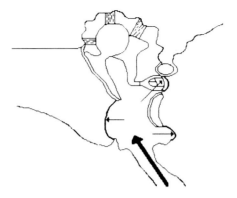

Intratympanic Pressure Increased By Barotrauma

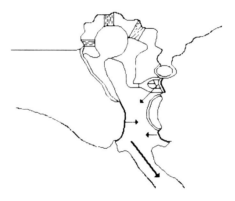

Intratympanic Pressure Decreased By Eustachian Tube Obstr uction

Fig. 2.4-7. Mechanism for labyrinthine window rupture. (Redrawn from Goodhill, V.: *Ear Diseases, Deafness and Dizziness,* P. 671. Harper & Row, Hagerstown, 1979.)

view of evidence that other viruses produce sudden deafness, the absence of a positive titer in each patient does not detract from the possibility that the mumps virus is responsible for a substantial percentage of all cases of sudden deafness. Histopathologic examination of a number of the available temporal bones from patients who died soon after sustaining sudden onset of sensorineural hearing loss revealed changes compatible with viral endolabyrinthitis described after rubella, mumps, and measles.

Appropriate laboratory determinations may document the presence of hyperlipidemia, diabetes mellitus, toxic drug levels, allergy, and endocrine causes. The FTA-ABS is the most widely recommended laboratory determination to rule out congenital syphilis which may present with hearing loss as a symptom in children and adults. The diagnosis of lymphocytic meningitis may require a diagnostic spinal tap.

In addition to the laboratory determinations described above, evaluation of a patient presenting with a sudden sensorineural hearing loss must, of course, include a complete otologic history stressing such factors as ear infections, ear surgery, familial hearing, and ototoxic drug exposure, as well as a history of trauma and exposure to hazardous noise levels. A history of barotrauma (diving, snorkeling, scuba diving, or aircraft flight) should be specifically sought, and any relationship of hearing loss onset to physical stress factors such as lifting, coughing, sneezing, and straining at urination or defecation should be carefully noted. A complete otoneurologic/audiologic examination should include otoscopy, standard audiologic tests, special site of lesion auditory test battery, tympanometry, stapedius reflex, vestibular studies, cranial nerve and basic neurologic examination, as well as screening Schüller and Stenver radiographic views of the petrous bone. If a cochlear anomaly is suspected, computerized imaging of the temporal bone may be indicated.

Usually, otoscopic examination reveals normal tympanic membranes, and audiologic findings show moderate, severe, or total sensorineural hearing loss (SNHL). In a large study of sudden deafness, Sheehy classified his patients into four groups: low-tone, flat, high-tone, and total hearing loss. A flat type of hearing loss was found in 41 percent of his patients. Studies of the natural history of this disease revealed that approximately one-third of patients have a return of normal hearing, one-third are left with a moderate to severe loss (40 to 80 dB), and one-third have total loss of useful hearing. Spontaneous recovery to normal hearing is more likely to occur if the deafness is not associated with severe vertigo and if the deafness is not total initially.

Empiric therapeutic regimens for those cases not associated with fistulas have included, in addition to bed rest, various pharmacologic agents deemed helpful in overcoming the supposed microvascular spasm in the cochlea. Histamine phosphate and nicotinic acid have been popular therapies in adults, but there is no documented evidence of their pharmacologic effectiveness in increasing cochlear blood flow, and potential side effects would, in the author's opinion, make their use unacceptable in children. In an elegant series of experiments assessing the effects of various agents on cochlear blood flow, Snow demonstrated that inhalation of carbon dioxide did, in fact, produce dilatation of cochlear blood vessels and increase flow, but the author is unaware of any reports of its use with pediatric populations.

A rational approach to the management of children with sudden SNHL should include a high index of suspicion of labyrinthine membrane rupture and viral etiologies, as well as a careful search for associated systemic disease processes such as congenital syphilis, diabetes, and hyperlipidemia. Surgical exploration of the middle ear should be carried out if labyrinthine membrane tears are suspected and appropriate medical therapy for underlying systemic disorders initiated. The risk/benefit relationship in the pediatric age group for the other empiric therapies described in the literature for adult patients would seem sufficiently unfavorable to preclude their use with children.

Sound Trauma to the Ear: Acoustic Trauma and Noise

A relationship between hearing loss, usually accompanied by tinnitus, and occupational noise exposure has been appreciated for a long time as reflected by such epithets as "boilermaker's" deafness. Hearing loss resulting from acoustic trauma and prolonged noise exposure cannot be effectively reversed, but it can be prevented or minimized by taking appropriate precautions.

Acoustic Trauma

Acoustic trauma is a term used to describe the type of hearing insult represented by acute exposure to high-intensity noise often accompanied by an explosive or percussive blast. Depending on the severity of the insult, the tympanic membrane may rupture, in some cases providing at least some sound attenuation and protection for the sensitive structures of the inner ear. If the drum remains intact, the severity of the resultant sensorineural hearing loss may vary from mild frequency-limited losses to total absence of measurable hearing. It is postulated that mechanical damage to the organ of Corti results from excessive vibratory energy and is initially most noticeable in the outer hair cells of the basal turn of the cochlea near the oval window. This would correspond to the 8- to 10-mm region of the basilar membrane, which represents the 4,000-Hz pitch area. Vasoconstriction undoubtedly plays a part in the pathophysiology of the injury, leading to loss of hair cells and support structures secondary to prolonged hypoxia. Generalized cellular swelling and pyknosis of hair cell nuclei have been observed in experimental animals immediately after exposure to high-intensity sound. Such damage may progress to massive destruction of the cochlear structures with rupture of the endolymphatic system in the face of prolonged exposure to high-intensity sound. No changes are ordinarily found in the bones, ligaments, nerves, blood vessels, stria vascularis, spiral ligament, limbus, or basilar membrane.

The mechanism of cochlear injury resulting from a blow to the head is substantially similar to that sustained from exposure to an explosion. The explosion produced waves of vibratory energy transmitted through the ear canal, tympanic membrane, and ossicular chain to the labyrinthine system. In the case of head trauma, inertia delays movement of the ossicular chain relative to movement of the skull in response to a blow. As the skull is set in motion by a blow to the right side of the head, for example, the left temporal bone moves more rapidly than the ossicular chain, effectively driving the stapes into the vestibule, whereas on the left side the skull movement results in an outward pull on the stapes away from the oval window. Interestingly, the resultant hearing loss on the contralateral side is generally more severe than on the side ipsilateral to the trauma.

Chronic Noise Exposure

In experimental animals exposed daily to levels of noise ranging from 105 to 110 dB sound pressure level (SPL) for variable periods of up to 2 years, histologic changes observed were essentially similar to those described previously for lesser degrees of acute acoustic trauma. Progressive destruction of outer hair cells, followed by inner hair cells and supporting cells, and ending with nerve fiber and spiral ganglion degeneration has been observed.

It is thought that the 4-kHz area of Corti's organ is most sensitive to damage because of the tendency for a particular segment of basilar membrane to vibrate in response not only to the frequency to which it is most sensitive but also with vibratory energy representing lower tones as well.

Intensity and Time

Factors determining the degree of damage, if any, sustained by a human ear exposed to loud sounds over an extended period of time may be categorized as intensity of the sound, duration of the average exposure episode, and recurrence rate of episodes of exposure. Most data collected concerning noise hazards relates to adults and exposure in the work place. The Occupational Safety and Health Administration (OSHA) has issued guidelines regarding damage risk criteria for noise exposure developed in conjunction with otolaryngologists and audiologists. Equivalent "doses" of loud sounds (80 dB and greater in intensity) have been computed in relation to time of exposure. Because the decibel scale is logarithmic, the "rule of fives" applies, so that as the intensity of sound increases by 5 dB above 80 dB the exposure time must be halved to maintain sound dose equivalency. Representative examples are:

Weighted sound level (dB)	Duration (hr)
80	32
90	8
110	0.5
120	0.063

The relative hazard posed by even recurrent short-duration exposure to high-intensity sound should be apparent. Some reports have suggested that the ears of infants and children may have a different degree of susceptibility to noise damage than those of adults, but this impression is not supported by conclusive data. Because no universal program of hearing testing and conservation has been implemented for children, the incidence of noise-induced permanent hearing loss in this population is unknown. As Mills noted in his excellent review of the literature regarding noise and children, noise-induced hearing loss in children should be of more than academic interest. Many sound sources with which infants and children come in contact, often on a daily basis, have noise levels which are capable of producing an acoustic injury to the adult ear and temporary, chronic, or permanent hearing losses. Common devices with high noise levels to which children are commonly exposed include firecrackers, power mowers and trimmers, snow blowers, motorcycles, snowmobiles, model airplane engines, and firearms, both toy and real (Fig. 2.4-8). The risk posed to children's hearing by exposure to rock music amplified to high-intensity levels (either in person through large speakers or through stereo earphones) has been given a considerable amount of media attention. Some surveys of adolescents reveal a higher incidence of typical 4-kHz "noise notch" hearing losses than was true during past decades. There is also some evidence that noise exposure and certain ototoxic drugs, e.g., kanamycin, may act synergistically to damage hair cells.

Initially, a period of exposure to potentially hazardous levels of noise produces the ear equivalent of system fatigue resulting in a temporary threshold shift (TTS), often accompanied by tinnitus, meaning that auditory acuity for certain sounds will be decreased temporarily. If the noise exposure continues and adequate precautions are not taken to protect the ears, as well as to limit the duration and frequency of exposure, a permanent decrease in auditory acuity may result. The initial loss is usually in the region of 4,000 Hz, but the damage may progress to involve higher and lower frequencies as exposure continues. A subjective awareness of tinnitus in the young child may be difficult for him to express but should not be ignored. Once

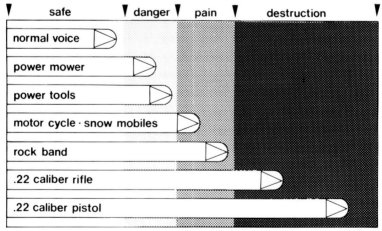

Thought about your hearing lately?

Listening to loud sounds may cause a loss of hearing. Damage to your hearing, in many cases, is permanent.

Exposure to loud, explosive noises can cause either immediate or gradual hearing loss. Less abrupt, less intense sounds can also damage your hearing, but it happens more slowly. Many of the day-to-day sounds in our lives are more dangerous than one might realize. Even listening to music at high sound levels can damage your hearing. The following chart illustrates the degree of stress some sounds impose upon your hearing.

Fig. 2.4-8. Hearing conservation poster for adolescents. (Adapted from Boys Town National Institute brochure.)

other otologic disease has been ruled out, the possibility of noise exposure in the child's environment should be explored and the parents made aware of potential noise hazards. A hefty dose of prevention is the best answer to the increasing levels of noise exposure in the child's environment. If they are made aware of the hazards, provided with ear plugs, and instructed in their use, most children comply. Although different levels of susceptibility to noise damage appear to exist among individuals, there are no reliable test instruments to identify those most at risk. High-frequency audiometric testing and recording of cochlear emissions are promising research pathways now being explored for their predictive value.

"Knocked-Out": Physical Trauma to Ear and Skull

Traumatic Tympanic Membrane Perforation

Trauma to the tympanic membrane and middle ear structures can result from such diverse etiologies as a slap in the ear, a foreign body (e.g., cotton swab) inserted too deeply, impact of the ear against water while diving, and in conjunction with skull trauma as discussed below. As a general rule, the infant's ear is more prone to damage from foreign bodies than the adult's because of its foreshortened canal, whereas other sources of trauma are more common with increasing age. The older child should be able to describe the traumatic incident and a constellation of symptoms including acute pain, often bloody discharge from the ear, hearing loss, tinnitus, and possibly vertigo. On visual inspection, the examiner may find blood clots and debris in the canal which should be carefully removed aseptically to allow adequate inspection of the tympanic membrane. The size and location of any resultant tympanic membrane perforation should be noted as well as the status of the edges of the tear. If substantial portions of the tympanic membrane have been reflected into the middle ear, it may weigh on the otologist's decision regarding management of the injury. The ear should be kept dry with sterile cotton inserted into the external meatus until audiologic evaluation can be carried out.

The most commonly observed audiometric pattern is a mild to moderate conductive hearing loss, occasionally accompanied by a high-frequency sensorineural component reflecting acoustic trauma sustained by the labyrinthine structures. Greater degrees of conductive loss suggest possible damage to the ossicular chain, and a more substantial sensorineural component should raise suspicions of possible labyrinthine membrane ruptures including fistulas of the round window and annular ligament around the stapes. The use of evoked-response audiologic techniques may be necessary if behavioral thresholds cannot be obtained. Impedance audiometry should not be used in the face of recent traumatic perforation of the tympanic membrane for fear of further damaging the middle ear and labyrinthine structures.

The uncomplicated traumatic performation will heal, over a period of several weeks, with surprisingly little residual scarring. If the ear has not been contaminated by foreign material, e.g., dirt, sand, or water, the ear should be kept dry and the patient followed expectantly. Significant foreign body contamination may require cleaning of the ear under anesthesia and the use of prophylactic antibiotic coverage. Large perforations, those in which severe infolding of the drum edges has occurred, and those accompanied by ossicular damage or a suspected labyrinthine fistula are best managed by otosurgical intervention. Usually the flaps of the torn tympanic membrane are reflected back to anatomic position and held in place with an absorbable packing material (e.g., Gelfoam). Severe ossicular damage may require ossicular repositioning techniques or the use of ossicular homografts to effect repair. Repair of labyrinthine fistulas requires the use of autografts such as fat from the ear lobule or perichondrium from the tragus. The sensorineural component of the loss is usually permanent in character, and some progression may be seen over time if the trauma has been severe.

Temporal Bone Fractures

Head trauma, particularly as related to motor vehicle accidents, constitutes a major health concern of children and adolescents. The addition of motorized cycles, such as mopeds and mini-bikes, to the usual array of pedal-driven cycles and skateboards available to youngsters increases the risk of injury, particularly head trauma. Safety helmets for children are receiving renewed emphasis as protective devices to be worn even when riding nonmotorized vehicles.

Serious head injury, of course, can pose a threat to life, and neurosurgical concerns regarding possible intracranial injury must take precedence over otologic considerations. On the other hand, bloody otorrhea had long been stressed as a cardinal sign of basilar skull fracture, and its presence should alert emergency physicians to the possible coexistence of specific damage to the contents of the temporal bone.

Although fracture lines can assume many possible axes with relation to such skull base features as the petrous pyramids, temporal bone fractures are broadly classified into those which are longitudinal and those which are transverse with respect to the long axis of the petrous portion of the temporal bone. Longitudinal fractures account for 70 to 90% of temporal bone fractures and are usually caused by blows to the temporal or parietal areas rather than to the occipital or frontal regions. The fracture usually begins in the squamous portion of the temporal bone, coursing along the posterosuperior external bony canal wall, often causing noticeable separation and displacement, before it runs across the roof of the tympanic cavity along the carotid canal in front of the bony labyrinth to end in the middle cranial fossa (Fig. 2.4-9). The course of this fracture is most likely to disrupt the skin of the external ear canal, the posterior superior portion of the tympanic membrane, and the ossicular chain, specifically the incudomalleal and incudostapedial articulations by displacing the incus from its fossa. Bleeding from the ear after head injury is the most common presenting sign, ususally accompanied by hearing loss, which should lead to a careful examination of the external ear canal.

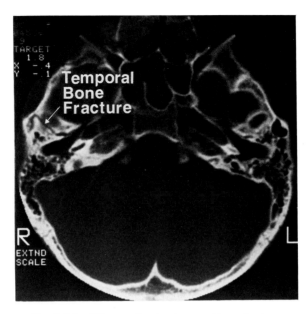

Fig. 2.4-9. CT scan showing temporal bone fracture.

Once the patient's general condition permits, careful aseptic technique should be used to clean debris from the canal sufficiently to allow assessment of the damage to the underlying canal, tympanic membrane, and ossicular chain. Bleeding may be significant in some cases, and concurrent CSF leakage can occur as a result of dural tears along the fracture line. Because longitudinal fractures usually spare the inner ear structures, conductive hearing loss (bone conduction better than air conduction) is most often demonstrated by tuning fork tests and audiologic evaluation. Concussion injury to the structures of the inner ear may occur from any blow to the head with or without skull fracture and may result in a coexistent sensorineural component with the conductive hearing loss usually observed in longitudinal fracture cases. Although the facial nerve in its bony fallopian canal courses near the posterior superior portion of the bony canal, reports of large series of temporal bone fractures indicate only a 20 to 25% incidence of facial nerve injuries. Symptoms of vestibular system injury are much less common in patients with longitudinal fractures than is apparent with transverse fractures. Bilateral temporal bone fractures can occur, and this possibility should not be overlooked.

Fractures which have a transverse course with relation to the long axis of the petrous pyramid account for approximately 20% of temporal bone fractures. This type of fracture usually begins in the posterior cranial fossa near the foramen magnum, extending transversely across the petrous pyramid through the labyrinthine system and/or the contents of the internal auditory canal to the middle cranial fossa. Traumatic interruption of the labyrinthine capsule may result in functional destruction of the vestibular system and the cochlea along with damage to the closely associated facial nerve.

Signs and symptoms associated with transverse temporal bone fractures include vertigo with associated spontaneous nystagmus, hearing loss (primarily sensorineural rather than conductive), facial paralysis in approximately 50% of cases, and hemotympanum without rupture of the tympanic membrane. Because the tympanic membrane is not ruptured, bloody otorrhea is less likely to be present, although fractures involving the temporomandibular joint/anterior bony canal wall may produce blood in the canal in the presence of an intact ear drum.

Because the patient with a suspected temporal bone fracture is often evaluated after a period of unconsciousness or intensive care for intracranial injury, a thorough history is important. Temporal bone fractures are notoriously difficult to see on routine radiographic views of the temporal bone and may even be missed with polytomographic or CT imaging techniques. The inability to demonstrate such a fracture radiographically should not decrease the examiner's index of suspicion. The patient should be questioned and evaluated for nystagmus, facial palsy, and objective hearing loss including careful audiometric tests. Collections of blood and fluid in the middle ear may superimpose a conductive hearing loss on an underlying sensorineural impairment in cases of transverse fracture. CSF otorrhea may be seen in either variant of fracture, and the possible existence of such a leak should lead to the administration of appropriate systemic antibiotic prophylaxis. Surgical repair of middle ear damage is not an urgent necessity and often a period of careful observation while the middle ear clears itself of fluid and debris is indicated before a final surgical treatment strategy is defined.

In cases of suspected or confirmed temporal bone fracture the otolaryngologist should be consulted early in the course of the patient's management. A good rule for the primary care physician to follow in the interim is to place sterile cotton in the external auditory canal, avoid putting any eardrops or foreign substance into the ear canal, and administer an appropriate systemic antibiotic prophylactically. The otolaryngologist should clean the ear aseptically, utilizing the otosurgical microscope in most cases, before deciding the appropriate audiologic testing to be undertaken. It may be desirable, for example, to forego any acoustic impedance testing for fear of displacing a damaged ossicular chain or reopening a CSF leak. Paralysis of the facial nerve should be carefully assessed and followed by the otolaryngologist utilizing electrodiagnostic testing procedures. In cases where the facial nerve innervation to the periorbital musculature and the lacrimatory system has been interrupted, special care must be directed toward avoiding damage to the cornea. Spontaneous recovery of facial function is more common after longitudinal fractures than those of the transverse type and in most cases begin to occur within the first 5 days. If recovery is not evident after 6 weeks, there probably will never be a complete functional return; tics, spasms, mass movements, and synkinesis are common late sequelae. Corticosteroid and surgical decompression are indicated in some cases of facial nerve injury depending on the degree of damage as documented by electrodiagnostic testing.

An obvious break in the posterior superior bony canal wall is frequently observed and is the presenting sign of a longitudinal temporal bone fracture. This fracture line can be seen running from its extension into the middle ear near the notch of Rivinius obliquely, posteriorly, and laterally on the canal wall.

Middle ear pathologic findings resulting from closed head injuries may be conveniently divided into the following categories: (a) incudostapedial joint separations; (b) marked dislocation of the incus; (c) fracture of the stapedial arch; (d) fracture of the malleus; and (e) hyperostosis and concomitant disease.

Selected Reading

Ballenger, J. J. (1985): *Diseases of the Nose, Throat, Ear, Head and Neck.* Lea & Febiger, Philadelphia.

Bieber, F. R. and Nance, W. E. (1979): Hereditary hearing loss. In: *Clinical Genetics: A Sourcebook for Physicians.* Wiley, New York.

Bluestone, C. D., and Stool, S. E., editors (1983): *Pediatric Otolaryngology.* Saunders, Philadelphia.

Bordley, J. E., editor (1973): The effect of viral infection on hearing: A state-of-the-art report with special emphasis on congenital rubella. *Arch. Otol.*, 98:217–276.

Bordley, J. E., Brookhouser, P. E., and Worthington, E. L. (1972): Viral infections and hearing: A critical review of the literature, 1969–1970. *Laryngoscope*, 82:557–577.

Bordley, J. E, and Kapur, Y. P. (1972): The histopathological changes in the temporal bone resulting from acute smallpox and chickenpox infection. *Laryngoscope*, 82(8):1477–1479.

Borkowski, W., Goldgar, D., Gorga, M., Brookhouser, P. E., and Worthington, D. A. (1985): CSF parameters and auditory brainstem responses following meningitis. *Pediatr. Neurol.*, 1:134–139.

Boughman, J. A., and Shaver, K. A. (1982): Genetic aspects of deafness: Understanding the counseling process. *Am. Ann. Deaf.*, 393–400.

Boughman, J. A., Shaver, K. A., and Nance, W. E. (1981): Responsibilities in genetic counseling for the deaf. *Am. J. Hum. Genet.*, 32:72A.

Brookhouser, P. E. (1979): Early recognition of childhood hearing impairment. *Ear Nose Throat J.*, 58:288–292.

Brookhouser, P. E., and Bordley, J. E. (1973): Congenital rubella deafness. *Arch. Otolaryngol.*, 98:252–257.

Brookhouser, P. E., and Bordley, J. E., editors (1980): Childhood communication disorders: Present status and future priorities. *Ann. Otol. Rhinol. Laryngol.* [*Suppl. 74*], 89:1–184.

Brookhouser, P. E., Hixson, P. K., and Matkin, N. D. (1979): Early childhood language delay: The otolaryngologist's perspective. *Laryngoscope*, 89:1898–1913.

Compere, W. E., and Valvassori, G. E. (1964): *Radiographic Atlas of the Temporal Bone.* H. M. Smyth, St. Paul, Minnesota.

Davis, L. E., and Johnson, R. T. (1976): Experimental viral infections of the inner ear. I. Acute infections of the newborn hamster labyrinth. *Lab. Invest.*, 34(4):349–356.

Eviatar, L., and Eviatar, A. (1981): Aminoglycoside ototoxicity in the neonatal period: Possible etiologic factor in delayed postural control. *Otolaryngol. Head Neck Surg.*, 89:818–821.

Eviatar, L., and Eviatar, A. (1982): Development of head control and vestibular responses in infants treated with aminoglycosides. *Dev. Med. Child Neurol.*, 24:372–379.

Fee, W. E. (1980): Aminoglycoside ototoxicity in the human. *Laryngoscope*, 90 (Suppl.):24:1–19.

Fraser, G. R. (1976): *The Causes of Profound Deafness in Childhood.* Johns Hopkins University Press, Baltimore.

Goodhill, V. (1979): *Ear Diseases, Deafness and Dizziness,* Harper & Row, Hagerstown, Maryland.

Hardy, J. (1973): Fetal consequences of maternal viral infections in pregnancy. *Arch. Otolaryngol.*, 98:218–227.

Harper, P. S. (1981): *Practical Genetic Counseling.* John Wright, Bristol.

Hemenway, W. G., and Bergstrom, L. B. (1971): Forward to symposium on congenital deafness. *Otolaryngol. Clin. North Am.*, 4:221.

Konigsmark, B. W., and Gorlin, T. J. (1976): Genetics and deafness. In: *Genetic and Metabolic Deafness.* Saunders, Philadelphia.

Levin, L. S., and Knight, C. H. (1980): Genetic and environmental hearing loss: Syndromic and nonsyndromic. *Birth Defects,* 16(7).

Matkin, N. D. (1979): The audiologic examination of young children at risk. *Ear Nose Throat J.,* 58:297–302.

Mills, J. H. (1975): Noise and children: A review of the literature. *J. Acoust. Soc. Am.,* 58(4):767–779.

Mouney, D. F. (1979): Differential diagnosis of hearing loss in children. *Ear Nose Throat J.,* 58:293–296.

Paparella, M. M., and Shumrick, D. A., editors (1980): *The Ear,* Vol. II. Saunders, Philadelphia.

Pinsky, L. (1979): Penetrance and variability of major malformation syndromes associated with deafness. *Birth Defects,* 15:207–226.

Quick, C. A. (1980): Chemic and drug effects on the inner ear. *Otolaryngology, Vol. II: The Ear,* edited by M. M. Paparella, and D. A. Shumrick, pp. 1804–1827. Saunders, Philadelphia.

Schuknecht, H. F. (1974): *Pathology of the Ear.* Harvard University Press, Cambridge.

Sheehy, J. L. (1960): Vasodilator therapy in sensory-neural hearing loss. *Laryngoscope,* 70:885–914.

Smith, D. W. (1982): *Recognizable Patterns of Human Malformation.* Saunders, Philadelphia.

Snow, J. B., (1977): Vasodilators of the inner ear. In: Shambaugh, G. E., and Shea, J. J., editors: *Proceedings of the Shambaugh Fifth International Workshop on Middle Ear Microsurgery and Fluctuant Hearing Loss,* edited by G. E. Shambaugh, and J. J. Shea, pp. 406–411. Strode Publishing Co. Birmingham, Alabama.

Stagno, S., Pass, R. F., Dworsky, M. E., Henderson, R. E., Moore, E. G., Walton, P. D., and Alford, C. A. (1982): Congenital cytomegalovirus infection: The relative importance of primary and recurrent maternal infection. *N. Engl. J. Med.,* 306(16):945–949.

Thompson, J. S., and Thompson, M. W. (1980): *Genetics in Medicine.* Saunders, Philadelphia.

Worthington, E. L. (1973): *Handbook of Ototoxic Agents, 1966–1971.* Johns Hopkins University Press, Baltimore.

The Ear

Section 5: Measurement of Hearing

Behavioral Audiologic Testing 151
  Behavioral Observation Audiometry 151
  Visual Reinforcement Audiometry 153
  Conditioned Play Audiometry 153
  Tangible Reinforcement Operant Conditioning Audiometry 154
Auditory Discrimination 155
Audiogram Interpretation 156
Objective Measures of Auditory Function 159
Auditory Evoked Potentials 160
  Use of ABR in the Intensive Care Nursery 162
  Use of ABR in Postmeningitic Children 163
  Use of ABR in Children with Other Problems 164
Acoustic Immittance Measurements 164
  Tympanometry 165
  Acoustic Reflexes 167
Importance of Early Identification 169
Philosophy of Hearing Aid Selection 169
Preschool Counseling 170
Educational Options for the Hearing-Impaired Child 172
  Major Questions to Ask a Parent 173

Hearing is essential for the normal development of speech and language. It is evident that the child who does not hear the spoken word will not acquire normal receptive or expressive language. In fact, impairment of hearing poses a serious handicap to the child's entire psychosocial development. Alleviation of the handicap or minimizing its effect is best begun at the earliest possible age, and ideally within the first year of life. Obviously, this requires early identification, diagnosis, and habilitation. Unfortunately, hearing impairments in children frequently are not detected until the child is 2 to 3 years of age.

In a study of 150 students from a state residential school for the deaf, the average age at the time of identification was found to be 30 months; however, the trend with regard to the age of suspicion and confirmation of the hearing loss was encouraging. That is, the difference between the age of initial suspicion and subsequent confirmation was shorter for the younger age groups than for the older age groups. This still represents a delay of approximately 8 to 10 months during a critical developmental period. Possible reasons for this delay are:

1. Parents delay in contacting professionals.
2. Parents are apprehensive about wanting to know the truth.
3. Parents do not know whom to contact for professional consultation.
4. Family physicians and/or pediatricians do not recognize the problem and therefore do not make the necessary referrals.

This chapter reviews the essential ingredients of a pediatric audiologic evaluation. Evaluation of cooperative adults and older children involves a behavioral response, e.g., pushing a button or holding up a finger, to signify that they have heard an auditory stimulus. The inability or unwillingness of infants and young children to voluntarily cooperate in the evaluation requires utilization of different strategies. Technologic advances and the clinical utilization of known behavioral, auditory testing techniques can be combined into a pediatric test battery sufficiently powerful to dispel two outdated philosophies espoused by some health care specialists: (a) wait and see, the child will outgrow the problem; and (b) the child is too young to be tested. Reliable behavioral and electrophysiological techniques for obtaining valid auditory thresholds with infants under 1 year of age are available and should be used as an integral part of the diagnosis and treatment of ear disorders in children.

In general, more, not less, testing should be undertaken with children than with adults. If an adult experienced a hearing loss, otolaryngologists and audiologists would complete extensive testing to determine not only the degree of impairment but also the site of the lesion in the auditory system. Yet when a child is suspected of having a hearing loss, some professionals use gross screening measures (e.g., hand-clapping, noisemakers, loud speech) to assess hearing sensitivity. Use of these high-intensity, broad-frequency spectrum sounds serve only to rule out a severe-to-profound hearing loss, thereby missing less severe, but developmentally significant, degrees of impairment.

Basic measures which should be included in a pediatric audiologic test battery include:

1. Comprehensive case history
2. Measures of middle ear function (acoustic immittance)
3. Measures of auditory sensitivity
   a. Pure tone thresholds
      (1) Air conduction
      (2) Bone conduction

b. Speech awareness/reception thresholds
c. Electrophysiological measures (auditory brainstem response, etc.)
4. Measures of auditory discrimination
a. Speech
(1) In quiet
(2) In competition
b. Non-speech signals

Equally as important as the measures listed above are the specific clinical techniques used to obtain them. These are summarized below.

BEHAVIORAL AUDIOLOGIC TESTING

To evaluate the auditory sensitivity of infants and young children, an understanding of early childhood development is essential. Considerable time and research has been expended in pinpointing the normal developmental milestones in the areas of motor, intellectual, language, social, and emotional development. The normal developmental stages of auditory behavior are not as well known or recognized. Furthermore, most of the developmental work on auditory skills has been done by disciplines other than audiology, otolaryngology, or pediatrics.

Behavioral Observation Audiometry

In order to evaluate an infant, one must understand the sequence of normal development and recognize the type of response that is age-appropriate and the stimulus most likely to elicit a response. The primary behavioral test methodology for use with most infants less than 6 months of age is behavioral observation audiometry (BOA), which does not require conditioned or voluntary behavior on the part of the infant. With this technique, a variety of test signals are presented and the minimal sound intensity at which behavioral changes are observed is determined (e.g., Moro response, alerting, scanning, aural–palpebral reflex, cessation of activity, increase in activity, flexion or extension of limbs, grimacing, change in sucking, change in breathing pattern). These responses primarily are reflexive in nature, are dependent on the physiological state of the child at the time of the stimulus presentation, and can be quite subtle. As a result, well-trained observers working in teams are needed to evaluate the very young infant.

When using BOA, even a trained observer can rule out only severe and profound losses, as relatively high sound intensities are required to elicit unconditioned responses even in normal-hearing infants. Untrained observers may become confused by what they consider to be inconsistent responses. Initially, the child may respond appropriately but soon ceases to exhibit stimulus-related behavioral changes. This rapid habituation of an unconditioned response is normal behavior for this age and is unrelated to the level of auditory sensitivity. Although noisemakers have been advocated by some as a suitable sound stimulus for screening infants' hearing, results obtained by this method should be interpreted with caution. The frequency spectrum of these stimuli are not usually as narrow as identified by the accompanying specifications. In addition, the intensity (loudness) can vary considerably depending on the distance from the subject, the method of test administration, and the noise-maker used. These errors can result in underestimating the degree of hearing loss and/or completely misdiagnosing a high-frequency loss.

More controlled stimuli can be presented via a loudspeaker through a calibrated system, but all behavioral observation techniques with neonates are, at best, gross measures of their responsiveness to sound. The response observed is reflexive in nature, and if the infant fails to respond one can only say that he does not respond; it cannot necessarily be inferred that he does not hear.

With increasing age, a normal child generally becomes more responsive to all stimuli, including sound. Responses, which are in part learned behavior, can be observed to a wider variety of sound stimuli presented at lower intensities. Infants and toddlers usually respond best to familiar sounds, with their ability to localize sound also undergoing developmental changes. At 3 to 4 months, there is usually a rudimentary head turn toward a sound. By 4 to 7 months, children turn their heads from side to side in a horizontal plane, and by 13 to 16 months they turn to a sound source that is located directly to either side, below or above. By 21 to 34 months, they can localize a sound signal coming from any angle. A similar but more rapid course of development occurs in response to sound intensity (loudness). The human voice provides the best stimulus for eliciting both a quick response and a response at lower intensity levels. The human voice or speech, however, is a complex signal with a broad frequency spectrum which provides little information about auditory sensitivity at specific frequencies.

When testing a child from birth to approximately 6 months of age several points must be remembered:

1. The spectrum of the stimuli being used to elicit a response must be selected carefully.

2. Intensity of the stimulus must be recorded.

3. Stimuli must be presented outside the visual field.

4. Stimuli should be presented in an ascending approach and should be varied frequently because of the rapid habituation of response.

5. Multiple stimuli must be available.

6. Caution must be exercised to ensure that the child does not respond to a vibrotactile stimulus when auditory stimuli are being presented.

With children older than 6 months, one can generally employ behavioral operant conditioning techniques so long as the task to be performed is within the cognitive and motor developmental levels of the child. A hierarchy of conditioning tasks should be included in the pediatric audiologic battery including, at a minimum, visual reinforcement audiometry, conditioned play audiometry, and tangible reinforcement operant conditioned audiometry.

All of these methods can be used to assess auditory sensitivity (air conduction and bone conduction), speech reception thresholds, and speech discrimination abilities. In addition, they can be used for testing under earphones, in sound field (in cases where the child will not accept earphones), and/or with hearing aids.

Visual Reinforcement Audiometry

Visual reinforcement audiometry (VRA), as used clinically for assessing auditory sensitivity, involves visual reinforcement (with flashing lights, toys, etc.) of a child's head-turn response toward a sound source which can be varied in frequency and intensity to obtain threshold measures. Infants turn their heads reflexively toward a novel auditory stimulus, and the use of visual reinforcement takes advantage of the baby's heightened visual awareness. As initially described, the procedure required the child to turn correctly to one of several sound sources before being reinforced. This approach causes confusion with an infant who cannot localize the source of a sound either because of developmental factors or a hearing loss. In such cases, a child can be conditioned to respond to sound without demonstrating precise localization. If he turns to the same location regardless of the sound source, the baby's behavior should be reinforced because the goal of any task used in behavioral audiometry is to measure a consistent response to sound, the exact nature of that response being of secondary importance. The application of VRA to the assessment of hearing sensitivity in infants and young children has increased since the mid-1970s, and it is the principal technique presently being utilized for the evaluation of young children.

Systematic variation of stimulus and reinforcement parameters has revealed that infants as young as 5 months (developmental age) can be tested by reinforcing localization behavior using complex visual stimuli (moving toy and flashing lights). Thresholds obtained for infants are very close to those obtained for adults, and the range of thresholds for a normal population of presumed normal-hearing infants is small. Thus VRA offers both a valid and reliable means of assessing auditory sensitivity in young children particularly as they approach 1 year developmentally. Either broad-band or frequency-specific auditory stimuli can be employed to obtain a more accurate estimate of the degree and slope of a hearing loss. Because many infants initially may not accept earphones, it may be necessary to present stimuli in a sound field with loudspeakers so that responses reflect only the sensitivity of the better-hearing ear, possibly causing one to miss a unilateral hearing loss.

Conditioned Play Audiometry

In conditioned play audiometry (CPA), a conditioned bond is established between the presentation of an auditory stimulus and some play activity (e.g., putting rings on a peg, blocks in a bucket, marbles in a container, or pegs in a peg board). The play activity and social interaction during the test phase serve as the reinforcement. So that learning is not a factor in test performance, the reinforcing activity should already be within the infant's behavioral repertoire. Motor activity such as grasping, moving, placing, and releasing requires a higher level of coordination than simply hitting a large object. Observation of a child's motoric skills before beginning testing should help the examiner select an appropriate task that is reinforcing to the child from the variety of play activities which should be available. Too often audiologic test results read, "could not test, could not condition." More accurately, they should state, "Could not test, clinician too rigid." Although some children do condition easily to any task, failure to condition could result from selection of an inappropriate task. CPA is of limited usefulness for children under the age of 24 months and for older children with significant developmental delays. Like VRA, CPA can be used in conjunction with any frequency-specific stimulus, including sound field testing if the child refuses to wear earphones.

With CPA, the social reinforcement provided by the examiner may be of more interest to the child than the actual play activity, and determination of the amount of social reinforcement to provide comes with experience. The clinician must recognize when a specific play task is no longer of interest to the child and quickly change to another appropriate task without a break in the test session and without the need for laborious reconditioning. With the proper task selection and motivation, CPA can be used to obtain a wide variety of data in a short amount of time.

Tangible Reinforcement Operant Conditioning Audiometry

With tangible reinforcement operant conditioning audiometry (TROCA) a conditioned bond is established between the auditory stimulus and motoric act, e.g., button pressing. The actual reinforcement is a tangible item which may be edible (e.g., candy, sugar-coated cereal, crackers) or nonedible (e.g., stickers, tokens, toys). As with CPA, the tangible reinforcement must be selected carefully so that it is a positive reinforcer to the child. Not all children like sugar-coated cereal or "M & M" candy, and satiety may play a role in limiting the test session. With TROCA, presentation of sound stimuli of decreasing intensity is the most effective strategy; a potential drawback is the complexity and cost of the equipment required for best results. To lessen the cost the clinician can dispense the tangible item by hand, although a mechanical dispenser is preferable.

TROCA has proved particularly useful for testing older mentally retarded children, hyperactive children, and other difficult-to-test patients who have a short attention span. It is not used clinically as frequently as BOA, VRA, and CPA, but inclusion of TROCA in the pediatric audiologic test battery provides a powerful alternate conditioning technique with appropriate patients if the child tires of the play task before all necessary test data have been obtained. The success rate with TROCA is highest when used with children over 30 months of age, but the clinician must be aware of signs of satiation, e.g., an increase in response latency, a decrease in response strengths, or a sudden lack of interest in the reinforcer. When this occurs, there should be a change in the task or the reinforcer.

AUDITORY DISCRIMINATION

The preceding section described the use of behavioral techniques in the auditory evaluation of infants and children, particularly the measurement of sensitivity to broad-band or frequency-specific signals as a means of determining the degree and configuration of any hearing loss. It also is important to determine a child's ability to discriminate between sounds, and the identical behavioral techniques (VRA, CPA, and TROCA) can be used to obtain measures of auditory discrimination. Too frequently, clinicians or technicians believe that all necessary information for predicting a child's ability to use his residual hearing is provided by the basic pure-tone audiogram; experienced clinicians realize that more information is required. Children with identical pure-tone audiograms function very differently, suggesting the need for more extensive testing, including some measures of functional discrimination ability, to determine how well the child uses his residual hearing.

Material for assessing auditory discrimination must be within the child's receptive vocabulary to avoid confusing a receptive language deficit with a deficit in auditory discrimination ability. A hierarchy of discrimination measures must be included in the test battery, ranging from open-set vocabulary word lists to closed-set response tasks using pictures or objects (Table 2.5-1). For children with extremely limited discrimination abilities, simple syllable recognition or nonspeech recognition materials may be needed.

Mindful of the need to assess not only auditory sensitivity but the child's ability to process information presented at suprathreshold levels, one should be aware that existing test instruments available to clinicians are limited. There is a need to further standardize and refine an auditory discrimination test battery for children so that age-dependent levels of expectation can be established. This must be based on a more thorough understanding of the limitations imposed by a particular auditory impairment and of the negative influence of hearing loss on general communicative development.

TABLE 2.5-1. *Auditory discrimination testing based on receptive vocabulary age*

RVA (years)	Test material
Over 12	Adult word lists
6 to 12	PBK-5 word lists
4 to 6	Word Intelligibility by Picture Identification (WIPI) Northwestern University Children's Perception of Speech (NU-CHIPS)
Up to 4	Selected words
	Environmental sounds
	Sound Effects Recognition Test (SERT)
	Auditory Numbers Test (ANT)
	Pediatric Speech Intelligibility Test (PSI)
Nonverbal	Phoneme limitation and differentiation

AUDIOGRAM INTERPRETATION

The ear is a delicate, intricate, amazing system that can detect sound waves so small that the tympanic membrane is moved only a distance one-tenth the diameter of a hydrogen atom. The range that is covered between the faintest audible sound and sounds intense enough to elicit pain is enormous. The latter is 10 million times as powerful as the former. In addition, the range of audible frequencies extends from 20 to 20,000 Hz. Of this range, the ear is most sensitive from 500 to 3,000 Hz, which is also the most important range for understanding speech.

To determine the magnitude and extent of an individual's hearing, measurement standards had to be established. Because the dynamic range of the ear for intensity was so large (10 million times), numbers expressed in watts or dynes per square centimeter were unmanageable. Therefore a logarithmic system was adopted to provide a range of values that were manageable. The logarithmic system (to the base 10) was named bel, in honor of Alexander Graham Bell. Subsequently, to avoid fractional values of a bel, the decibel, which is one-tenth of a bel, was employed. The term decibel (dB) is used to express the level of sound which generally is measured as an acoustic pressure by a sound level meter.

In order to establish the normal limits of hearing at different frequencies, psychophysicists measured the intensity level required for an individual with no known hearing loss to detect the presence of the signal. By testing a number of individuals with normal hearing, they were able to establish an acceptable standard for threshold sensitivity (American National Standards Institute, ANSI). Whereas the absolute intensity required to reach threshold varied as a function of frequency, the pure-tone audiometer is calibrated so that its zero reading at each frequency corresponds to the median hearing level for healthy, young adults.

It should be kept in mind that "normal hearing" is a statistical concept and represents a range of hearing rather than a single level. The zero hearing level on the dial of an audiometer represents the average threshold level of a particular segment of the general population. Because this is a statistical concept and represents a restricted sample of the population, normal hearing is considered to include minor deviations above and below the zero reference. Consequently, a person's hearing is considered normal if his threshold level does not exceed 25 dB (ANSI) at the test frequencies, as shown in Fig. 2.5-1.

The audiogram can be very valuable in assessing the severity of a person's hearing handicap. The Committee on the Conservation of Hearing of The American Academy of Otolaryngology—Head and Neck Surgery recommends dividing hearing handicaps into degrees and classes based on an individual's ability to hear everyday speech.

We have found that the categories of hearing loss associated with the degree of loss, as shown in Fig. 2.5-1, to be more representative of the difficulty a person will have in hearing speech than a single percentage disability figure. Table 2.5-2 shows a convenient way of categorizing a person's loss by degree.

Table 2.5-3 provides a guide to the educational significance of various degrees

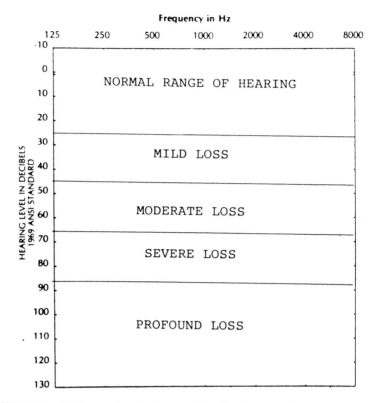

Frequency in Hz

FIG. 2.5-1. Audiogram showing degree of hearing loss as a function of intensity.

of hearing impairment and program needs. This information is a compilation from several sources. Recent research has demonstrated that children with less severe hearing loss than those indicated in Table 2.5-3 are underachieving in the regular classroom setting and should be monitored carefully. This is true especially of young children with repeated episodes of middle ear problems (otitis media).

TABLE 2.5-2. *Degree of hearing loss as a function of threshold average at 500, 1,000,and 2,000 Hz*

Degree	Threshold average (dB)
Normal	0–25
Mild	26–45
Moderate	46–65
Severe	66–85
Profound	>85

TABLE 2.5-3. *Relationship of degree of hearing impairment[a] to educational needs*

Average of the speech frequencies (500, 1,000, 2,000 Hz) in the better ear (dB)	Effect of hearing loss on the understanding of language and speech	Educational needs and programs
27–40	May have difficulty hearing faint or distant speech. May experience some difficulty with the language art subjects.	Child should be referred to special education for educational follow-up. May benefit from a hearing aid. May need attention to vocabulary development. Needs favorable seating and lighting. May need lip-reading instructions. May need speech therapy.
41–55	May not hear conversational speech at a distance of more than 3–5 feet (face to face). May miss as much as 50% of class discussions if voices are faint or not in line of vision. May exhibit limited vocabulary and speech anomalies.	Child should be referred to special education for educational follow-up. Individual hearing aid by evaluation and training in its use. Favorable seating and possible special class placement, especially for primary children. Attention to vocabulary and reading. Lip-reading instruction. Speech conservation and correction, if indicated.
56–70	Conversation must be loud to be understood. May have increased difficulty in group discussions. Is likely to have defective speech. Is likely to be deficient in language usage and comprehension. May have limited vocabulary.	Child should be referred to special education for educational follow-up. Resource teacher or special class. Special help in language skills; vocabulary development, usage, reading, writing, grammar, etc. Individual hearing aid by evaluation and auditory training. Lip-reading instruction. Speech conservation and correction. Attention to auditory and visual situations at all times.
71–90	May hear loud voices about 1 ft from the ear. May be able to identify environmental sounds. May be able to discriminate vowels but not all consonants. Speech and language defective and likely to deteriorate.	Child should be referred to special education for educational follow-up. Full-time special program for deaf children, with emphasis on all language skills, concept development, lip-reading, and speech. Program needs specialized supervision and comprehensive supporting services.

TABLE 2.5-3. *Continued*

Average of the speech frequencies (500, 1,000, 2,000 Hz) in the better ear (dB)	Effect of hearing loss on the understanding of language and speech	Educational needs and programs
91 or more	May hear some loud sounds but is aware of vibrations more than tonal pattern. Relies on vision rather than hearing as primary avenue for communication. Speech and language defective and likely to deteriorate.	Individual hearing aid by evaluation. Auditory training with individual and group aids. Part time in regular classes only as profitable. Child should be referred to special education for educational follow-up. Full time in special program for deaf children, with emphasis on all language skills, concept development, lip-reading, and speech. Program needs specialized supervision and comprehensive supporting services. Continuous appraisal of needs in regard to oral and manual communication. Auditory training with group and individual aids. Part time in regular classes only for carefully selected children.

[a] Medically irreversible conditions and those requiring prolonged medical care.

OBJECTIVE MEASURES OF AUDITORY FUNCTION

Although a behavioral test battery can effectively assess auditory function in most patients, 5 to 10% of the pediatric population require additional evaluative techniques. This figure may be higher for a clinic that specializes in multiple handicapped children.

The difficult-to-test child might include but not be limited to:

1. The neonate at risk for a hearing loss
2. The child with severe mental retardation
3. The child with significant developmental delays
4. The child with multiple handicaps, e.g., cerebral palsy
5. The autistic child
6. The child who is hyperactive or emotionally disturbed
7. The well baby from hearing-impaired parents

Behavioral evaluation techniques are fraught with problems if the child is uncooperative and/or noncommunicative. For these children, objective tests of hearing are needed. The goal of such tests is to eliminate the need for a child to provide a voluntary, behavioral response, relying instead on the measurement of physiological variables, e.g., heart rate, respiratory rate, electrodermal response, and audio-ocular responses. Individual investigators have reported success with these measures, but none have been universally accepted as an accurate estimator of auditory sensitivity.

Sound is delivered to the ear in the form of acoustic energy (sound waves). At the eardrum, the acoustic energy is transformed into mechanical energy, which is transmitted via the ossicular chain to the oval window. At the oval window the mechanical energy is transformed into hydromechanical energy as a fluid pressure wave is established in the inner ear (cochlea). This fluid pressure wave stimulates the hair cells (sensory structures within the inner ear), and the mechanical motion is converted or transformed into electrical activity (neural discharges). This neural activity is transmitted up the auditory pathway through the brainstem to the cortex, and only recently have we been able to measure it.

Neural discharges in response to auditory stimuli cannot be recorded by external electrodes regardless of the stimulus intensity or recording amplification because of their small size in comparison with the large amount of nonauditory neural and environmental electrical "noise." This problem can effectively be overcome, however, by employing a device referred to as a signal-averaging computer. The function of this instrument is to record all electrical activity from electroencephalogram (EEG)-type electrodes placed on the scalp in response to a series of acoustic stimuli. Because the auditory neural activity is essentially time-locked and all other electrical "noise" tends to occur randomly, the computer's function of adding all electrical activity following each stimulus presentation yields a result in which activity from auditory centers is amplified and all other unwanted information is diminished.

AUDITORY EVOKED POTENTIALS

Early work with auditory evoked potentials (AEPs), utilizing EEG potentials occurring about 100 to 300 msec after signal onset, revealed that these potentials were state-of-consciousness-dependent (significant degradation occurred with sleep, either natural or sedated), showed considerable variability both within and between subjects, and were poorly defined near threshold. The problems precluded use of these techniques with pediatric cases.

As mentioned previously, measurement of the electrical activity of individual auditory nerve fibers, consisting of very brief electrical pulses, can only be accomplished with an electrode in contact with the nerve fiber. Clinically, this is not feasible except during surgery, which allows access to the auditory nerve. Alternatively, if a sound is presented which causes a large number of nerve fibers to fire simultaneously, the summed voltage can be recorded by an electrode in either the ear canal or the middle ear. This measurement of responses from the auditory nerve has been termed electrocochleography (ECOG).

Initially, ECOG measurements were recorded with an electrode inserted through the eardrum (transtympanic) and placed on the promontory (bone overlying the first turn of the cochlea). This invasive recording procedure restricted its clinical utility. Placement of the electrode was critical, requiring a patient to remain motionless either voluntarily or using sedation or general anesthesia. Thus recordings were made only in medical settings with a restricted population.

During the mid to late 1970s, surface electrodes placed in contact with skin in the external auditory canal were used to record the ECOG. Although it minimizes the risk to the integrity of the eardrum or middle ear, the more distant electrode placement is not as sensitive. Electrode impedances are higher, the response amplitude is reduced, and recording artifacts are increased. Although there is excellent correlation between audiometric thresholds and whole nerve responses (ECOG) when the transtympanic recordings are used, ear canal recordings do not appear to be satisfactory for the purpose of estimating audiometric thresholds below 4,000 Hz.

Measurement of the early auditory brainstem potentials (ABR), a less invasive procedure, provides similar information in most cases. On the other hand, ECOG has been shown to provide excellent diagnostic information for localization of the size of the lesion, particularly in Meniere's disease or endolymphatic hydrops. When ECOG is combined with ABR, considerably more information can be obtained about processing within the cochlea and about pathology affecting the auditory nerve.

Attempts to utilize auditory electrophysiological responses were equally problematic until Jewett and Williston's 1971 description of an early component of the AEP in man, occurring within the first 10 msec after onset of the auditory stimulus. This response, colloquially referred to as the auditory brainstem response (ABR), has since become a cornerstone of objective audiometry for difficult-to-test patients.

In the procedure referred to as ABR, the recording electrode array consists of metallic discs placed on the top (vertex) of the head, the forehead, and the mastoid of the ear to be tested. The sound delivered to the ear is called a click and sounds like a finger-snap. The clicks are presented at various loudness levels beginning with a relatively loud level and decreasing until a response is no longer seen. The actual response that is measured represents a synchronous discharge of nerve cell populations within the cochlea and brainstem. During the testing session, which usually lasts about an hour, measurements are made of the latency (time interval from stimulus onset to peak deflection) of wave V, the largest and most consistently present wave. Plots are constructed of stimulus intensity versus wave V latency. Using normative data, threshold determinations can usually be ascertained to within 10 to 20 dB of behavioral methods, and distinctions can be made between conductive and sensorineural types of hearing loss. In addition, interwave latency information can help in detecting neuropathology that affects the auditory neural pathways through the brainstem.

The ABR has been shown to be stable both within and between subjects, whether awake, asleep, or sedated; and it reliably approximates behavioral thresholds for at least the higher frequencies. Figure 2.5-2 shows a typical ABR recorded from

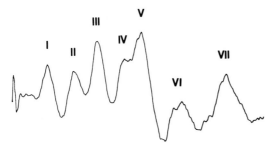

FIG. 2.5-2. Typical ABR in a child with normal hearing.

a child with normal hearing, illustrating a waveform composed of as many as seven components or waves labeled with Roman numerals.

Although precise neuroanatomic generators of the ABR have not been completely defined, current concepts are based on lesion data obtained from animal and human studies. In general, the ABR reflects the caudal-rostral progression of electrical activity in the auditory pathways of the brainstem. Wave I definitely reflects the response from primary afferent fibers in the eighth nerve. An eighth-nerve origin for wave II has also been hypothesized. Waves III and IV are thought to originate in the pons, wave V in the mid-brain, and waves VI and VII possibly arising in the thalamus. In humans several potential generators may be active at any given time; thus a combination of this electrical activity recorded at the surface of the scalp comprises the ABR. Although experimental confirmation of the putative origins appears imprecise compared with current knowledge of auditory neuroanatomy, it is sufficient for the technique to have considerable relevance as a clinical tool in audiology, otolaryngology, and neurology.

Use of ABR in the Intensive Care Nursery

Galambos and his colleagues pioneered use of the ABR for evaluation of intensive care nursery (ICN) graduates. ABR abnormalities observed in ICN survivors fall into two general categories: those presumed to reflect either neuropathy and/or neuromaturational delays and those presumed to reflect the presence of a significant hearing loss (conductive, sensorineural, or mixed). The reported incidence of abnormalities among this population has ranged from 9 to 45%, but a number of these studies did not consider variables such as the infant's physiological status, gestational age at the time of test, and artifacts introduced by background noise or electrical interference from other equipment located in the test environment.

The ABR can provide consistent and diagnostically helpful information if the evaluation is delayed until a good feeding status has been established and the high-risk neonate is ready for discharge from the ICN, free of systemic illness, and able to breathe room air without evidence of respiratory distress, apnea, or bradycardia. These precautions ensure that the infant is at least relatively stable physiologically. If possible, evaluations should be carried out in a sound-treated room utilizing a diagnostic approach to testing and interpretation of results.

TABLE 2.5-4. *Cases grouped into specific diagnostic categories on the basis of ABR results*

Category	Normal (%)	Conductive (%)	Sensori- neural (%)	Mixed (%)	Neuropathology and/or neural maturational delays (%)
Normal	64	11	1	0	2
Conductive		12	0	0	3[a]
Sensorineural			2	0	2[a]
Neuropathology and/or neural maturational delays					10[a]

[a] Includes children with hearing loss plus neuropathology.

Table 2.5-4 summarizes results collected from 225 infants referred from one ICN over a 2-year period. Sixty-four percent of the infants demonstrated normal peripheral auditory sensitivity in both ears with no evidence of neuropathology/neural maturational delays. An additional 14% appeard to have normal findings in at least one ear, and 22% showed abnormal results in both ears. Of the 16% suspected to have a bilateral hearing loss, 12% were conductive, 2% cochlear, and 2% mixed. Unilateral hearing loss was noted in 12%. If these two groups are combined, 5% of the infants showed cochlear involvement and required special follow-up including early intervention and remediation. Interestingly, approximately 25% were suspected of having a conductive hearing loss. This percentage is consistent with the reported incidence of middle ear effusion in ICN infants. The practicing clinician should be aware, however, that collapsing ear canals are not uncommon in the neonate's ear and may introduce a fictitious conductive hearing loss into test results.

The reported ABR data also indicate the presence of neuropathology and/or neural maturational delays in the auditory pathways of some ICN graduates. If the neonatal ABR is predictive of problems associated with general maturational delays, as some studies suggest, infants thus identified could be provided with early intervention to help mitigate the effects of other developmental handicaps.

Use of ABR in Postmeningitic Children

Hearing loss is known to be a serious residual impairment following meningitis in some children, but identification of hearing loss in the postmeningitic population is complicated by the relatively young age of these patients, together with the frequent coexistence of compounding neuropsychological sequelae. In spite of these problems, independent studies have demonstrated the feasibility of evaluating postmeningitic cases with the ABR and reported some rather startling findings.

Based on ABR and impedance data, approximately 47% of 101 postmeningitic patients in this series exhibit some form of hearing loss (conductive, mixed, or sensorineural). Furthermore, three-fourths of these hearing impairments were in the severe-to-profound category, and none of the cases with presumed cochlear loss in a large well-documented study showed any evidence of recovery on subsequent evaluations. These results emphasize the necessity of evaluating the hearing of any child with meningitis. Obviously, the sooner the presence of a hearing loss can be diagnosed, the higher is the probability of alleviating at least some of the subsequent psychological and educational delays.

Use of ABR in Children with Other Problems

In addition to high-risk infants and postmeningitic children, the efficacy of using the ABR as part of the audiologic test battery has been further demonstrated in evaluating:

1. Children with suspected neurologic disease or disorders
2. Unintelligible or noncommunicative children
3. Multiple-handicapped children
4. Mentally retarded children
5. Autistic children

Although the ABR is a clinically effective, objective test of auditory sensitivity, it is not a stand-alone procedure; it is most valuable in providing information about peripheral auditory sensitivity for the high-frequency region (above 1,000 Hz). The use of ABR as an isolated test of auditory function can provide a misleading impression of hearing ability with serious errors in diagnosis. For example, peripheral effects (i.e., conductive hearing loss, severe high-frequency cochlear hearing loss) must be ruled out before an abnormal ABR can be considered indicative of neuropathology affecting the auditory brainstem pathways. Likewise, the presence of concomitant central nervous system involvement may also render ABR results ambiguous when attempting to predict auditory sensitivity. The ABR can only provide information about the integrity of the brainstem auditory pathways and should not be considered a test of central auditory processing because hearing, by definition, requires processing and the actual perception of sound is a higher cortical function. The importance of behavioral evaluation and follow-up cannot be overstated, especially when dealing with young children.

ACOUSTIC IMMITTANCE MEASUREMENTS

Measurement of acoustic immittance or impedance of the middle ear was first described as a diagnostic tool by Metz in 1946, but initial acceptance of its clinical utility in the United States was slow. The advent of new electroacoustic equipment allowed a more simplified and objective measure of aural immittance so that acoustic immittance measures now are widely utilized as a clinical diagnostic tool in otologic,

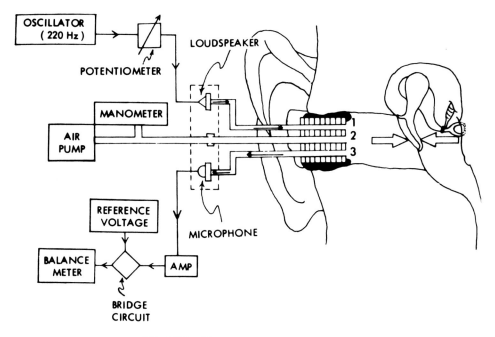

FIG. 2.5-3. Electroacoustic impedance bridge.

audiologic, and pediatric clinics. Immittance measures provide an objective means of assessing the integrity and function of the peripheral auditory mechanism.

A diagram of an electroacoustic immittance device is shown in Fig. 2.5-3. An airtight seal is obtained with a small probe which is inserted into the external auditory canal of the patient. The probe has three small holes. From one hole a 220-Hz probe tone is emitted; a second hole is an outlet for an air pressure system which is capable of creating positive, negative, or atmospheric air pressure in the cavity between the probe tip and the tympanic membrane; and the third hole leads to a pick-up microphone which measures the sound pressure level of the 220-Hz probe tone in the canal cavity. The sound pressure level of the 220-Hz tone in the external auditory canal cavity is determined by the compliance of the tympanic membrane and integrity of the middle ear system. The pick-up microphone quantifies the sound pressure level of acoustic energy that is reflected back into the external auditory canal.

Tympanometry

The most common method of assessing the compliance of the eardrum is to plot a tympanogram. The tympanogram reflects changes in eardrum compliance (measured reflected sound pressure level) as air pressure is varied in the external canal.

In effect, this graph is a pressure-compliance function showing relative changes in compliance as a function of pressure.

As the air pressure is changed from high positive ($+200$ mm H_2O) through atmosphere pressure (0 mm H_2O) to negative pressure, resulting compliance changes at the eardrum are recorded. Figure 2.5-4 shows a tympanogram for a normal eardrum and middle ear. Note that compliance is low at both high positive and high negative pressure. As pressure decreases toward zero (0 mm H_2O), compliance increases, reaching a maximum at near the zero pressure. The overall pattern is one of an inverted V.

Different otopathologic conditions tend to have their own tympanometric patterns, reflecting their effect on the status of compliance of the eardrum and middle ear. Not every pathology has its own distinct pattern, nor does a particular pattern by itself diagnose a disease. Tympanometry, however, is more objective than the otolaryngologist's eye, and the air pressures involved are small compared with those generated with a pneumatic otoscope.

Figure 2.5-5 show the five basic patterns that emerge from testing with a 220-Hz probe tone. These include the system for categorizing tympanograms suggested by Jerger. Type A corresponds with a normal tympanogram showing normal middle ear compliance and pressure. Type As shows normal middle ear pressure but suggests reduced compliance or a stiff system. This condition or pattern can occur with a stiff or thickened eardrum or reduced mobility of the ossicular chain. Hearing may be normal or can show a significant conductive loss (50 dB) with this pattern. Type Ad shows normal middle ear air pressure but increased compliance. This pattern is generally associated with a very flaccid eardrum or disarticulation of the ossicular chain. Sometimes this pattern demonstrates the presence of a single layer membrane covering an old perforation in the eardrum known as a monomeric membrane.

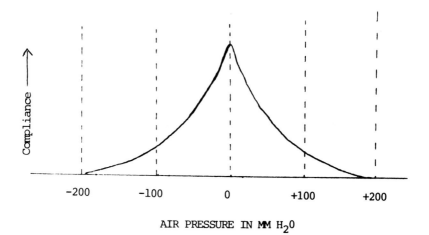

FIG. 2.5-4. Normal tympanogram.

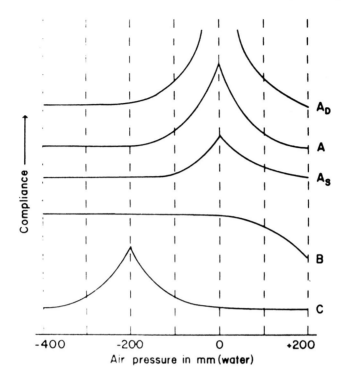

FIG. 2.5-5.   Synopsis of the Jerger tympanogram types.

Type C is the pattern observed in cases of abnormal negative middle ear pressure. This pattern denotes eustachian tube dysfunction. Although not common, middle ear fluid has been reported in cases with a type C tympanogram.

In the type B tympanogram, compliance is reduced and there is not a distinct point of maximum compliance. This tympanogram is very characteristic of middle ear fluid. However, one must be cautious, as several other conditions can result in a type B tympanogram as well. These include wax impaction in the external auditory canal, stenosis of the ear canal, perforation of the eardrum, or an open, functioning tympanostomy tube. These conditions can be distinguished on the basis of measuring the volume. If there is a hole in the drum (either from a perforation or an open PE tube), the volume will be large. If, on the other hand, there is either wax impaction or stenosis, the volume will be extremely small. Therefore whenever a type B tympanogram is obtained, a volume measurement must be made.

Acoustic Reflexes

Additional diagnostic information can be obtained by measuring the presence or absence of the acoustic reflex. This reflex is contraction of the stapedius muscle elicited by a loud sound. When the muscle contracts, it increases the stiffness of the ossicular chain, thereby decreasing compliance at the eardrum. This change in compliance results in a deflection on the meter of the electroacoustic immittance device. The diagnostic interpretation of the presence, absence, or strength of the muscle contraction is complicated and requires careful study. A detailed description of the complicating factors is not within the pervue of this volume, but it must be remembered that the inclusion of acoustic reflex measures in the immittance battery is extremely important. A positive response also indicates an intact facial nerve.

Numerous texts and articles have been written describing in detail the basic physics of sound and principles involved in immittance measures and the clinical utility of these measures. Table 2.5-5 summarizes the information which can be obtained in appropriate cases if one uses an acoustic immittance test battery consisting of (a) tympanometry, (b) static acoustic immittance (volume measures), and (c) intra-aural muscle reflexes.

Most clinicians are aware of how middle ear function (Table 2.5-5, items 1 through 6) is assessed with immittance measures; however, some clinicians underestimate or misunderstand information gained by accurately testing for the presence of the acoustic reflex. Two of the most important uses deal with items 7, 8, and 9 of Table 2.5-5: objective inference of hearing sensitivity and its use in a site of lesion battery. If the acoustic reflex is present, one can use acoustic reflex thresholds to roughly predict the degree of hearing loss, although they do not accurately establish pure tone sensitivity.

If the tympanogram is normal and the acoustic reflex is present, one can feel confident that the middle ear is functioning normally. On the other hand, if the tympanogram is normal but the acoustic reflex is absent, one cannot infer that the child is deaf or even that he has a sensorineural hearing loss. Caution must be exercised because the acoustic reflex can be absent in some individuals with normal hearing. In fact, the presence of a measurable acoustic reflex is age-dependent and is much more difficult to measure in the newborn or young infant. In addition, an air–bone gap (conductive loss) as small as 5 to 10 dB can obscure measurement of the acoustic reflex. Although the absence of a measureable acoustic reflex in young children must be interpreted with caution, acoustic immittance measures can and should be used in the audiologic evaluation of all children. Clinical results can

TABLE 2.5-5. *Information obtained from immittance test battery*

1. Existing middle ear static pressure
2. Tympanic membrane mobility
3. Eustachian tube function
4. Continuity and mobility of the ossicular chain
5. Patency of tympanostomy (ventilation) tube
6. Integrity of the tympanic membrane
7. Prediction of hearing loss
8. Integrity of the peripheral afferent portion of the auditory pathway (eighth nerve at least to the brainstem)
9. Integrity of the peripheral efferent portion of the facial (seventh) nerve

be interpreted only in combination with other measures of auditory function, either from the behavioral test battery or from the auditory evoked response measures.

As a final note, some clinicians have advocated the use of acoustic immittance measures to the exclusion of pure-tone testing. To do so would cause one to fail to detect either a pure sensorineural loss or a mixed-type loss. When assessing patients with mixed losses, bone conduction thresholds are necessary to ascertain the degree of cochlear damage (sensorineural component). Isolated use of immittance measures in school screenings would detect most medically treatable problems but could miss educationally significant hearing losses. Again, acoustic-immittance measures are essential as part of a test battery but must be used in conjunction with other audiologic tests.

IMPORTANCE OF EARLY IDENTIFICATION

At a very early age, perhaps from the moment of birth, a child begins the learning of language, which forms the basis for other aspects of development. Language development is important in the development of auditory, psycholinguistic, and academic skills. For the infant with adequate hearing, language learning apparently occurs primarily through auditory experiences. Vocabulary is learned because words are heard and associated with objects, events, or experiences. One learns to combine words into meaningful phrases and sentences based on how others use speech and language.

Acquisition of reading and writing skills depend on one's previous knowledge of spoken language. Because hearing is so essential to the natural learning of language, it follows that a hearing impairment at birth or early in life (before linguistic skills are learned) seriously interferes with most important areas of development. Therefore hearing loss must be identified as early as possible, so that its handicapping effects (physiological, educational, psychological, and social) can be minimized.

PHILOSOPHY OF HEARING AID SELECTION

Identification of a sensorineural hearing loss demands prompt action to begin aural habilitation of the child. The following discussion details the steps followed by the authors in responding to the needs of the young hearing-impaired patient and his/her family.

Once a sensorineural loss is identified, no matter at what age, immediate steps should be taken to fit the infant or child with amplification. Often sensitivity for only high test frequencies is known, via ABR, for a very young infant or child. Ear impressions should be taken for custom ear molds and, within 2 weeks, the infant/child will be able to wear an amplification device. A loaner aid can be provided for a trial period, and the family should be provided with an in-depth explanation of amplification and instructions in caring for the aid. The parents are told that they play a very important role in helping the audiologist serve the child's needs. They are asked to alternate the loaner aid from ear to ear every 4 to 7 days and observe their child's response or lack of response to sound. A diary is kept for approximately 4 weeks, at which time the parents and audiologist meet and determine whether there appears to be an ear preference by the infant/child.

Hearing aid selection takes place when a child is approximately 8 to 10 months of age. A number of aids are tried on the child and he/she is tested behaviorally to assess the benefit of the aid. Although one aid is initially recommended to facilitate familiarization, most children are candidates for binaural aids. The second aid is recommended at the time of the hearing aid recheck session, 1 month after selection of the initial aid. An infant with an identified hearing loss may wear loaner amplification for several months prior to behavioral testing and hearing aid selection. The child undergoes monthly audiologic sessions for the first year so that informal monitoring of hearing aid benefit can be accomplished and auditory thresholds assessed to detect any threshold shift that might be attributable to excessive amplification by a high-gain hearing aid. If a threshold shift is detected, the aid may be removed for several days to allow recovery and the hearing reevaluated so that the most beneficial but safest level of amplification can be determined. Parental questions and concerns can also be dealt with as they are expressed. The key premise, which is often forgotten, is that more, not less, testing should be completed with the young child.

PRESCHOOL COUNSELING

It is our practice to discuss the issue of programming as early as the second or third session after identification of the hearing loss. The devastating effect that hearing loss has on speech and language development must be presented to the parents clearly and seriously enough to stimulate their thinking toward finding a program as soon as possible. Through provisions of Public Law 94-142, programming should be available in most areas for hearing-impaired children, even newborns. Typically, programming is arranged through the local school district. The John Tracy Clinic Home Study Course for parents of hearing-impaired preschoolers is a resource to keep in mind.

Most often, parents ask about using sign language with their child. The avenues of aural-oral programming or total communication programming are widely discussed and debated as to appropriateness of language stimulation of the hearing-impaired child.

Although audiologists and educators of the hearing-impaired should be involved in counseling the parents regarding educational alternatives for their child, it is difficult to overestimate the importance parents attach to opinions expressed by a physician (particularly an otolaryngologist) regarding the most appropriate habilitation plans for their child. The otolaryngologist should be aware of the issues involved and have a general familiarity with the several communication modes used by the deaf adult population listed in Table 2.5-6.

TABLE 2.5-6. *Philosophical/educational approaches for teaching the hearing-impaired*

American sign language
  Standard signs
  Language in own right/does not follow English syntax
  Supplemented by finger spelling
  Has unique grammar and syntax
  Used widely by adult deaf population
Aural/oral
  Amplification and exploitation of residual hearing
  Speech reading
  Speech
  Unisensory in "purest" form
Manual English
  Seeing essential English
  Signed English
  Signed exact English
  Linguistics of visual English
    Includes finger spelling
    A standard sign often used as a root
    Creation of new signs for inflections, endings, tense, affixes, articles
    Follows English syntax
Cued speech
  Eight hand configurations; form facial positions: cue speech reading of ambiguous
    phonemes
Total communication
  Combines all potential avenues and stresses development of residual hearing, speech,
    and speech reading but is supplemented by signs and finger spelling

---

While counseling parents regarding educational alternatives, it is important to educate them about all alternatives, pro and con. Parents are advised to observe a program that uses each of the communication modes before they make a decision as to which they want for their youngster. It is appropriate to share your own bias so long as you speak from clinical experience and inform the parents that it is a bias. Many otolaryngologists favor a trial of aural-oral programming for all young hearing-impaired children, reserving total communication programs only for so-called oral failures. Most important of all is to stress to the parents that decisions made about programming are not irreversible. It is possible to change, supplement, or in some way determine an alternative to language stimulation if the child does not make expected progress. Determining when a change should be made can be an emotionally charged experience for some teachers, parents, and physicians. With this in mind, it is also important to monitor communication progress with standardized test instruments that can evaluate general development, receptive and expressive language, auditory communication, cognitive skills, and so on (the communication assessment).

A communication assessment should be carried out at least annually, preferably by clinicians not directly involved with the child's educational program. It is often difficult for the teacher with a substantial emotional investment in the child's communicative development to assess objectively language development or lack thereof.

Standard intelligence test instruments, which rely heavily on verbal skills, are not valid for children with severe to profound hearing impairment. These tests significantly underestimate the child's intellectual potential and could lead to serious errors in educational placement. A psychologist who is experienced in testing hearing-impaired children should conduct the evaluation, and he or she must be prepared to communicate with the child in the child's preferred mode: oral, sign, or total communication.

EDUCATIONAL OPTIONS FOR THE HEARING-IMPAIRED CHILD

In 1975 the Advisory Council for the deaf recommended a range of options for educational programming to meet the unique needs of hearing-impaired individuals. As a child progresses educationally, options may change. As changes occur, the concept of the least restrictive environment for each stage in a child's development should operate. The most common options are the following:

1. *Complete mainstreaming.* The child's educational needs are met by a regular classroom teacher. This may suit a very limited number of severely hearing-impaired children. The teacher will require consultative services as well.

2. *Mainstreaming with supportive services.* Many hearing-impaired children can function in regular classrooms with the tutorial assistance of a teacher of the hearing-impaired. The teacher-tutor acts as the child's advocate and coordinates a team approach.

3. *Resource room.* Staffed by teachers of the hearing-impaired, a resource room provides specialized approaches, equipment, and so on for partially mainstreamed children. These are usually located in a public school, and the child spends varying portions of the school day in the resource rooms as his needs dictate.

4. *Special class.* A self-contained class of hearing-impaired children may be located in the public school. This approach is appropriate for those students who require more educational assistance than that provided by a resource room. The special class provides the child with an educational environment favorable to his unique handicap. Usually limited mainstreaming is primarily completed in non-academic areas.

5. *Day schools.* Day schools focusing on hearing impairment are available in some geographic locations. They provide highly specific programs, equipment, materials, teacher supervision, and support staff. Some children's unique needs are best met in such a setting.

6. *Residential schools.* The role of residential schools in providing an educational option for some hearing-impaired children has changed. Nevertheless, many children's needs are best met through this placement. Provision for family interaction is made on weekends. Some residential schools are providing reverse integration.

7. *Home programs.* Teachers of the hearing-impaired with an appropriate background in parent and early childhood education are guiding parents in making the home environment educationally valuable, especially during the preschool years.

Major Questions To Ask a Parent

On regular visits to the otolaryngologist, it is not uncommon for parents to raise questions about their child's educational progress. The physician should avoid becoming embroiled in controversies between the parents and school system unless he/she is thoroughly versed in all issues involved in the case. We have found the following questions helpful to parents in thinking through the pros and cons of their child's educational plan:

1. Is the program involving you as well as the child?
2. How often is the child receiving support service?
3. How much is the child mainstreamed?
4. Does the program nurture the use of residual hearing, speech, and communication?
5. Are reasonable options available to you?
6. What is the preferred mode of communication, and are you satisfied with the youngster's progress?

The otolaryngologic management of the congenitally deaf child must be recognized as an ongoing multidisciplinary process involving skills in diagnosis, habilitation, parental counseling, and interaction with schools and other professionals.

SELECTED READING

Gerber, S. E., and Mencher, G. T. (1978): *Early Diagnosis of Hearing Loss.* Grune & Stratton, New York.

Glattke, T. J. (1983): *Short-Latency Auditory Evoked Potentials: Fundamental Bases and Clinical Applications.* University Park Press, Baltimore.

Jacobson, J.T. (1983): *Seminars in Hearing: Auditory Evoked Potentials,* Vol. 4. Thieme-Stratton, New York.

Jaffe, B. F. (1977): *Hearing Loss in Children: A Comprehensive Text.* University Park Press, Baltimore.

Jerger, J. (1975): *Handbook of Clinical Impedance Audiometry.* American Electromedics Corporation, Dobbs Ferry, New York.

Jerger, J. (1984), *Pediatric Audiology: Current Trends.* College-Hill Press, San Diego.

Jewett, D. L., and Williston, J. S. (1971): Auditory-evoked far fields averaged from the scalp of humans. *Brain,* 94:681–696.

Northern, J. L., and Downs, M. P. (1984): *Hearing in Children,* 3rd ed. Williams & Wilkins, Baltimore.

The Ear

Section 6: Vestibular Assessment

Overview of the Vestibular System 175
   Vestibular and Ocular Motor Function 176
Eye Movement Systems 177
   Ocular Motor System 177
   Visual Pursuit 177
   Saccades 178
   Optokinetics 178
Current Methods of Vestibular Assessment: Limitations 179
Pediatric Vestibular Test Methods 180
Pediatric Test Modifications 182
   Caloric Testing 183
   Eye Movement Examination 184
   Visual Pursuit 184
   Optokinetic Testing 186
   Positional Tests 186
   Rotational Tests 186
   Computerized Rotational Tests (Harmonic Acceleration) 188
Summary 190

The vestibular system, interacting with the visual system and with proprioceptors in the neck, trunk, and limbs, provides critical information for the maintenance of head/body posture, eye position/movement, muscle tonus, and equilibrium. In addition, interaction among these three systems, together with the control exercised by the brainstem and cerebellum, is critical to the acquisition of developmental reflexes and postural control. Such specific functions as eye position and movement, muscle tonus, and developmental reflexes are also necessary for acquisition of visual motor skills and are needed for academic abilities including reading and writing.

Abnormal function or immature development of the vestibular end-organs has been incriminated not only as a primary factor in delayed acquisition of motor milestones and visual motor coordination, but also as a primary cause of dizziness, dysequilibrium, balance problems, and vertigo.

The theory that vestibular dysfunction may be a potential factor in learning disabilities (e.g., dyslexia) has gained widespread support. Investigations have suggested that: (a) disordered muscle tonus (secondary to peripheral vestibular end-organ pathology) may contribute to abnormal visual perception in children with learning disabilities; (b) abnormal output from the inner ear vestibular apparatus adversely affects coordinated, conjugate eye movements needed for reading; and (c) peripheral vestibular lesions create uncoordinated eye–hand movements needed for writing.

Objective assessment of the maturation and function of the vestibular end-organs is more complex than often realized. Even with cooperative adult patients, the most commonly used clinical procedure (electronystagmography) evaluates only a portion of the inner ear vestibular organs (horizontal semicircular canals and the superior branch of the vestibular nerve) and the neural pathways to the lateral and medial rectus muscles of the eyes (vestibulo-ocular reflex). Vestibulospinal function, along with proprioceptive and visual input, are rarely evaluated specifically regarding their interaction with the vestibular system, a critical omission considering that these two systems may be as important in the maintenance of balance and body/head posture as the vestibular system.

When dealing with a pediatric population, even the most basic evaluation of peripheral (inner ear) vestibular function can be a monumental task, especially if some sort of objective measure of vestibular output is desired. This section discusses the modified vestibular assessment of children presenting with dizziness, dysequilibrium, balance problems, and motor delays.

OVERVIEW OF THE VESTIBULAR SYSTEM

The vestibular end-organs' primary function is to provide information to the brain for the detection of tilt, linear and angular acceleration, and static head position relative to gravity. The inner ear vestibular apparatus is also assumed to be the primary organ responsible for maintenance of balance, whereas the proprioceptive and visual systems may actually play a more critical role. The initial response to a loss of balance is a proprioceptive one. Because the proprioceptive system is able to detect velocity and acceleration (motion) at threshold levels lower than that of the vestibular system, it is the first to react to loss of balance. Inner ear vestibular responses do not take place until body movement of approximately 2 to 3 degrees occurs, adding credence to the assertion that the vestibular apparatus of the inner ear may not be the primary system for the maintenance of balance. Proprioceptive and visual inputs may be more important than initially realized, whereas vestibular function may relate more to control of eye and head movement and position. The proprioceptive response to loss of balance is mediated at the spinal level, whereas vestibular and visual responses are mediated at the brainstem, midbrain, and cortical levels. In other words, the reaction to loss of balance follows the hierarchy of central nervous system development, i.e., spinal cord, brainstem, midbrain, and cortex.

Vestibular and Ocular Motor Function

Following introduction in 1939 of Jung's noninvasive procedure for measuring eye movements, a series of subtests employing various types of vestibular stimuli were developed and standardized to evaluate the peripheral vestibular end-organs and their central connections via the vestibulo-ocular pathways. This standardized battery, called electronystagmography (ENG), permits objective assessment of at least a portion of the peripheral vestibular system and vestibulo-ocular pathways, as well as assisting in the identification of a variety of pathologies presenting with dizziness or vertigo.

When the vestibular mechanism of the inner ear or brainstem is stimulated or inhibited (either externally by rotating the head or internally as a result of an irritative or suppressive vestibular lesion), a compensatory eye movement occurs. This ocular response usually takes the form of either a rhythmic, back-and-forth movement called a nystagmus, or a counter-rolling action of both eyes in the opposite direction of the head tilt. Lesions more "central" to the vestibular end-organs, specifically those within the brainstem, may interrupt normal eye movements, producing a variety of ocular tracking aberrations including random eye jerks, disconjugate eye movements, and breakup of smooth visual tracking ability. Identification of these types of eye movement abnormalities is accomplished while concurrently stimulating the vestibular end-organs.

Ever since the human caloric response was described in the latter part of the nineteenth century by Brown-Sequard, the caloric test has been the primary component of the peripheral portion of the ENG battery. The first clinical utilization of the caloric test by Barany consisted of stimulating the vestibular system by the introduction of ice water into the external ear canal and simultaneously observing the resultant ocular movements (nystagmus). This caloric procedure was modified during the 1940s by Fitzgerald and Hallpike to include bithermal stimulation of each external ear canal with warm and cool (not icy) water, 7°C above and below body temperature. This "bithermal" caloric test is the most commonly used and sensitive subtest within the ENG battery for evaluating the peripheral vestibular end-organs, specifically the horizontal semicircular canals.

Another commonly used method of stimulating the peripheral vestibular end-organs employs a horizontally spinning chair (Bárány chair), which moves the patient in a circle from right to left and from left to right. Nystagmic activity is observed and measured after rotation to the right and then compared to the nystagmic activity following rotation to the left. As initially described, the "Bárány rotational test" utilized the "after-nystagmus" as the measured response (postrotary nystagmus). That is, the nystagmus was observed and measured in a variety of ways following rotation of the patient. Subsequent procedural modifications have dealt with recording and measurement of *per*rotary nystagmus (during rotation), a more sensitive and reliable measure of peripheral vestibular function than *post*rotary nystagmus.

EYE MOVEMENT SYSTEMS

The central vestibular regions of the brainstem have been evaluated with a series of ocular tracking tests devised for inclusion in the ENG test battery. These tests comprise measures of slow ocular movements called "pursuit movements," fast ocular movements called "saccades," and optokinetics (an involuntary nystagmus created by watching moving stripes or other repetitive stimuli in the visual field). These eye movement subsystems relate to a series of eye movements initially classified by Dodge to include saccadic, slow continuous, coordinate compensatory, reactive compensatory, and convergence or divergence movements.

Ocular Motor System

The ocular motor (eye movement) system has been described as a dual system consisting of a vergence mode and a version mode. Stimuli for the version mode include ocular fixation and refixation, after-image, optokinetic, motion, volition, audition, and vestibular output. These stimuli result in slow and fast eye movements called pursuits and saccades. Vergence stimuli include retinal blur and diplopia and consist of disconjugate or opposing eye movements. For the purposes of this discussion, the types of version stimuli to be considered include fixation, refixation, and optokinetic motion. These are discussed below as visual pursuit movements, saccadic movements, and optokinetic movements, respectively.

Visual Pursuit

Visual pursuit (fixation), resulting in a slow eye movement, functions to stabilize retinal images by matching the angular velocity of the eye with the angular velocity of a moving target. Such eye–target velocity matching results in smooth eye pursuit of an image moving in space and is typically not seen until a child is 4 to 6 months old. Smooth ocular pursuit movements are often affected by lesions in the central vestibular system, primarily in the brainstem. Peripheral vestibular pathology may also affect visual pursuit, as smooth pursuit is improbable in the presence of intense spontaneous nystagmic activity resulting from an acute unilateral peripheral vestibular weakness.

Saccades

Saccades (refixation) are the most rapid eye movements within the ocular motor system, their primary purpose being to redirect the eyes from one target in the visual field to another target in the shortest possible time. This eye movement system is operational shortly after birth. During most saccadic movements, visual acuity is markedly reduced. When the eyes have reached the intended target, visual acuity returns to its presaccadic state (refixation). By a series of separate high-velocity jumps, saccadic eye movements act to maintain the image of an object on the fovea of the retina, the area of best visual acuity, which is critical for reading. Abnormalities in the velocity, gain, and latency of saccadic eye movements are often seen with brainstem pathology and during the early phases of demyelinating diseases such as multiple sclerosis. In general, saccades are not affected by peripheral vestibular lesions. However, saccadic eye movements can be induced by electrical stimulation of the frontal and occipital cortex, superior colliculus, cerebellum, and paramedial pontine reticular formation (PPRF). As a result, they can be measured but are very difficult to trace electrophysiologically and neurotopographically.

Optokinetics

Optokinetic (compensatory) movements allow for maintenance of visual fixation on a fixed target when the head is in motion; they consist of two phases: a slow-pursuit eye movement in one direction and a fast saccadic eye movement in the opposite direction. Asymmetrical responses are often seen in central vestibular pathologies that unilaterally affect the optokinetic system, such as cortical space-occupying lesions or cortical infarctions. When the entire visual field of a subject is filled with a moving stimulus (e.g., alternate black and white stripes), an involuntary optokinetic nystagmic response occurs. The morphology of the resultant nystagmic waveform and the symmetry of the nystagmic response with target motion from right to left and from left to right are the parameters used to judge normalcy. The optokinetic test, as an isolated indicator of cortical disease, is not totally satisfactory because of the effect produced by peripheral vestibular impairments. For example, optokinetic asymmetry can be observed in the same direction as a peripherally induced spontaneous nystagmus. This has been noted during optokinetic stimulation and following optokinetic stimulation, called "after-nystagmus" (OKAN).

Outputs from the vestibular and visual systems are integrated centrally, thus coordinating head and eye movements during visual search, whether the individual is in motion relative to the environment or the environment is in motion relative to the individual. This interaction, the vestibulo-ocular reflex (VOR), can modify the above-mentioned visual effects. The VOR can enhance visual pursuit when the head is turning rapidly by generating compensatory eye movements which stabilize the "image" on the retina, or it can inhibit visual pursuit and fixation by causing an inappropriate nystagmus as in unilateral labyrinthitis, Meniere's disease, or benign paroxysmal vertigo. In other words, an intact vestibular system can enhance visual pursuit, eye positioning, and other types of eye movements, whereas an abnormal vestibular system can detrimentally affect eye/head movement and positioning.

In view of the above, present methods for evaluation of the vestibular end-organs and their ascending neural pathways seem somewhat less than definitive. Consideration must be given to the interaction between vestibular and ocular motor systems to investigate the effect of each on the other, especially for determination of the status of head and eye position, and for posture in general.

CURRENT METHODS OF VESTIBULAR ASSESSMENT: LIMITATIONS

A sensitive measure of vestibular function is requisite for delineating the interaction between vestibular output and ocular motor movements needed for skills such as writing or reading. Assessment of peripheral vestibular integrity is also essential for determining the cause and site of a lesion in children presenting with dizziness, balance problems, or delayed motor development.

Examination of vestibular function via postural reflexes (tonic neck, Moro, extensor thrust, parachute, etc.) is used fairly extensively in the fields of occupational and physical therapy. This type of testing, relying on intact muscular and central nervous systems, incorporates proprioceptive and visual inputs, making it difficult to separate the vestibular response from the proprioceptive and/or visual responses. Similar problems exist when using consistency boards and posture platforms designed to evaluate the vestibulospinal tracts. Nevertheless, postural reflex testing continues to be a useful tool in the assessment of suspected vestibular abnormalities. Although postural reflex testing is discussed in greater detail later, the reader is referred to the Selected Reading (Fiorentino, 1978) for a more detailed description of a postural reflex battery.

Attempts to elicit vestibular evoked potentials have been relatively unsuccessful. The vestibular system is a complex series of neural pathways with numerous afferent and efferent connections involving vestibular, visual, and proprioceptive systems. These inputs exist not only within the peripheral end-organs but also within the spinal cord, brainstem, midbrain, and cortex. It is difficult to isolate a common vestibular pathway which would allow investigation of vestibular function using current evoked potential methodology, and thus vestibular evoked response testing is not clinically useful at this time.

Most rotational testing has relied on either postrotary stimulation, which is a highly variable procedure, or perrotary stimulation, which may yield either an invalid measure of peripheral vestibular symmetry or may not be able to distinguish central from peripheral vestibular lesions. During perrotary stimulation (slowly rocking the child from right to left and back), the number of observed nystagmic beats is influenced by factors such as the presence and intensity of a spontaneous nystagmus secondary to a lesion of the brainstem. Thus perrotational results may suggest a unilateral peripheral vestibular weakness when such is not the case. A computerized rotary chair has been developed which is sensitive to subtle peripheral vestibular pathologies and has the capability of eliminating effects of a spontaneous nystagmus by canceling extraneous noise via a signal-averaging computer. This test, referred to as Harmonic Acceleration, is discussed in more detail later in the text.

Binocular and monocular counterrolling of the eyes has also been proposed as a method to evaluate peripheral vestibular output. This has been studied during dynamic head tilt and rotation, as well as with static studies using photographic methods. However, this procedure primarily evaluates otolith (utricular) function and, as a result, yields limited information. The procedure is difficult to administer to young children.

The ENG evaluation is currently considered one of the more sensitive and complete measures of peripheral vestibular and vestibulo-ocular function. However, this procedure's subtests still measure only a fraction of the peripheral vestibular apparatus, specifically the horizontal semicircular canal, the utricle, and the superior branch of the vestibular nerve. The remainder of the vestibular end-organ, including posterior and inferior branches of the vestibular nerve, the saccule, and the posterior and superior semicircular canals, is not evaluated. Furthermore, the caloric portion of the ENG utilizes cool- and warm-water stimuli, which produce a vestibular response much greater than is typically encountered by the organism on a daily basis. The caloric test consequently becomes so "nonphysiological" that its contribution to evaluating physiological processes involved in maintaining head and body posture, as well as eye control, is limited. Still, the ENG remains the most commonly used test procedure for evaluating peripheral vestibular function through the vestibulo-ocular pathway.

Of the newer peripheral vestibular evaluation methods currently available, the most sensitive measure appears to be a computerized rotary chair system referred to as Harmonic Acceleration. Phase shift (reaction time within the entire peripheral and central vestibular system to motion) and eye velocity versus head velocity (strength of the overall output from both inner ear vestibular systems combined) are the primary response parameters. Low-frequency harmonic acceleration (HA or the rotary chair test) can be used to assess minor unilateral peripheral deficits, and the results agree with caloric findings on the ENG. However, responses to the rotary chair test are less variable, more sensitive, and more "physiological" than the caloric responses and permit the physician to monitor changes within the vestibular system over time.

PEDIATRIC VESTIBULAR TEST METHODS

The ENG procedure initially gained widespread acceptance for evaluation of an alert and usually cooperative adult population, so that virtually all of the normative data reported in the literature were compiled from adults. Only a limited amount of available information is specifically related to ENG findings in infants and young children.

On the other hand, clinical reports from the disciplines of pediatrics, physical therapy, occupational therapy, neurophysiology, pediatric otolaryngology, and child neurology describe various methods (other than ENG) for evaluating the pediatric vestibular system. For the most part, that literature is concerned with reflexive response to postural change, per- and postrotary stimulation, or ice-water calorics. One can marvel at the unique complexity and redundancy of the vestibular system, but it is not safe to assume that young children possess neurologically intact central vestibular connections or that their peripheral vestibular systems are mature and developing in an orderly fashion. Investigation of the maturational level of the central vestibular system must precede any assumptions regarding peripheral vestibular function. This can be accomplished, in part, with an evaluation of developmental reflexes with sites of origin ranging from the spinal cord through the cortex of the brain.

Four levels of central nervous system development are examined via a postural reflex evaluation: spine, brainstem, midbrain, and cortex. Spinal and/or brainstem development results in an apedal, prone, or supine infant. Although these reflexes are primarily primitive, further development of the midbrain region results in a quadrapedal, crawling, or sitting child, with the development of head and body "righting" reactions. Finally, integration of the cortical level of development produces a bipedal, standing, and walking child, with the emergence of equilibrium reactions during the latter stage of maturation. If, for instance, a child is dominated by the spinal and/or brainstem reflexes and his overall central nervous system has not developed beyond that point, the emergence of righting reactions, e.g., crawling, walking, and sitting, are not observed because the lower-level reflexes dominate the motor actions of this child. As maturation of the central nervous system proceeds to involve ever higher levels, those higher neural mechanisms inhibit reflexes mediated from the lower brain and spinal cord. That is, once the midbrain begins to develop, very primitive responses such as the Moro response and extensor thrust reflex are inhibited.

Before discussing modification of the standard ENG battery for use with children, we should briefly deal with the question, "Why perform an ENG on a young child or infant?" It is not unusual in neuro-otologic practice to discover patients with unrecognized vestibular defects that occurred during childhood. As far back as 1938, the importance of identifying vestibular disease during childhood was described along with some of the resultant psychological sequelae. Since that time, extensive literature has dealt with the incidence of childhood vestibular disorders such as pediatric benign paroxysmal vertigo and vertiginous epilepsy. However, little has been written regarding objectively measured vestibular responses in children with unilateral or bilateral sensorineural hearing loss, postviral disease—measles and mumps, head trauma, or infectious diseases—pneumonia, meningitis, or osteomyelitis—necessitating the administration of ototoxic antibiotics. A pediatrician may find it useful to distinguish between bilateral peripheral vestibular dysfunction versus other postmeningitic sequelae as a cause for delayed walking in an

18-month-old postmeningitic child. Data from our vestibular laboratory suggests that nearly 95% of all postmeningitic children showing subsequent bilateral sensorineural hearing loss also have bilateral peripheral vestibular hypoactivity sufficient to cause significant delays in motor milestone development. Not only postmeningitic children but also children with congenital deafness may present with delayed postural control as the result of bilateral peripheral vestibular weaknesses. Identification of abnormal vestibular function in the deaf and hard-of-hearing population is critical for appropriate counseling regarding employment options, recreation limitations, and related issues.

The standard ENG procedure in adults and older children can help determine whether the vestibular system is functioning outside the normal range and, on many occasions, can specify the site of the lesion, i.e., peripheral versus central vestibular involvement. However, this procedure alone cannot effectively specify the actual pathologic condition. The physician must rely heavily on the case history and symptom complex to reach an appropriate diagnosis. Children can seldom communicate history or symptoms, thus reinforcing the need to supplement the medical examination with an objective measurement of vestibular function within this young population.

PEDIATRIC TEST MODIFICATIONS

Data have been published regarding vestibular responses in infants and young children secondary to rotation in a chair or by ear canal stimulation with ice water. Vestibular response to ice water stimulation in infants has usually been measured by duration of the nystagmus, a questionable means of quantifying vestibular system activity. The temperature of the ice water stimulus is difficult to control, and minor changes in water stimulus temperature can significantly affect the resultant vestibular end-organ response. Also, an ice water stimulus can feverishly drive the vestibular system in a manner far different from everyday physiological vestibular functioning and, as a result, is probably not a very effective means of determining actual vestibular response to subtle changes in posture or acceleration. Finally, the ice water stimulus does not appear to be the least bit comfortable judging by the reactions of the patients. Because ice water calorics produce less accurate results when compared to cool- and warm-water stimulation, the ice-water caloric test is today used only on a limited basis in most clinics, although it is able to provide suggestive results regarding the status of the inner ear vestibular system. The paucity of published pediatric research utilizing a more controlled caloric stimulation (warm and cool water or air) and an objectively measured nystagmic response is likely due to difficulty in adapting the standard adult ENG procedure for use with this younger population. The following discusses modifications of the adult battery currently employed with children at the Boys Town National Institute for Communications Disorders in Children.

Caloric Testing

The most effective method of caloric irrigation with infants and young children is the closed-loop caloric irrigator consisting of a closed-loop balloon which fits into the ear canal (Fig. 2.6-1). Air inflates the balloon to a mild pressure, and water circulates through the balloon at a fixed flow rate. The balloon fills the ear canal

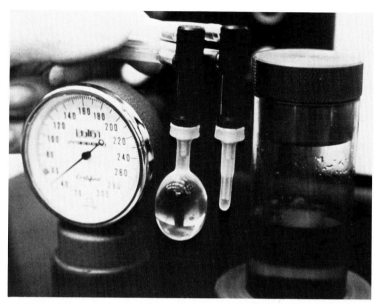

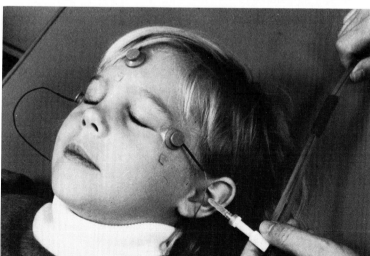

FIG. 2.6-1. Closed-loop caloric irrigator with and without inflated balloon.

and is held firmly in place even if the child should move rapidly. This stimulus produces a caloric response similar to the standard warm/cool-water irrigation and does so in a safe and painless fashion. Another acceptable caloric method utilizes a water-filled balloon in each ear for simultaneous binaural, bithermal irrigation, referred to as the SBB test. The sometimes unpleasant calorically induced vertigo usually experienced by patients undergoing standard unilateral caloric stimulation is minimized with the SBB test if the two inner ear vestibular systems are fairly equal in sensitivity. Theoretically, the calorically induced neural discharge from one labyrinth cancels the discharge from the simultaneously stimulated opposite labyrinth. Because no information is then transmitted up the medial longitudinal fasciculus to the extraocular muscles, nystagmus and resultant vertiginous sensations, nausea, and occasional vomiting are not induced. This situation is much less frightening to a child than standard unilateral stimulation. Simultaneous binaural, bithermal caloric testing removes the necessity of calibrating between caloric presentations because both ears are being compared under the same degree of ENG recorder sensitivity. It should be emphasized that a "no-response" SBB test indicates only that the vestibular end-organs are equal: equally active, equally hyperactive, or equally hypoactive. Therefore one must stimulate at least one ear independently to ensure that there is function from at least one system.

Eye Movement Examination

If the child is at least 3.5 years old, calibration of the ENG recording unit, as well as examination for gaze or spontaneous nystagmus, can be accomplished using a standard calibration light bar. For very young children, an effective calibrating system consists of two painted lamp shades mounted on a horizontal bar (Fig. 2.6-2). Each of the lamp shades is painted with cartoon characters and may be manipulated to produce sound, light, or motion to alternately attract the gaze of children as young as approximately 6 months of age. Any properly spaced pair of colorful or lighted objects can be used for this purpose provided the testing is performed in a room with few visual distractions or, more effectively, in a totally darkened room. Detection of a spontaneous/gaze nystagmus aids in determining whether a lesion is peripheral or central to the vestibular end-organs.

Visual Pursuit

Pendular eye tracking (visual pursuit) can be accomplished using a modified "doll's eye" maneuver with the infant or youngster in the parent's arms. The parent holds the child in a rocking chair in a horizontal position perpendicular to the parent, while the child's eyes are fixed on a lighted toy directly above him (Fig. 2.6-3). As the infant rocks, the eyes move from side to side, permitting inspection of the

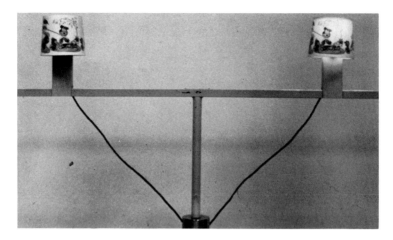

FIG. 2.6-2. Calibrating system for use with young children.

slow pursuit motion as well as determining the degree to which movements of the two eyes are conjugate. Because the visual pursuit system makes up the slow component of nystagmic beat (the other component being a fast saccadic eye movement), an intact pursuit ability is prerequisite to any assumptions regarding a calorically or rotationally induced nystagmus. In addition, it is important to distinguish pathologic gaze nystagmus on this test caused by antiseizure medication or by a lesion within the vestibular system from benign, ocular nystagmus that is seen in a fair percentage of the pediatric population. Congenital benign ocular nystagmus rarely produces difficulties with balance or visual tracking.

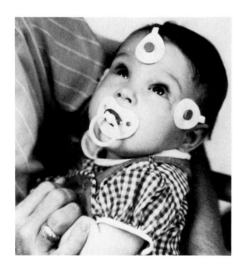

FIG. 2.6-3. Visual pursuit with eyes fixed on target above.

Optokinetic Testing

Optokinetic tracking can be measured in very young children with any suitable stimulus that fills a majority of the child's visual field, such as a large test drum which fits over the child's head with test stimuli projected on the interior surface (Fig. 2.6-4). Cartoon characters projected on the wall can be used with very young children provided the room is dark enough to prevent peripheral distractions. Optimally, one employs a full-field optokinetic stimulus that revolves around the child in a visually isolated room. It is essential to be able to fill the entire visual field of a patient if a true optokinetic response is to be elicited. All too often in optokinetic testing of children, examiners use a hand-held drum of alternating stripes or a tape measure with lines that fills only a small portion of the child's visual field. Such an approach in actuality may be testing the visual pursuit system rather than the optokinetic system. A patient confronted by this type of optokinetic stimulus may possibly fixate on points peripheral to his center gaze, visually pursuing the optokinetic stimulus relative to those fixed points. This is especially important if one is attempting to elicit an optokinetic response in infants under the age of 3 months. In order to accomplish this task, a full-field optokinetic stimulus is mandatory.

Positional Tests

Positional testing of the otolith organs (utricle and saccule) can be accurately performed in a completely darkened room or with the child blindfolded. In either case, it is important that the child be tested in absolute darkness to rule out visual suppression of nystagmus. Children can detect small amounts of light even in a room that is 95% dark and can effectively suppress a caloric, rotational, or spontaneously induced nystagmus. Current procedure in our laboratory is to enclose the child and parent in a totally darkened room while an infrared camera observes the eye movements. Total darkness can frighten some toddlers so that blindfolding is more feasible in some cases.

Rotational Tests

Vestibular assessment may also be accomplished using a torsion swing chair in a darkened room or with the child blindfolded. The child sits upright in the chair or on the parent's lap as the chair rotates in a 180 degree horizontal arc. A nystagmic burst generated by interaction of both inner ear vestibular systems is recorded with surface electrodes taped near the outer canthus of each eye while the chair swings to the right and to the left. A right beating nystagmus (fast component to the right) is normally observed when the chair turns to the right, and a left beating response is produced when the chair swings to the left (Fig. 2.6-5). The number of beats occurring in each direction of rotation are then counted at serial points in time. The

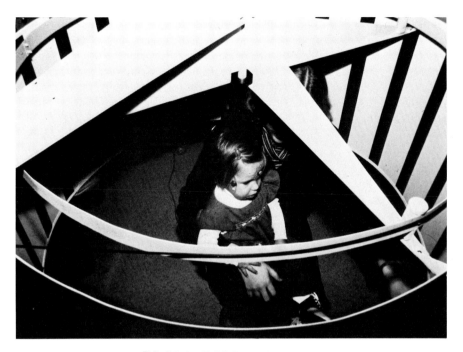

FIG. 2.6-4. Full-field optokinetic drum.

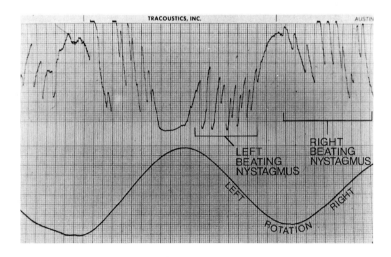

FIG. 2.6-5. Right beating and left beating nystagmus from torsion swing stimulation.

results must be interpreted cautiously, as they do not always agree with caloric results. The torsion swing test shows an increased nystagmic response with rotation in the same direction as a coexisting spontaneous nystagmus. For example, if a child has a right beating, direction-fixed spontaneous nystagmus generated by a space-occupying lesion of the brainstem, rotation of the chair to the right increases the strength of the right beating spontaneous nystagmus, whereas rotation to the left decreases the strength of the right beating spontaneous nystagmus. As a result, the torsion swing chair suggests a weakness of the left inner ear mechanism even though the lesion is central to the end-organ and has nothing to do with the integrity of the peripheral mechanism. Ruling out a true unilateral peripheral weakness versus a spontaneous nystagmus secondary to a peripheral or central vestibular disease is a difficult task with this rotational test procedure. The test is effective, however, in determining the presence or absence of peripheral vestibular output, especially in the detection of a bilateral peripheral vestibular weakness. Again, it is extremely important to rotate the child in the absence of any visual fixation to avoid mistaking an optokinetically (visually) induced nystagmus for one produced by the peripheral vestibular system.

Computerized Rotational Tests (Harmonic Acceleration)

A computerized sinusoidally rotating chair that relies on slow-moving harmonic rotation has proved very effective in our laboratory for evaluating the vestibular system in pediatric patients, including infants as young as 2 months of age (Fig. 2.6-6). The procedure permits measurement of vestibular asymmetry, as well as output and reaction time of each peripheral vestibular end-organ, in a pleasant, slowly rocking motion that children and infants readily accept.

When evaluating children for positional, spontaneous, caloric, and rotational nystagmus, mental alerting tasks must be used to prevent central neural suppression of the nystagmic response. Mental tasking can be accomplished with infants and young children during the computerized rotary chair test by playing taped music or nursery rhymes over speakers in the visually isolated test enclosure. When evaluating slightly older nonoral children with severe to profound hearing impairment, it is often necessary to have the patient manually finger-spell or sign a story, e.g., during positional, rotational, or caloric tests. Our laboratory evaluated 166 youngsters (ages 3 to 19 years) from the state school for the deaf and determined that a significant number of students would have been misidentified as having bilateral peripheral vestibular hypoactivity if they had not been appropriately tasked with finger-spelling and sign language. Approximately one-half of the children who demonstrated bilateral vestibular weaknesses during the initial evaluation without tasking eventually had normal and symmetrical responses when appropriate tasking was utilized. This population, more than any other previously evaluated in our laboratory, was capable of marked suppression of peripherally induced nystagmus. The tandem Romberg test in the Jendrassik position (Fig. 2.6-7), with eyes open

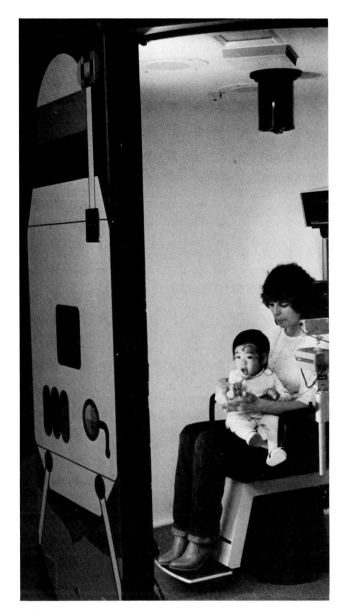

FIG. 2.6-6. Computerized pediatric rotary chair system.

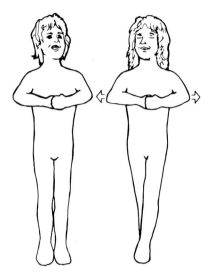

FIG. 2.6-7. Standard and tandem Romberg testing used in Jendrassik position with eyes open and closed.

and eyes closed, proved to be most predictive of the final results of the peripheral vestibular output battery for these older children.

SUMMARY

Numerous problems exist with current methods for evaluating vestibular functions, particularly in infants, toddlers, and special-needs children. The standard adult battery has significant limitations which are further magnified when the procedure is used with young patients. It may be just as essential to realize that the vestibular system controls other important functions specifically related to academic achievement and to the development of motor milestones. Given the system's complexity, a multidisciplinary approach to vestibular evaluation, including otoneurologic examination, ENG, and postural reflex testing, as well as a variety of rotational and ocular tracking tests, should be employed. A possible key to the complexities of vestibular and ocular motor performance rests in analysis of the interaction between the vestibular and ocular motor systems, rather than with observation of each system independently.

Whatever method is employed to evaluate vestibular function, the question that needs to be asked is, "What information do I want to obtain from a pediatric vestibular test?" If concern is for overall maturation of vestibular pathways and the central nervous system in general, postural reflex testing may be the most appropriate method to use. If concern is for a peripheral vestibular lesion that may be responsible for a sudden attack of dizziness, vertigo, or ataxia, a pediatric ENG with positional, rotational, caloric, and ocular tracking tests is needed. For detecting the presence of bilateral peripheral vestibular disease as a potential cause of delayed motor development (especially after meningitis), a caloric or rotational test in a dark environment may be most efficient. One must, at the same time, be mindful that a total loss of one inner ear vestibular system rarely causes motor delays, whereas bilateral vestibular weakness definitely causes such problems depending on the age of the patient. If concern is for the presence of a space-occupying lesion of the brain or brainstem, the ocular tracking battery (visual pursuit, optokinetics, ocular saccades, and gaze nystagmus detection) is important to the overall evaluation. Coupling objective vestibular test results with history and physical examination, plus a basic knowledge of the manner in which the vestibular system contributes to and affects balance and eye movements in general, will become the initial step in the diagnosis and potential treatment of young children and infants with dizziness, vertigo, balance problems, and delayed development of motor milestones.

SELECTED READING

Beddoe, G. M. (1977): Vertigo in childhood. *Otol. Clin. North Am.,* 10:139–144.

Black, F. O., Wall, C., and O'Leary, D. P. (1978): Computerized screening of the human vestibulo-spinal system. *Ann. Otol. Rhinol. Laryngol.,* 87:853–860.

Brookhouser, P. E., Cyr, D. G., and Beauchaine, K. A. (1982): Vestibular findings in the deaf and hard of hearing. *Otol. Head Neck Surg.,* 90:773–778.

Coats, A. C. (1975): Electronystagmography. In: *Physiologic Measures of the Audio-Vestibular System,* pp. 37–85. Academic Press, New York.

Cyr, D. G. (1980): Vestibular testing in children. *Ann. Otol. Rhinol. Laryngol.* [*Suppl. 74*], 89:63–69.

Eviatar, L., and Eviatar, A. (1978): Neurovestibular examination of infants and children. *Adv. Oto-rhinolaryngol.,* 23:169–191.

Eviatar, L., and Eviatar, A. (1979): The normal nystagmic response of infants to caloric and per-rotary stimulation. *Laryngoscope,* 89:1036–1044.

Eviatar, L., Eviatar, A., and Naray, I. (1974): Maturation of neurovestibular responses in infants. *Dev. Med. Child Neurol.,* 16:435–446.

Finestone, A. J. (1982): *Evaluation and Clinical Management of Dizziness and Vertigo.* John Wright–PSG, Boston.

Fiorentino, M. (1978): *Reflex Testing Methods for Evaluating C.N.S. Development, 2nd ed.* Charles C Thomas, Springfield, Illinois.

Robinson, D. A. (1964): The mechanics of human saccadic eye movement. *J. Physiol. (Lond.),* 174:245–264.

Robinson, D. A. (1965): The mechanics of human smooth pursuit eye movement. *J. Physiol. (Lond.),* 180:569–591.

Wolfe, J. W., Engelken, E. J., and Kos, C. M. (1978): Low-frequency harmonic acceleration as a test of labyrinthine function: Basic methods and illustrative cases. *ORL Trans.,* 86:130–142.

Wolfe, J. W., Engelken, E. J., Olson, J. W., and Kos, C. M. (1978): Vestibular responses to bithermal caloric and harmonic acceleration. *Ann. Otol. Rhinol. Laryngol.,* 87.

The Ear

Section 7: Speech and Language Disorders: A Clinical Perspective

Normal Language Development 194
    Communicative Development Landmarks.....................195
Developmental Language Disorders 197
Voice Disorders 201
Disorders of Speech Sound Production......................202
Stuttering 203
Cleft Palate and Related Disorders 205
Hearing Loss and Language Development 207

With relative ease, the normally developing child learns and begins to utilize, at a predictable time and rapid rate, the complex symbolic system for communicating meaning called language. Employing his/her intact vocal tract and neuromotor control systems, the child learns to pair sounds with meaning, producing the modality of language expression referred to as speech. This developmental feat belies the interactive role played by a multiplicity of constitutional and environmental factors in normal language and speech development (Fig. 2.7-1).

Building on the sensory experience gained through the auditory and visual system during the first year of life, the infant by 12 months of age evidences understanding of the meaning of simple words and uses his/her first words expressively. By 18 months of age, most normal infants have a vocabulary of 50 words and have begun to combine words into simple two-word phrases usually to express desires or needs. During the next 1.5 years up to age 36 months, the child demonstrates significant language growth both vertically, in the number of words he knows, and horizontally, in his ability to link words together in more complex groups (sentences) to reflect his/her developing cognitive abilities.

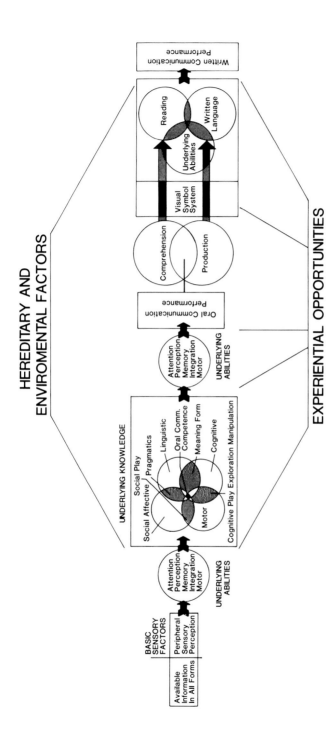

FIG. 2.7-1. Constitutional and environmental factors in normal language and speech development. (Adapted from McLean, J. E., and Snyder-McLean, L. K.: *A Transactional Approach to Early Language Training.* Merrill Communication Development and Communication Disorders Series; Columbus, Ohio, 1978.)

A significant delay in language acquisition can seriously hamper social and educational development. Delay in language development may be associated with an underlying anatomic, neurosensory, or psychological disorder, e.g., deafness, cerebral palsy, cleft palate, autism, or mental retardation. A condition called specific developmental language delay may occur in children devoid of any other identifiable disorder or developmental delay.

NORMAL LANGUAGE DEVELOPMENT

A developmental delay can be defined only with reference to the normal course of development. Modern language research has focused on the preconditions for language learning. The child must have the cognitive abilities to relate intellectually to the physical and social events encoded in language, as well as the ability to process, organize, and store linguistic information. In addition, the child must be exposed to the thing or event to which the speech/language refers simultaneously with the word(s) to be learned.

Some researchers suggest that the human brain is in some way uniquely prepared to learn language, whereas others believe that a basic set of mental operations is used by the child in structuring all sensory input including auditory language.

Language behavior may be broadly categorized as comprehension and production. Comprehension, also called receptive language ability, involves identification of a sound phonemically, recognition of the sounds previously identified, discrimination of one sound from another, and a final decoding process requiring a knowledge of syntax, semantics, and the rules for communicative appropriateness.

On the oral output side, one can enumerate 10 functional components of the vocal tract which generate or valve the speech air stream, together with five aerodynamic variables that allow inferences to be made concerning malfunction of these components (Fig. 2.7-2).

Oral communication performance can be seen as involving both comprehension and production abilities. Reading is viewed as a language-based activity built on preexisting oral comprehension and production skills. Reading and written expression involve processing of visual information and association of this information with the underlying auditory base. Therefore certain higher level abilities involving attention, perceptual memory, integration, and motor skills interact with the underlying oral language comprehension and production abilities to produce reading and written expression skills. These higher-level abilities involve the capacity to treat language analytically, which is fundamental to learning to read.

Underlying visual and auditory-visual skills assume greater importance at this stage. Reading is seen as being related to oral language comprehension, whereas written expression is seen as related to oral language production. This relationship is not absolute, however, and certain types of expressive language deficits may interfere with specific reading skills, particularly those involved in oral reading.

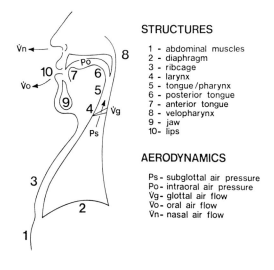

STRUCTURES

1 - abdominal muscles
2 - diaphragm
3 - ribcage
4 - larynx
5 - tongue/pharynx
6 - posterior tongue
7 - anterior tongue
8 - velopharynx
9 - jaw
10- lips

AERODYNAMICS

Ps - subglottal air pressure
Po - intraoral air pressure
Vg - glottal air flow
Vo - oral air flow
Vn - nasal air flow

FIG. 2.7-2. Physiological and aerodynamic variables in speech production. (Adapted from Netsell, R., and Daniel, B.: Dysarthria in adults: Physiologic approach to rehabilitation. *Arch. Phys. Med. Rehabil.*, 60:502–608.)

These factors—oral language comprehension and production, and reading and written expression—interact to form basic written communication.

The role of environmental factors in language development, although important, is poorly defined. A child raised in an environment deficient in sensory stimulation, including auditory, visual, and tactile experiences, demonstrates impaired development of linguistic skills. To associate such environmental deprivation only with families of lower socioeconomic status may be overly simplistic. Some children from impoverished backgrounds develop communication skills at normal or above-normal rates. Poor parenting skills rather than simple economics appear to be a critical element. A developing child must be exposed to language which is related to significant events, and this ordinarily requires the active participation of another individual, usually the child's mother, who helps to focus attention on the critical experiential event to be paired with a linguistic concept.

The following list of developmental landmarks are useful for assessing the child's growing communicative capacity.

Communicative Development Landmarks

Early Infancy

Receptive: Child listens mainly to patterns and intonation of language. Attends to faces and voices; distinguishes friendly/angry, male/female, familiar/unfamiliar voices.

Expressive: Child vocalizes small, throaty sounds. Grunts, sighs, and coos. Gives vocal expression to feelings.

7 to 9 Months

Receptive: Child begins to distinguish between questions, commands, and statements on the basis of intonation. Gestures mean more than speech. Child may lift arms to "come up" gesture.

Expressive: Babbles two syllables on one breath. Vocalizes to gain attention or in recognition. Alters voice to express displeasure or satisfaction.

9 to 12 Months

Receptive: Child comprehends individual words. "No!" "Bye-bye." Gives a toy on request in response to a gesture plus speech.

Expressive: True babbling. Wide range of sounds developing. Babbles four or more syllables. Imitates speech and gestures. Attempts to command and comment (vocalizes and points).

12 to 14 Months

Receptive: Understands words in usual context. Comprehends simple commands pointing to key word. "Where?" is answered by pointing.

Expressive: First words; only 25% intelligible. Still relies on babbling and gestures to communicate. Develops a range of meanings and functions in his/her language. May be echolalic (often imitates what is heard).

13 to 15 Months

Receptive: Child continues to acquire new words. Responds to simple commands and answers "yes/no" and "where" questions. Can name a picture when asked "What's this"? May echo in response to question.

Expressive: Jargon stage. Child jabbers freely. Attempts to produce adult-like utterances, and vocalizations sound very "conversational" but totally unintelligible.

15 to 18 Months

Receptive: Child enjoys simple stories. Listens to language for sake of listening. Rapid acquisition of vocabulary (50 to 300 words emerge).

Expressive: Child uses many more words. He/she uses words to communicate physical needs or answer questions. There is a decrease in babbling and jargon. The child may "chain" two words together.

18 to 24 Months

Receptive: The child is able to process longer sentences but not complex ones. He/she follows more complex directions. Begins to understand the use of objects. (What goes on your foot?)

Expressive: The child develops rules to put words together. Two-word combinations stage. He/she begins to use pronouns (mine, me).

2 to 3 Years Old

Receptive: The child is skilled in answering a variety of questions and recognizes actions. He/she follows directions with prepositions and remembers sequences of simple stories. Concepts emerge (e.g., big).

Expressive: The child learns that the *order* of words is important. He/she produces sentences of three to five words, containing key words in order, but often lacks smaller function words (articles, tense changes, etc.). (For example: "Me throw ball table" instead of "I threw the ball under the table"). Vocabulary 600 to 1,000 words. Ask who? And what?

3 to 4 Years Old

Receptive: The child understands class words (show me the animals) and comprehends needs. He/she follows two-step commands, identifies some colors, and begins to answer "why" and "how" questions.

Expressive: The child uses simple, grammatically complete sentences often. He/she can communicate experiences more intelligibly but still makes grammar errors. He/she begins to use pronouns and articles and to ask many questions.

4 to 5 Years Old

Receptive: This period is characterized by rapid acquisition of vocabulary. The child is curious about time concepts and other abstract words. He/she asks the meaning of words and continues to asks many "why" questions.

Expressive: Complex sentences emerge. The child begins to define objects and describe actions in a picture. The degree to which he/she can engage in a genuine exchange of ideas remains limited. Language may be used in "make believe" play.

5 to 6 Years Plus

During this period connected language develops and is refined. The child's conversational skills are related to his/her cognitive and social competence. He/she learns to see other's viewpoints and to analyze and make judgments. The child also learns to use language to suit the context, learns the rules for refined social interactions, as well as academically related abstract concepts (left, right; before, after).

DEVELOPMENTAL LANGUAGE DISORDERS

Development of language skills is a complex process which extends far beyond the use of the first words. When a child learns that the word *dog* refers to a four-legged animal which barks, this is only the beginning of the use of a vocabulary related to dog(s). The child must then learn that *puppy, Rover,* and *canine* may also refer to that animal, but that *fox, wolf,* and *coyote* do not equal *dog.* In addition, all of these can be called *animals.* Word naming or vocabulary development is only one of the aspects of language. There is also a complicated system of linguistic rules that combine words into related sequences and meaningful sentences. Rules also govern designations such as possession, pluralization, and tense.

Rule-governed language emerges in regular stages of development in the child and is maintained in the adult so long as neurologic and cognitive abilities are unimpaired. A child's linguistic competence develops from: (a) cognitive/perceptual abilities experiences, i.e., how sensory input is organized; (b) linguistic experiences—how verbal information is used to order, predict, and control the environment; and (c) nonlinguistic experiences—how nonverbal information is coded into language.

Children do not have formal instruction in development of language skills. They learn language as they hear it, and many encounter problems. Delayed and disordered language development may be related to a variety of factors or combination of these factors, e.g., environmental deprivation, psychosocial deficits, hearing loss, cognitive (learning) deficits, trauma, and pre-, post-, and perinatal factors, such as fetal alcohol effects, prelingual tracheostomy, and neurologic impairment. After suffering a stroke, an adult often manifests disordered language as a result of the neurologic impairment. Aphasia or reduction in the ability to process symbolic stimuli may exist in auditory, visual, and tactile input modalities and in spoken, written, and gestural output modalities. In particular, damage to the left hemisphere leads to the greatest deficits in language function. Neuroanatomic explanations of aphasic symptoms are based on assumptions that the parts of the brain responsible for these functions have been damaged or the communication between parts of the brain have been interrupted. Major contributors to speech–language function lie in the region surrounding the sylvian fissure in the language dominant hemisphere and include the primary auditory cortex, the auditory association area, the premotor cortex of the frontal lobe, and the arcuate fasciculus. Damage in these areas may selectively involve deficits in word recognition, word comprehension, repetition, syntax, sound selection, and sequenced movements needed for spontaneous speech production.

Children, as well as adults, may suffer language impairment following closed head injuries, strokes, and other cerebral insults. There are also other forms of neurologic impairment, some of which are so subtle that language or speech problems may be the only manifestation. When neurologic impairment is congenital or early in onset, it poses considerable difficulty for the child who has not yet developed language skills. It is also possible for a child to experience neurologic disorders superimposed on preexisting developmental language delay. Children are determined to have specific developmental language delay by excluding coexisting sensory, neurologic, or other developmental deficits. On the other hand, attention must be directed toward delineating those subtle factors in the patient's heredity, health history, physical examination, or environment which may provide clues to the etiology of this disorder.

A substantial body of research has explored the relationships between prenatal events, neurologic damage, and behavior and learning difficulties. Maternal and fetal factors have been related to a broad array of subsequent disorders extending from fetal death through a range of impairments, e.g., cerebral palsy, epilepsy, mental deficiency, behavior disorders, and reading disability. A significantly greater number of poor readers has been found in groups of neonates with histories of low birth weight, shortened gestational period, or other perinatal complications such as eclampsia and placental abnormalities when compared with normal controls. Several longitudinal studies have found that children who were premature (1,550 to 2,250 g) had reading abilities which were not significantly different from those of a control group at ages 7 to 8. At ages 11 to 12, however, the control group read significantly better. The British National Child Development Study showed a correlation between reading performance at age 7 and mother's age at delivery, maternal smoking history during pregnancy, and birth weight.

The author and co-workers in 1979 evaluated the importance of high-risk factors and other developmental indicators in the histories of 24 children who manifested preschool language delay significant enough to require remedial intervention. A scale of 13 potential risk factors was developed based on prenatal, birth, and postnatal histories (Fig. 2.7-3). The background of all 24 children contained at least one of 13 possible factors, with 87.5% of subjects demonstrating two or more factors. The only factor which showed a significant relationship to the severity of receptive language delay was a history of severe childhood illness with a fever of 104°F or greater for a period of 24 hr.

Studies of families in which a specific reading disability appears to be inherited through several generations in an autosomal dominant fashion strongly suggest that

H History in family of communication disorders

E Ear, nose or **throat** deformities

A Anoxia at birth or low **apgar** score

R Rx — Ototoxic or teratogenic drugs during pregnancy

I Maternal **illness** during pregnancy including "infections" or pre-eclampsia

N Neonatal intensive care or prolonged hospital stay for infant

G Growth retardation — prematurity or full term low birth weight

'S Stress factors in delivery

R Recurrent otitis media beginning before 2 years of age with surgical intervention and/or hearing loss

I Serious childhood **illness** with a fever of 104° F for a period greater than 24 hours

S Seizures, diminished **sucking** reflex, or other signs of CNS dysfunction

K "Knocked out" — head trauma with loss of consciousness or bloody otorrhea

S Subjectively difficult to test audiologically

FIG. 2.7-3. Potential risk factors for speech language delay. (Adapted from Brookhouser, P. E., Hixson, P. K., and Matkin, N. D.: Early childhood language delay: The otolaryngologist's perspective. *Laryngoscope,* 89:1898–1913.)

a gene playing a major etiologic role in one form of reading disability is on chromosome 15. If this presumption is confirmed in further studies, it may provide a means for early prediction of children at risk for reading disabilities and perhaps for early developmental language delay.

The physician frequently is the first professional who comes in contact with the language-impaired child. Using interview and observation, the physician may determine whether referral for evaluation is appropriate. Although observation of a child's language may be difficult in the medical setting and require an unreasonable amount of time from the busy practitioner, parental concerns and questions should be heeded, and if parents suspect problems referral is indicated. Children who do not meet the developmental guidelines as outlined in Table 2.7-1 or whose progress appears to be stagnated or slow should be referred for further screening or for evaluation. Children's progress through stages of language acquisition is rapid, and thus early referral is important. Although children may appear to "grow out of" early obvious language delay, more subtle sequelae may be evidenced later in academic areas, taking the form of a learning disability, or in deficits in social interactions. Prompt referral and intervention can prevent or minimize such complications.

A speech–language pathologist employs standardized, norm-referenced tests and procedures to determine the presence of a delay or disorder. The extent of the problem, the specific areas of problems, and responsiveness to treatment are investigated. When language delay or disorder is discovered, remedial speech–language services should be initiated as soon as possible. For most children, carefully planned and sequenced language skills are introduced, practiced, and reinforced through play and social interactions. Sometimes augmentative communication devices such as electronic communication systems and manual language (signing) may be used to facilitate language development. Severely impaired children may need life-long augmentative communication. The school-age child may require special assistance

TABLE 2.7-1. *Criteria for referral for evaluation of language problems*

Time	Criteria
12 months	No differentiated babbling or vocal imitation.
18 months	No use of single words; the child has difficulty understanding common requests.
24 months	10 words or less used spontaneously and appropriately.
30 months	100 words or less; no evidence of two-word combinations; speech unintelligible.
36 months	200 words or less; no use of subject–verb–object sentences; speech intelligibility 50% or less.
48 months	600 words or less; no use of simple sentences; speech intelligibility 80% or less.
Older children	Difficulty formulating and expressing thoughts in a cohesive way; predicting, hypothesizing, and verbal explanations are difficult; word retrieval problems (tip of tongue phenomena) are frequent.

in the development and application of language skills in reading, writing, and verbal reasoning. Early assistance helps to prevent the complications which may ensue as communication attempts fail, academic problems develop, and the child recognizes the deficits. Most school systems now not only provide speech–language remedial services but also have preschool and school-age language classrooms as well as resource personnel to provide additional support.

VOICE DISORDERS

Problems in phonation (voice) result from abnormal patterns of closure and vibration of the vocal folds, including closure with excessive force, failure to attain complete closure, asymmetrical vocal fold vibration, excessive vocal fold tension, and use of unusual modes of vibration. Laryngeal dysfunction may be caused by vocal fold pathologies such as papillomas, carcinoma, and laryngeal web. Patients attempting to override the dysfunction in order to achieve functional or improved voice may significantly aggravate the problem prior to, during, and following medical intervention. In concert with necessary medical intervention in these cases, a speech–language pathologist can alleviate detrimental compensatory behaviors and vocal abuses, as well as assist the patient in redeveloping normal communication skills.

For those patients who become aphonic for any period of time, the speech–language pathologist can prepare the patient for an alternative communication system, select or develop a communication system appropriate for the patient, and assist the patient in learning to use the system. For some patients alternative speech systems, e.g., esophageal speech or prosthetic speech devices used with adults following laryngectomy, become a permanent system for expressive communication. For those with temporary tracheostomy or after laryngeal injury, augmentative or alternative communication systems may be used temporarily until normal vocal function returns.

Vocal misuse and abuse may result in vocal fold pathologies including vocal nodules, certain polyps, and contact ulcers. The etiologic basis of these lesions is reflected in the colloquial descriptors applied to them, e.g., screamer's or singer's nodules. By modifying aspects of abusive vocal behavior, the speech–language pathologist can, in most cases, eliminate the vocal fold pathology and restore normal vocal fold function. In such cases, surgical intervention is not generally a procedure of choice. If abusive vocal behaviors continue, the laryngeal pathology is likely to reappear. Thus aside from the attendant surgical risk, surgical excision of such vocal fold pathology will be only temporarily successful unless the phonatory patterns are changed. Well-motivated patients respond easily and quickly to remedial speech services, and vocal nodules, even large firm nodules of long standing, generally demonstrate reduction and finally disappear within relatively short periods of time. Some patients, however, find satisfaction in deviant phonation and are resistant to management. In young children, behavioral problems resulting in tantrums, screaming, yelling, or use of a loud voice can be the chief cause of vocal abuse. These patients have a poor prognosis for permanent elimination and/or reduction of both laryngeal pathology and the deviant phonation, whether this is through remedial speech services or surgery. For such children and their parents psychological counseling along with behavioral management may be of assistance when used in conjunction with remedial speech services.

When evaluating a voice disorder, the speech–language pathologist studies the parameters of pitch, loudness, and quality of voice as utilized in speaking situations and considers the implication of these aspects of voice in terms of the mechanics of voice production. Behaviors and attitudes which may contribute to vocal abuse and vocal fold dysfunction are also investigated.

Phonation is a complex process, carefully controlled and timed to interact with all aspects of speech production. Instrumentation such as ultra high speed motion picture photography, stroboscopic laminography, and endoscopy permit viewing of laryngeal function during speech conditions. Ultrasonic scanning and tomography are among procedures used to investigate the dimensions of laryngeal function. Protocols for speech production elicited during such examinations should be developed by the speech–language pathologist, who also should assist in interpretation of the findings in terms of the influence of laryngeal function on speech. Aerodynamic pressure–flow techniques provide measures of subglottal, glottal, and supraglottal airflow and pressure, thus providing objective information which assists in definition of phonation problems. Similarly, spectographic data provide acoustic descriptions of phonatory interactions with other dimensions of speech production. This instrumentation is most likely to be available to clinical speech–language pathologists located in hospital and university diagnostic centers. The findings are increasingly being translated and applied to augment standard clinical procedures. Evaluation and management of voice problems has moved far beyond the days of the speech and voice teachers and is now based on a rapidly expanding body of scientific knowledge. Effective management of voice problems requires cooperative professional interactions among otolaryngologists, speech–language pathologists, and psychologists, as well as other specialists.

DISORDERS OF SPEECH SOUND PRODUCTION

Vowel sounds are produced by lingual shaping of the oral cavity which produces change in the acoustic characteristics of the emerging phonated (voiced) airflow. Consonant sounds result from velar, lingual, dental, and labial contacts and releases, timed with orally and nasally directed airflow, which may be phonated or non-phonated according to the requirements of the particular consonant being produced. These speech sound productions are made with incredible speed, as well as exquisite motor planning and timing which are interactive with linguistic rules and organization. Disorders in production of speech sounds may result from problems in the child's learning, organization, and selection of the rules for speech sound production. On the other hand, disorders may be due to aural, oral, and neural pathologies which result in impaired input or output.

Children as young as 6 weeks of age demonstrate differentiation of speech sounds that they hear. These differentiations are based on timing and method of production of the sounds. Maturation of the child's developing nervous system allows increasingly finer differentiations to be made, and speech sound development begins long before the first word appears. Early in the first year of life, the child begins to operate on his environment by use of voice and gesture. As the child matures, speech sound productions, which at first are general approximations of adult productions, are gradually refined. This process of refinement continues until about the age of 7 or 8 years, by which time the child's speech sound productions closely match those of adults. Children systematically change their speech sound systems as their neuromotor and auditory analysis skills develop.

Children exhibit speech sound production deficits if they have structural impairments such as hearing disability. Through analysis of their speech sound repertoire and aspects of production, the clinician is able to categorize the errors in order to determine approaches to intervention. Treatment approaches must take cognizance of the patterns of the child's physiological abilities, as well as the level of organization of his phonologic and language system. Treatment takes the form of production and comprehension programs which help the child monitor his or her speech and learn production strategies which preserve and increase information transmission. A few children may not be able to produce intelligible speech despite intensive remedial efforts. For these children, speech communication devices may be selected and adapted to a particular child's needs and skills by the speech–language pathologist. All children should be given the opportunity, however, of becoming oral speakers.

STUTTERING

One of the most widely used definitions of stuttering is as follows: Stuttering is an interruption in the ongoing flow of speech which calls attention to itself and interferes with the transition from one word to the next in a sentence. The term *stammering* is generally used interchangeably with *stuttering*. These interruptions in the flow of speech may take a variety of forms: (a) erratic, sudden blockages or interruptions in the ongoing flow of speech; (b) secondary behaviors which may involve excess tension in the speech musculature (tongue, lips, pharynx, larynx, thorax) and facial or body musculature; and (c) psychological reactions to the stuttering events. Not all stutterers present the same collection of behaviors or the same degree of severity. Normal speakers may experience fluency breakdowns similar to those of the stutterer. These are called normal dysfluencies and are differentiated from stuttering by the frequency, severity, and degree to which they interfere with the speaker's communication. The incidence of stuttering in the U.S. population is about 0.7%. Up to 4% of adults report having stuttered at some point in their lives. Although these figures vary for different population groups, the patterns of onset, maintenance, and recovery are similar.

Parents sometimes are concerned about the sudden appearance of whole word repetitions and other dysfluency phenomena in their child's speech between the second and fifth years. Most children go through a period of normal dysfluency, with the most frequent onset being during their second and third years. Approximately 80% children with normal dysfluency have normal speech patterns by their seventh birthday. Table 2.7-2 provides some guidelines for differentiation of incipient stuttering from normal dysfluency, which will diminish with maturation and increasing language skill. Incipient stuttering can be controlled through treatment by a speech–language pathologist experienced in childhood stuttering.

A reliable relationship for predicting stuttering is apparent between sex, environmental, and familial factors. Stuttering has been found to be more common among males, 9% of whose daughters and 22% of whose sons may also be stutterers. For the fewer women who have stuttering problems, 17% of their daughters and 36% of their sons will likely be stutterers. A monozygotic twin is more likely to share stuttering with his same-sex twin than a dizygotic twin of the same sex. Stutterers as a group demonstrate normal intellectual function.

For many years it was believed that stuttering was associated with underlying neuroses or anxiety states. There is no support in the literature for this theory, as stutterers consistently perform similarly to normals on assessments of psychological status. However, anxiety is associated with the act of stuttering. The success of intervention methods employing instrumental conditioning techniques has led to a theory that stuttering is a learned behavior embodying instrumentally and classically conditioned components. Although some behaviors manifested by the stutterer may be learned responses, studies of sex differences, familial incidence, and environmental patterns among stutterers suggest that stuttering behavior, as it originally appears in the child or the adult, is not primarily a learned response.

It is well known that stuttering is reduced under several special speaking con-

TABLE 2.7-2. *Development of stuttering*

Normal dysfluency
 1. Appears between 2 and 3 years of age.
 2. Frequently is limited to repetitions of whole words or syllables.
 3. Seldom interferes with the ongoing flow of speech.
 4. Usually begins to diminish by 4 years of age.
 5. Seldom is associated with audible or visible tension while speaking.
 6. Child is generally not aware of a problem.
Stuttering
 1. May appear between 2 and 3 years of age, 5 through 7 years of age, or 9 through 12 years of age.
 2. Involves repetitions of syllables, sound prolongations, or struggle interfering with the ongoing flow of speech.
 3. May occur through the phrase or sentence.
 4. May involve visible or audible tension associated with the initiation of voice.
 5. Child may be aware of and frustrated by difficulty in talking.
 6. While cyclic, remains stable or increases in severity with age.
 7. Dysfluencies are increased in severity/frequency with increases in conversational or speech pressures.

ditions: whispering, choral speech, singing, rhythmic or metronymic speech, speaking under auditory masking, or with delayed auditory feedback. Speech production in general is monitored by a self-feedback system and changed to satisfy self-perceptions. Stutterers may have difficulty utilizing the feedback used by fluent speakers to maintain control.

Speech theorists postulate a reduced capacity in stutterers for utilizing feedback on the current status of the speech mechanism in order to make effective transitions from one speech movement to the next in a sequence. Thus conditions such as singing or rhythmic organization appear to assist self-monitoring. Treatment procedures employing fluency shaping and prolonged speech techniques have been used successfully to achieve long-term fluency, with natural-sounding speech, in a wide variety of stutterers. With well-coordinated programs for transfer and maintenance, it is possible to produce fluent speech which is maintained successfully outside a clinical setting in a majority of child and adult stutterers.

CLEFT PALATE AND RELATED DISORDERS

A cleft palate has a significant negative impact on speech production. Ability to direct respiratory airflow in either an oral or a nasal direction and to control the air pressure in the oral cavity is required for normal speech. The velar muscles acting in concert with pharyngeal muscles provide this control which is precisely timed with all other aspects of speech sound production. The speech sounds *m, n,* and *ng,* as in *naming,* are produced with nasal airflow. All other speech sounds require oral airflow. The sounds *p, b, t, d, k,* and *g,* as in *pet, bed,* and *keg,* are known as plosives and are particularly sensitive to loss of oral air pressure. The sibilant sounds *s, z, sh, ch, zh,* and *dzh,* as in *sue, zoo, shoe, chew, vision,* and *pigeon,* are even more sensitive than plosives. The plosives and sibilants are referred to as pressure consonants. In the presence of an open cleft, the coupling at the oral and nasal cavities results in an inability to control oral airflow and increased nasal airflow, making normal production of the pressure consonants impossible. The oral sounds are then nasalized, and the escaping airflow may be audible. Velopharyngeal valving disorders and accompanying speech problems also occur when there is neuromotor dysfunction, submucous clefting, or a short palate.

Sometimes velopharyngeal incompetence is unmasked by an adenoidectomy. In such cases the speech may be relatively normal prior to the surgery, but abnormalities will be observed and persist after the surgery. When nasalized speech continues beyond 3 months postsurgery, referral should be made for evaluation by a speech–language pathologist and a head and neck surgeon who are specialists in cleft palate.

A primary reason for surgical closure of a palatal cleft or surgical management of noncleft conditions, e.g., the short palate, is to provide a functional mechanism which permits normal speech production. The word "functional" here is important. The alveolus and hard palate must be completely closed, as any connecting oronasal fistulas will permit nasal escape of airflow. The soft palate must be capable of elevating to the level of the hard palate while extending to make good contact with the pharynx to prevent nasal leak of the air. Even a small fistula can be extremely detrimental to speech production. An oronasal fistula is sometimes difficult to detect on visual examination. Velar elevation can be observed, but visual examination will not permit accurate determination of the adequacy of closure for speech production.

Evaluation of velopharyngeal competence for speech production is additionally complicated by behavioral factors. A child must learn to use the velopharyngeal mechanism for speech. Some children with no physical abnormality fail to do so. When there are velopharyngeal problems, children may develop compensatory speech patterns. For example, vocal fold valving may be used to create a glottal plosive as a substitute for conventional plosives, or the tongue may be positioned in proximity to the posterior pharyngeal wall to produce a plosive or fricative approximation. Even when the surgical repair of the palate has been successful, compensatory patterns may persist and remedial speech services will be required. Of course, surgical closure of a palatal cleft or repair of a noncleft palate may not always achieve a functional velopharyngeal mechanism for speech.

In the presence of velopharyngeal disorders, there is also concern for possible eustachian tube dysfunction and thus middle ear problems. Clefting which involves the alveolus and hard palate also may contribute to significant problems in maxillary and facial development. Syndromes with which palatal clefting may be associated, e.g., Pierre-Robin anomaly, Stickler's syndrome, Turner's syndrome, and velo-cardioifacial syndrome, adds factors which must be considered in management planning.

Team evaluation, planning, and management of velopharyngeal and craniofacial disorders is advised. The team environment facilitates multidisciplinary consultation and planning that is critical to effective management. The team usually is comprised of individuals of special interest, experience, and currency in management of these disorders. The interrelationships of the problems associated with craniofacial disorders is such that the individual practitioner who is working in isolation or who may be inexperienced with disorders of this type may actually contribute complications to the management of the problems. Team management of cleft palate begins at birth. Early assistance helps parents in their understanding of the problems and the causes of these problems, helps them with management of feeding, and prepares them for the projected course of treatment. Children with cleft palate should be followed by the team until maturity so that problems involving hearing, dental and speech development, and maxillary growth and development are given full consideration to achieve the best possible results.

Evaluation and definition of speech characteristics is critical to effective management of velopharyngeal problems. Observation and analysis of patterns of speech production provide a basis for: (a) identification of the presence and degree of velopharyngeal incompetence; (b) differentiation of velopharyngeal and other problems; (c) evaluation of the effectiveness of surgical management; (d) a determination of the timing and need for management procedures; and (e) selection among management options. Evaluation of velopharyngeal disorders can be assisted by specialized examinations such as cine(video)fluoroscopy and nasoendoscopy, which provide dynamic assessment by permitting visualization of the velopharyngeal mechanism under speech conditions. The speech–language pathologist's assistance is important in: (a) determining the protocol for elicitation of speech during these procedures; (b) the conduct of the evaluation; and (c) interpretation of the results of such studies. Aerodynamic pressure–flow measurements can be made by the speech–language pathologist to determine the amount of airflow and air pressure at the laryngeal, oral, and nasal ports. Spectrographic data permit acoustic analyses of the speech patterns and their timing and interactions. These procedures are of greatest value when used in the team setting. Instrumentation (pressure flow and spectrography) usually is available only through team programs.

Following surgery and/or prosthetic management, remedial speech services should be provided to help the patient learn to use the repaired velopharyngeal mechanism effectively and overcome compensatory patterns which may have developed. Response to remedial assistance determines the need for additional management of the valving mechanism. Remedial speech services should be provided by a speech–language pathologist who is experienced in work with cleft palate and velopharyngeal disorders.

HEARING LOSS AND LANGUAGE DEVELOPMENT

Studies of high-risk indicators and genetic linkage analysis hold future promise for further characterizing children with specific developmental language delay, but currently this disorder may present in an otherwise normal child. This finding is of considerable significance when weighing the relationship between hearing loss and deficits in the development of language and related academic skills. A child with an early-onset sensorineural hearing loss poses no problem because he/she would be determined to be hearing-impaired and excluded from the specific developmental language delay category. In contrast, fluctuating conductive hearing impairment, as seen with early-onset and recurrent otitis media with effusion, may cause confusion in categorizing a language-delayed child with respect to presumptive etiology—hearing loss versus specific developmental language delay.

The presence of a congenital, severe to profound bilateral hearing loss disrupts the normal process of language acquisition. Research has generally shown that the extent of language delay increases with the degree of hearing loss and that the gap between hearing-impaired children's language skills and those of their hearing peers widens with age. Delays have been reported for lexical/semantic skills, syntactic/morphologic skills, and pragmatics. Both receptive and expressive language skills are affected, with the greatest delays reported in the area of expressive language. Deficits in lexical/semantic skills result in limited work knowledge and verbal-conceptual skills in the hearing-impaired. Well-documented studies show the highest average score achieved by 8- to 20-year-old profoundly hearing-impaired students in a school for the deaf on vocabulary tests was equivalent to that of 8- to 10-year-old students with normal hearing. The assessment of syntactic/morphologic skills in the same study showed that the highest average score was equivalent to that of 6- to 7-year-old normal-hearing students.

In general, assessment of syntactic/morphologic skills has shown that students with severe and profound hearing losses acquire only the simplest sentences of English. Deficits in word knowledge, verbal-conceptual skills, and syntax/morphology pose serious problems for reading and academic achievement in this population. Hearing-impaired subjects had more difficulty than normals with complex verb constructions and tended to substitute simpler forms. Response patterns were compatible with those seen in normal children 4 to 5 years younger in chronologic age. Most recent studies have focused on the pragmatic or functional communicative aspects of severely and profoundly hearing-impaired children's language. These studies have shown delays and deviance in this area of linguistic performance which affects their discourse and related skills.

Children with early-onset, persistent conductive hearing impairments demonstrate delayed language development generally comparable to that experienced by children with similar sensorineural losses. The developmental consequences of fluctuating conductive hearing losses of less than 25 dB, associated with recurrent or chronic otitis media, is less well established, leading to extensive and sometimes heated debate in the current literature. Laboratory simulation studies have indicated that the presence of a 20-dB hearing deficit can cause loss of transitional information such as plural endings (e.g., *s* and *es*) and final position fricatives (e.g., *with, was, wish,* and *half*). Controversial studies have appeared in the otolaryngologic, pediatric, audiologic, speech/language, and learning disabilities literature suggesting that fluctuating conductive hearing loss during early childhood can significantly affect the development of language and related academic skills. Some authors have claimed that these deleterious effects can be irreversible, but there is little credible evidence to support these assertions.

The majority of studies have been retrospective in design and have focused on defining subtle linguistic and academic differences between groups of school-age children, some with positive histories for early otitis and others without. Care has been taken, in some instances, to rule out coexisting neurosensory or developmental deficits in the study children. On the other hand, little or no attention has been directed toward the potentially confounding variable posed by a preexisting specific developmental language delay in a child who concurrently develops otitis media with conductive hearing loss. If such an underlying developmental language delay went unrecognized, it could lead to specious conclusions regarding the nature and permanence of the effects of fluctuating hearing impairment.

A related concern involves identification of constitutional or environmental factors which may serve to minimize the effects of early-onset, recurrent otitis media on a child's language development. Clearly, not every young child affected with fluctuating conductive hearing loss suffers from delayed language development. Knowledge of such protective characteristics would be of great benefit to the pediatrician in arriving at a prognosis and treatment plan for the young otitis-prone child with respect to the development of language related skills. Thus far, no reliable indicators have been described which permit identification of a subset of children with recurrent otitis who are also suffering fron an intrinsic predisposition for a specific developmental language delay.

Longitudinal studies are presently underway in a number of centers aimed at understanding the relationship between preschool developmental language delay and later deficits in academic performance in school. Because communicative competence in oral language is a prerequisite for normal development of reading and written expression, children with language delay may later be labeled as learning-disabled based on academic performance.

The evidence for an association between otitis and language development is somewhat clouded by the failure of investigators to control for potential pitfalls posed by underlying factors that might predispose to both otitis media and developmental impairments, e.g., low socioeconomic status, impaired parenting, subtle unrecognized CNS disorders, and other types of chronic illness. The early and consistent medical management of children with histories of otitis media appears to mitigate the impact of the fluctuating conductive hearing impairment on language development. Delayed phonologic development observed in the children with a history of early-onset, recurrent otitis media appears to be a reversible phenomenon, so that the older children who have received early and consistent treatment came closer to the performance of the normal subjects.

An important void in the present knowledge of the effects of conductive hearing impairment, fluctuating or persistent, on the development of language would be filled by a longitudinal study focusing on preschool children. This study design would provide not only for documentation of the severity and frequency of otitis episodes with accompanying conductive hearing loss but also for on-going assessment of the developing child soon after the presumptive developmental insult. The otitis-prone preschool child may have more readily demonstrable deviance in language development than the more subtle linguistic deficiencies some investigators have found in school-age children with strong histories of early recurrent otitis. Such issues as the quality of parenting and the child's developmental progress in areas other than language could also be carefully evaluated.

A unilateral hearing loss, conductive or sensorineural, has failed to show correlation with any demonstrable deficits in vocabulary, language comprehension, syntax, and reading performance as has been was observed in children with persistent bilateral losses, assuming that the child had available compensatory strategies such as classroom seating which favors the better-hearing ear.

SELECTED READING

Aronson, A. E. (1973): *Audio Seminars in Speech Pathology: Psychogenic Voice Disorders*. Saunders, Philadelphia.
Aronson, A. E. (1980): *Clinical Voice Disorders*. Thieme-Stratton, New York.

Brookhouser, P. E., Hixson, P. K., and Matkin, N. D. (1979): Early childhood language delay: The otolaryngologist's perspective. *Laryngoscope,* 89(12):1898–1913.

Brookshire, R. H. (1978): *An Introduction to Aphasia.* BRK Publishers, Minneapolis.

Bzoch, K. R., editor (1979): *Communication Disorders Related to Cleft Lip and Palate.* Little Brown, Boston.

Dickson, D. R., and Maue-Dickson, W. (1982): *Anatomical and Physiological Bases of Speech.* Little Brown, Boston.

Hagen, C. (1981): Language disorders secondary to closed head injury: Diagnosis and treatment. *Top. Lang. Dis.,* 2:73–87.

McWilliams, B. J., and Philips, B. J. (1979): *Audio Seminars in Speech Pathology: The Velopharyngeal Incompetence.* Saunders, Philadelphia.

Skinner, M. W. (1978): The hearing of speech during language acquisition. *Otolaryngol. Clin. North Am.,* 11:631–650.

Chapter 3

Hearing-Impaired Child: The Pediatrician's Role

Foundations of Communication 211
Hearing Impairment in Childhood 213
   Factors Involved 213
   Sensorineural Hearing Loss: Effect on Development
      of Communication 218
   Conductive Hearing Loss: Effect on Development
      of Communication 218
   The Effect on the Child 219
   Early Identification 219
High-Risk Registry 220
History-Taking 221
Reaction to Sound 221
Physical Examination 222
Hearing Evaluation 223
Pediatrician's Role in Rehabilitation of the
   Communicatively Impaired Child 224

Probably the most complex learning period of childhood involves the development of communication skills. In addition to oral communication, there are other forms of communication for man. Communication distinguishes the human race from other mammals and is the foundation on which man's cultural development is based. Any failure to develop normal communication denies a child the chance to compete on equal terms with normal-hearing children socially or educationally.

FOUNDATIONS OF COMMUNICATION

Communication in man begins in infancy and continues to develop throughout life. Verbal communication in normal children is based on six functions: hearing, language development, speech development, storage, recall, and sight. Hearing and sight are the only communication functions present at birth.

Hearing continues its maturation for some time after birth, possibly not in the ear but in the registration of sound signals and their recognition in the brain. The evoked cortical responses to sound stimuli change in character between birth and age 3 years, when "mature waves" are recorded from the brains of normal children. The development of normal communication requires an auditory system capable of passing the mechanical energy of a sound stimulus through the middle ear into the fluids of the inner ear, where it is transduced into electrical impulses that are conducted along the auditory nerve through the auditory nuclei and up the brain relays to the auditory cortex. At this level, there must be correct recognition of the sound signal, and in the case of human communication, the combinations of word sounds must be integrated and understood. In short, all parts of the auditory system must be intact and in normal working order to permit the hearing and understanding of human speech. A child cannot learn speech until he learns to listen. Speech is more readily acquired and more easily understood by those children without visual problems but may be acquired by children without sight.

Language is the recognition that various sound combinations have significant meaning. As an example, the child who says "da da" repeatedly to his father is rewarded by the father with cuddling and pleasant sounds because the father thinks the child recognizes him and has addressed him as "Daddy." Eventually the child associates the happy man and the rewards for the "da da" sound and begins to use "da da" purposefully. It becomes the first word in his vocabulary. For a child, the recognition that sounds can be meaningful is the beginning of language. Language might be called recognition by association, but it also represents a learning skill.

Speech can be considered a learned process of imitation of significant sound signals. It involves the imitation of a set of signals representing a word, but the child must be able to recognize what that word means and to repeat it meaningfully before it can be said that he has acquired the word for his vocabulary. A child's vocabulary is the stock of words he can use meaningfully.

Storage is the ability a child has to retain words in his brain. Such storage consists of the sounds associated with their enunciation and recognition of their meaning.

Recall is a child's ability to take a word, a sentence, and/or an event out of storage and use it as speech whenever it is required for his communication.

If a child suffers impairment of any of the six major functions, or if he has acquired deformities of or injuries to the mouth, nose, or larynx through inheritance or injury, he will not develop what can be termed normal communication.

The following are some yardsticks by which to measure the normal acquisition of communication. The average child with normal hearing and with normal potential for speech development should meet these criteria.

Birth to 4 months: The infant emits sounds such as "ma ma" and "da da." These sounds are part of the physiological responses to pleasure and result from the infant opening and closing his lips or repeatedly placing the tongue against the hard palate while emitting a sound. At first they are without meaning and are not speech, but they do show the child's ability in basic phonation and articulation.

Four months to 1 year: Early development of language occurs during this period. The child becomes aware of variations of sounds and develops a pattern of listening.

Second year: The child begins to relate sounds to objects, listens to his own utterances, and experiments with inflection. Speech acquisition begins. Language acquisition is rapid.

Third year: The child should be using two- or three-word phrases and be adding to his vocabulary.

Third to fourth year: Speech becomes clear. The child demonstrates marked advances in sentence structure and a marked expansion of his vocabulary.

Vocabulary acquisition in the normal child based on normal speech stimulation by the family should approximate these figures: age 2, 200 words; age 2.5, 350 words; age 3, 800 words; age 4, 1,200 words.

HEARING IMPAIRMENT IN CHILDHOOD

Hearing loss during childhood can be expressed in a number of ways. The symptoms displayed by the child differ according to the age of onset, the severity of the loss, and the type of loss and determine the kind of program necessary for the family and child to undertake for his rehabilitation.

Factors Involved

The critical times for age of onset of hearing loss are at birth, 6 months, 2 years, and 4 years. The severity of loss may be total loss, total loss of high tones with partial loss of low tones, partial loss of high tones with no appreciable loss of low tones, partial loss of high and low tones equally, and inability to understand speech.

The types of hearing loss are: (a) Conductive hearing loss results from impairment to the middle ear mechanisms and causes suppression of hearing throughout both high and low tones. In conductive impairment, the loss is never total (Fig. 3-1). This type of impairment results from middle ear infections, trauma, or congenital maldevelopment of the middle ear structures. (b) Sensorineural impairment results from damage to the electrical transducing system of the inner ear, the auditory nerve, or the central auditory pathways of the brain and causes degrees of hearing loss from total to mild (Figs. 3-2 and 3-3). Any loss less than total is characterized by a loss in high tones that is more severe than that in the low tones. In the more severe cases, the high-tone loss (above 500 Hz) can be complete. In less severe cases, low tones may be normal, with medium loss of high tones. This results in hearing that distorts speech. Words are heard almost as a series of vowel sounds. This defect can be genetic in origin or can be the result of congenital damage, neurologic injury after birth, infection, or ototoxic drugs. (c) Combined or mixed

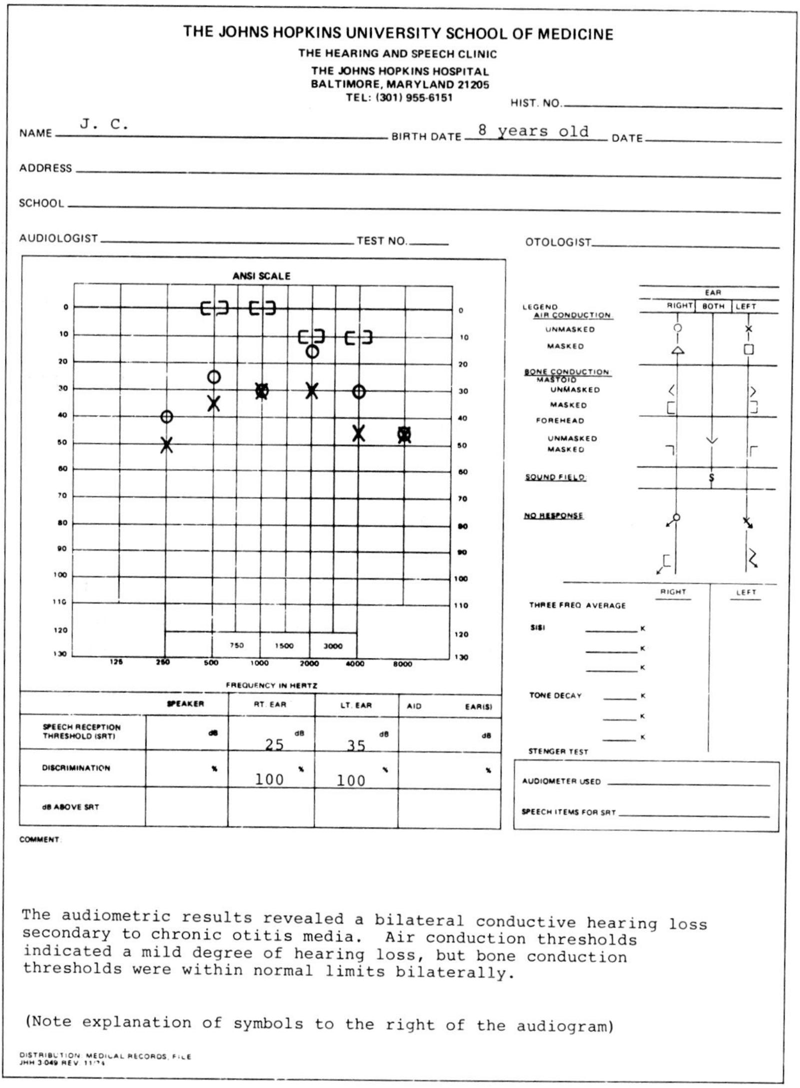

THE JOHNS HOPKINS UNIVERSITY SCHOOL OF MEDICINE

THE HEARING AND SPEECH CLINIC

THE JOHNS HOPKINS HOSPITAL

BALTIMORE, MARYLAND 21205

TEL: (301) 955-6151

HIST. NO. _____

NAME ___ J. C. _____ BIRTH DATE ___ 8 years old ___ DATE _____

ADDRESS _____

SCHOOL _____

AUDIOLOGIST _____ TEST NO. _____ OTOLOGIST _____

ANSI SCALE

FREQUENCY IN HERTZ

	SPEAKER	RT. EAR	LT. EAR	AID	EAR(S)
SPEECH RECEPTION THRESHOLD (SRT)	dB	25 dB	35 dB	dB	
DISCRIMINATION	%	100 %	100 %	%	
dB ABOVE SRT					

COMMENT

The audiometric results revealed a bilateral conductive hearing loss
secondary to chronic otitis media. Air conduction thresholds
indicated a mild degree of hearing loss, but bone conduction
thresholds were within normal limits bilaterally.

(Note explanation of symbols to the right of the audiogram)

DISTRIBUTION MEDICAL RECORDS FILE
JHH 3 049 REV 11-74

FIG. 3-1. Hearing tests illustrating a bilateral conductive loss of moderate degree in an 8-year-old child secondary to chronic otitis media. The bone conduction audiogram is better than the air conduction audiogram, and the discrimination score is normal.

FIG. 3-2. Severe sensorineural bilateral hearing loss in a 4-year-old child born prematurely weighing 3 lb 6 oz with severe hyperbilirubinemia secondary to Rh incompatibility. Language and speech were severely delayed.

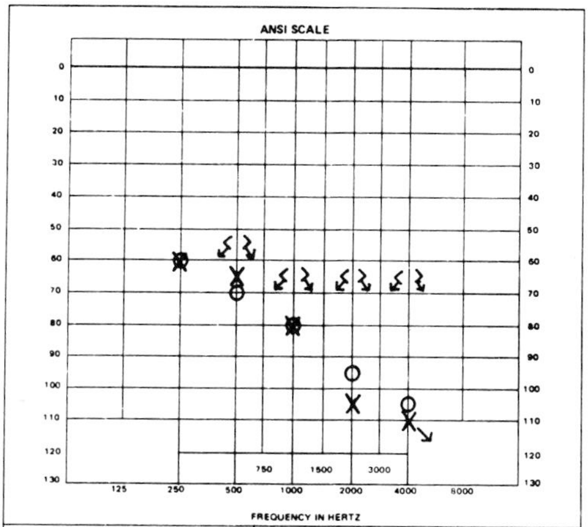

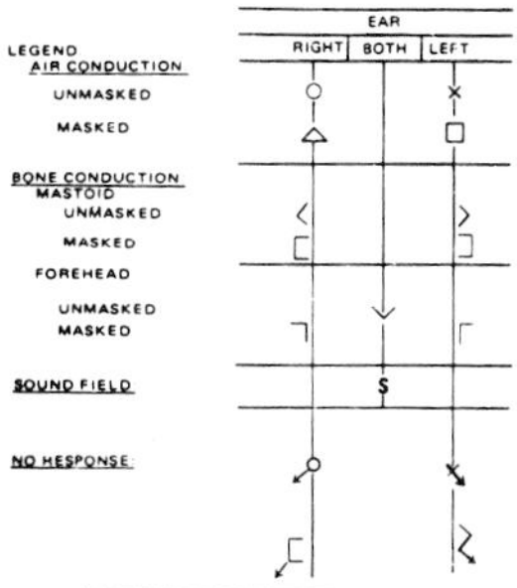

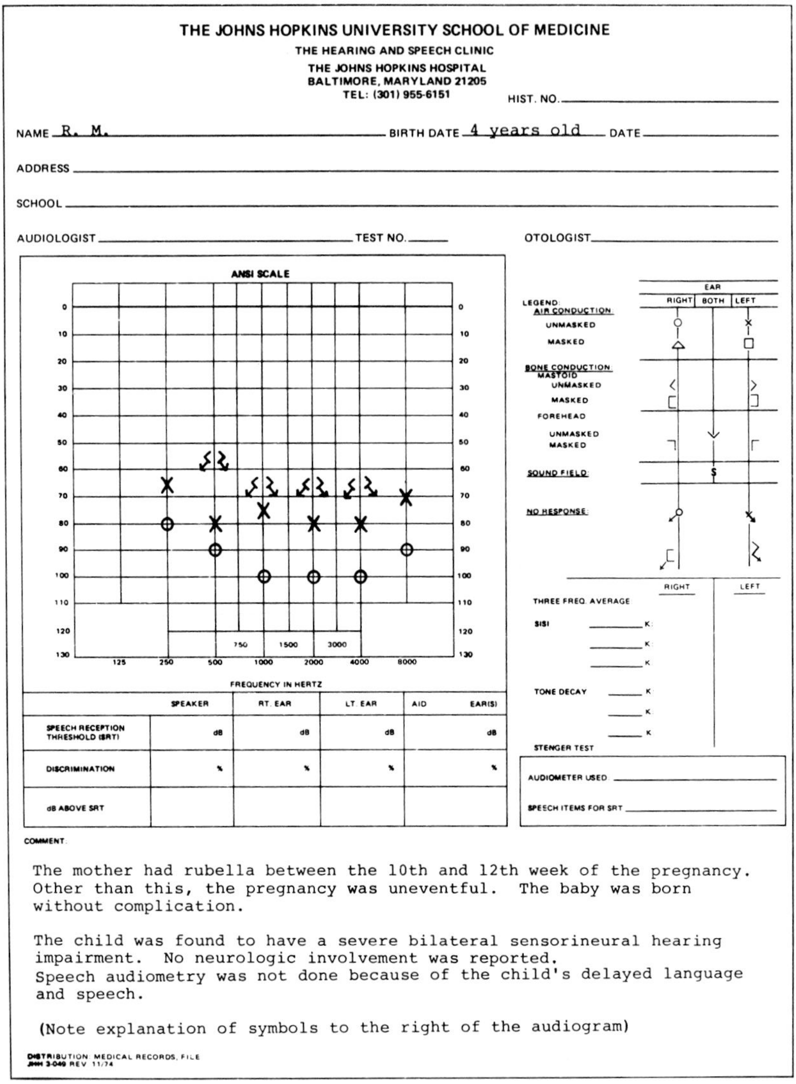

FIG. 3-3. Hearing of a 4-year-old child born of a mother suffering rubella infection during the 10th to 12th weeks of her pregnancy. Bone conduction is so reduced that it did not respond to the maximum intensity of the test tones; air conduction is severely reduced. The child had developed no useful speech.

THE JOHNS HOPKINS UNIVERSITY SCHOOL OF MEDICINE
THE HEARING AND SPEECH CLINIC
THE JOHNS HOPKINS HOSPITAL
BALTIMORE, MARYLAND 21205
TEL: (301) 955-6151

HIST. NO. ______

NAME T. B. BIRTH DATE 7 years old DATE ______

ADDRESS ______

SCHOOL ______

AUDIOLOGIST ______ TEST NO. ______ OTOLOGIST ______

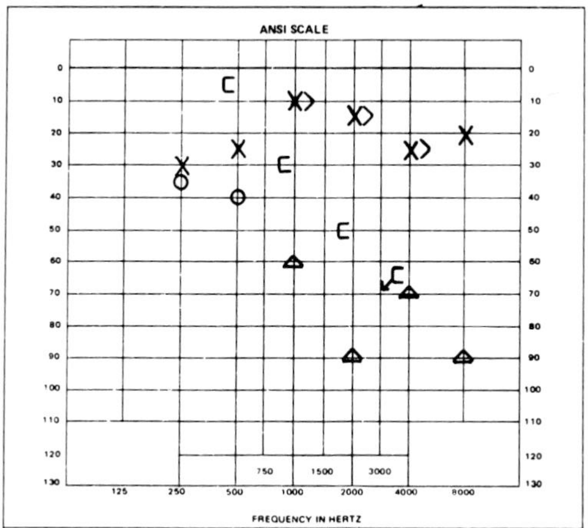

LEGEND

	RIGHT	BOTH	LEFT
AIR CONDUCTION — UNMASKED	O		X
AIR CONDUCTION — MASKED	△		□
BONE CONDUCTION MASTOID — UNMASKED	<		>
BONE CONDUCTION MASTOID — MASKED	[		]
FOREHEAD — UNMASKED		↓	
FOREHEAD — MASKED	┐		┌
SOUND FIELD		S	
NO RESPONSE			

	SPEAKER	RT. EAR	LT. EAR	AID	EAR(S)
SPEECH RECEPTION THRESHOLD (SRT)	dB	60 dB	20 dB		dB
DISCRIMINATION	%	28 %	100 %		%
dB ABOVE SRT					

	RIGHT	LEFT
THREE FREQ. AVERAGE		
SISI ___ %		
___ %		
___ %		
TONE DECAY ___ %		
___ %		
___ %		
STENGER TEST		

AUDIOMETER USED ______

SPEECH ITEMS FOR SRT ______

COMMENT

The child was a product of an uneventful, full term pregnancy but developed hypoxia at birth.

The test showed a moderately severe mixed type hearing loss in the right ear with type B tympanogram bilaterally. Speech discrimination of the right ear was poor.

(Note explanation of symbols to the right of the audiogram)

DISTRIBUTION: MEDICAL RECORDS, FILE
JHH 3-049 REV. 11/74

FIG. 3-4. Mixed-type right-sided hearing loss in a 7-year-old child born after a normal pregnancy but who developed severe hypoxia at birth. Air and bone conduction were reduced, and the discrimination score was very poor on the right. Language and speech were normal because the left ear functioned normally.

hearing loss can be described as a combination of conductive and sensorineural hearing loss (Fig. 3-4). (d) With central auditory disorders, the ear and auditory nerve are intact, and the damage lies in the auditory pathways from and including the auditory nuclei to the cortex of the brain and results in a failure to integrate the signals in a meaningful manner, which inhibits understanding of speech. This handicap in children can be confused with brain damage or mental retardation.

Sensorineural Hearing Loss: Effect on Development of Communication

The child born without hearing or with hearing so impaired that it cannot contribute to acquisition of language or speech is usually identified earlier because of his total lack of response than the child born with some residual hearing. The child with moderate low-tone loss and severe high-tone loss exhibits loss of ability to hear speech at a normal intensity and fails to develop normal speech. The child born with a mild high-tone loss and normal low-tone hearing may develop slightly deviant speech but can use his hearing in a relatively normal manner. His problem may not be identified until his hearing is screened in school.

The child who acquires a hearing loss shortly after birth has the advantage of having heard and so has a faint memory of sound. Identification here of even a moderately severe hearing impairment is thus delayed. The child who loses hearing after 6 months to 1 year has the support of having monitored his voice and having acquired some language and possibly some speech. The child who loses hearing after 2 to 3 years has a much better basis for rehabilitation than those described above. He will have language, speech, and relatively normal inflection. He will also have acquired some vocabulary and an ability to lip-read. Because of these skills, identification may not be made for many months.

The hallmark of the child suffering from sensorineural hearing impairment is imperfect speech. He cannot hear the entire phonetic structure of a word—only a skeleton composed of vowel sounds and none of the high-tone sibilants. He speaks as he hears, and even with excellent instruction, he seldom can achieve even relatively normal speech.

Conductive Hearing Loss: Effect on Development of Communication

Children, unless they have some congenital deformity involving the external ear or the middle ear, are not born with conduction impairment. In the great majority of individuals who acquire a conductive loss, it is secondary to middle ear disease, much of which is associated with upper respiratory infection and/or failure of eustachian tube ventilation of the middle ear. Onset may be prior to 2 years of age, and incidence of such impairment peaks during the years of primary school.

Conductive hearing impairment can be very subtle because it fluctuates and may even disappear for long periods, especially during the summer months, when there is a low incidence of upper respiratory infections. Because all tones are impaired neary equally and the inner ear functions normally, hearing is suppressed rather than distorted, so speech with enough volume is clearly heard and understood. The child hears conversation very well over the telephone because he has good bone conduction and the phone amplifies speech. Because his hearing is not distorted, his speech is not distorted. Identification of children with a moderate conductive loss is usually late, and many are missed until the middle school years unless there is a careful hearing-screening program in school.

The Effect on the Child

Children with hearing impairments are handicapped. They all have a slower than normal learning rate of language and speech, and when they enter school, they have greater difficulty than the normal child even when given special help. Sensorineural hearing loss results in poor speech, and the conductive handicap causes great difficulty in school because of an inability to hear the average classroom teacher and failure to develop normal communications with contemporaries and within the family circle.

As the child with impaired hearing advances into a more complicated communication environment, he encounters greater difficulty in keeping up with his contemporaries. He has to bluff more; he understands less and is subject to abuse for not being more attentive. His attempts to monitor a conversation visually are often mistaken for hyperactivity. Such stress often results in rebellion against the environment. The child stops trying to listen and isolates himself. He no longer makes an effort in school. Many such children react by becoming quite antisocial. Their presumed hyperactivity, their inability to communicate, and their combativeness are frequently mistaken for brain damage or mental retardation. The fact that some of the children born with sensorineural hearing impairment also have other neurologic defects may cause a physician who makes only a casual survey of the situation to overlook completely the diagnosis of hearing impairment.

Early Identification

The most important contribution a pediatrician or family physician can make in such situations is early identification of the hearing impairment. Such early identification may mean the difference between highly successful and poor rehabilitation.

The pediatrician and general practitioner are the individuals regularly attending such children and should be responsible for raising the first suspicion of possible loss, which should lead to establishment of the type and degree of the hearing loss. The tools necessary to identify a hearing problem in a child are available to all doctors and are very simple, but they must be employed by a physician with a high index of suspicion. When evaluating a communicatively handicapped child's mental capacity (IQ), it should be remembered that he may well fail a test planned for the child with normal hearing even though he has above-average intelligence.

Examination of a child suspected of having a hearing impairment should include determination of whether the child should be classified as belonging on a high-risk register, a careful history, a physical examination including a competent neurologic survey, and a hearing test. Of these, the most important for the physician who is not an otologist is the history. A high-risk registry and an outline for history taking in the case of a questionable hearing loss are outlined in the next sections.

HIGH-RISK REGISTRY

Repeated hearing studies were carried out in Baltimore between 1960 and 1971 on 1,182 selected children during their first 8 years of life. The children were born of women classified before delivery as threatening a high risk to their offspring because of their history or because of problems that occurred during their pregnancy (Table 3-1). Twenty-one percent of the children failed to give normal responses to pure-tone audiometry at age 8. Five percent presented findings of sensorineural loss, 11.6% of conductive hearing loss, and 3.6% of mixed loss. These figures far exceeded the national average of hearing-impaired children 8 years of age and thus emphasized the critical need of employing a high-risk registry when examining children suspected of hearing loss.

TABLE 3-1. *The high-risk registry*

Prenatal period	Delivery	Postnatal period
Family history of deafness	Birth injury	Unexplained high
Family history of anatomic	Breech	fever
maldevelopment of any	Forceps	Meningitis/encephalitis
kind	Prolonged engagement	Mumps
History of erythroblastosis	in the birth canal	Measles
Toxemia of pregnancy	Sever cyanosis	Scarlet fever
Prenatal viral infection of	Prematurity	Chickenpox
the mother		Influenza
Rubella		Otitis media
Chickenpox		Ototoxic drugs
Cytomegaly		Head injuries
Measles		
Unexplained high		
fever		
History of frequent		
miscarriages		
History of medication		
during pregnancy that		
could be considered		
ototoxic		

HISTORY TAKING

A complete personal and family history is an important part of any assessment. To optimize a physician's chances of being alerted to a hearing deficit, the history should include the data listed in the specimen history form illustrated in Table 3-2.

REACTION TO SOUND

A normal child's reactions to sound evolve with age. Table 3-3 shows normal responses to sound at 3, 6, 9, and 12 months of age along with landmarks of motor development.

TABLE 3-2. *Pertinent information to be obtained when studying a young child with possible hearing loss*

Sex
Birth date
Age (in years and months)
Family history
  Hearing impairment, age of onset in parents and grandparents
  Age of siblings (list any defects: bony, neurologic, hearing)
  Miscarriages
History of pregnancy
  Rh compatibility
  Mother's illness during pregnancy (particularly viral infections, high fevers, rashes, exposure to rubella)
  Immunization of mother before or during pregnancy
  Bleeding
  Toxemia
  Premature birth
Delivery
  Normal or prolonged
  Induced; forceps
  Drugs employed
  Delayed crying and breathing
  Cyanosis
  Jaundice
Postdelivery
  Appearance of baby (good color, cyanotic, head battered, rash, alert)
  Apgar rating
General health
  Growth rate
Serious illnesses
  Convulsions or loss of consciousness
  Children's diseases
  Unexplained high fevers
  Illness associated with immunization
  Serious injuries
  Exposure to high noise levels
  Neurologic defects
  Eye problems
  Cardiac defects

(continues)

TABLE 3-2. *(cont.)*

ENT
  Otitis media
  Mouth breathing
  Tonsillitis
  Frequent upper respiratory infection
  Allergies
  Previous operations
Drugs
  Medications received by the child that might be considered ototoxic
Development
  General
    Age of onset of walking
    Age of self-feeding
    Age of toilet training
  Speech and language
    Babble: Did it stop? When?
    Speech: age of onset; size of vocabulary
    When did child use two-word sentences?
    Is speech understandable?
    Does child understand mother's speech without pantomime?
    Is vocabulary development normal?
  Hearing
    Response to noises in the local environment
    Response to human voice, to being called—at what distance?
    Attention to radio/TV when screen cannot be seen
    Other indications of awareness of sound, not vibration
  Social maturity
    Self-management of clothes and toilet habits
    What are typical play activities?
    How adjusted toward other children?
    Temper tantrums
    Is there hyperactivity?
    Is he easily distracted?
    Does he endlessly repeat a single activity (perseveration)?
  Education or group activities
    Level
    Progress

PHYSICAL EXAMINATION

1. Glands should be examined. Any enlargement, especially that around the parotid or submaxillary salivary glands, should be noted.
2. The ear should be examined for a patent external canal and a normal-appearing tympanic membrane. Any fluid or bubbles behind the tympanic membrane should be noted.
3. Patency of both nostrils should be tested.
4. Nasopharynx should be examined for adenoid masses.
5. Size of tonsils should be checked for possible airway obstruction.
6. The palate should be checked for clefts and increased postpalatal space.

TABLE 3-3. *Reaction to sound and motor development*

At 3 months
  Can be startled by sudden loud sounds
  Stops feeding at sudden new sound
  Moves or jerks in sleep at sudden sounds
  (A brain-damaged child of this age can give the same responses to sound stimulation.)
  Motor activity: can lift head
At 6 months
  Turns toward sudden sound
  Will stop crying to listen
  Begins to recognize mother's voice
  Recognizes environmental sounds, e.g., preparing bottle, sound of bowl and spoon;
    searches (eye movement) for sound source
  Makes play sounds, enjoys vocalizing
  Motor development: can roll self over
At 9 months
  Responds to name
  Tries to form words
  Recognizes certain voices
  Motor development: can sit alone
At 12 months
  Uses consonants when he vocalizes
  Speaks words and uses word-like sounds for objects
Calls for attention
Motor development: can stand with self-support

HEARING EVALUATION

1. Check child's hearing by placing mother out of sight and let her address the child using familiar words at normal intensity; increase the intensity until the child responds.
2. Use rattles or strike spoons on a wooden block or use child's own noisy toys, unseen by child, at a distance of about 2 ft. Observe reaction.
3. A tuning fork of 512 Hz can be useful when moderately struck and slowly advanced from 2 ft to 1 to 2 inches from the ear when not seen by the child.

Note that any vibratory stimulus should be avoided when creating sounds. Remember that the vibration can travel through the floor to the child's feet and through a low- or mid-range tuning fork when struck hard and held near or in contact with the ear or skull.

Any child consistently failing to respond to sound stimuli at moderately increased intensity or failing a school hearing screening test or one who has a history of slow language and speech development, who has difficulty keeping up in school, or who becomes withdrawn and combative as communication becomes more complicated deserves a consultation with an otologist for definitive testing of the hearing.

The four most common causes for early failure to identify hearing disorders in children are mislabeling of the child's problem, dismissal of parental concern about a child's hearing, assumption that a child is too young to test, and a lack of information about available testing facilities. Such problems can be eliminated by contacting an otologist, a community health center, or a hearing and speech center at a large medical center.

PEDIATRICIAN'S ROLE IN REHABILITATION OF THE COMMUNICATIVELY IMPAIRED CHILD

After a hearing loss has been established, its type and degree determined, and the child's mental capabilities measured, the otologist, pediatrician, and individual in charge of rehabilitation should meet with the family and child to diagram a program for the child. The pediatrician should thoroughly understand the cause of hearing loss and the rehabilitation program. From that time, he should act in an advisory capacity. He should carefully check the child during any infectious disease and upper respiratory infections and determine the condition of the ears, especially to rule out serous or acute otitis media. He should counsel the family on the dangers of exposing the child to high noise levels and warn them against reckless underwater swimming and diving. He should take the greatest care to protect the child from the use of ototoxic drugs.

When planning rehabilitation, the first consideration should be to determine if the hearing can be improved through surgery or by amplification or both, because any gain in hearing efficiency, no matter how small, is extremely valuable for the child's future development of communicative skills. After such corrective measures have been completed, the final hearing level should be established and a course of training designed. This design depends on several factors: the level of hearing of the child and the age at which the hearing impairment occurred, the age and development of the child, and the family environment in which the child lives.

The young child (1 to 2 years) born with a severe hearing impairment requires a complete program of habilitation including basic training in lip reading, language, articulation, and speech. In such a program, plans must be made for the education of the family to prepare them for the special problems they will face when raising a hearing-impaired child because that child must be taught the rudiments of lip-reading language, speech, and vocabulary at home. Close consultation must be maintained through the developing years among the pediatrician, the family, and the teachers. After the child reaches 2.5 to 3 years of age, he may begin more formal instruction, as in kindergarten, where he can receive special instruction once or twice a week. Such formal instruction does not end the family's responsibilities for teaching at home, however, because home instruction is very necessary to reinforce any classroom work.

As the child approaches school age, a decision must be made about whether he should be placed in the regular school system (mainstreaming), in a special school, or in a special boarding school dedicated to the instruction of severely communicatively handicapped children. It should be emphasized that there are very real advantages for a child to live at home, especially if he has helpful parents and cooperative siblings. The family creates a normal environment in which to be raised and can contribute to the special teaching as well as furnish emotional security. Other children in the family may also be good teachers for their handicapped sibling. In "broken homes" or homes where there is little or no support given the child, especially when there are no brothers and sisters, the child may do better when placed in a boarding school where he will have contact with teachers acting as surrogate parents and other children with whom to interact.

Mainstreaming means entering the regular school system, where there is daily contact and competition with normal children. Here the hearing-impaired child receives additional special instruction to help keep up with the classwork and to help further develop lip reading, language, speech, and vocabulary skills. Mainstreaming has some advantages because the child lives in a normal environment and is in contact with normal children, which undoubtedly is excellent training for a youngster who must face a normal world when he grows up. However, it must be remembered that he has to work much harder than his normal-hearing fellow students to maintain the same level of school work. To succeed in such a program, the child must have above-average mental competence, and unless he gets along easily with other children and has determination, he may find difficulty in being accepted by his classmates, especially at recess time and in after-school activities because of the difficulty in communicating with them. Hearing-impaired children who have been mainstreamed require a great deal of support from family members who should frequently confer with teachers and always visit a new teacher and discuss any new program. Parents should insist on preferential classroom seating for the child and should take an active part in the local PTA.

Some hearing-impaired children, although of average intelligence, who suffer severe hearing loss are unable to meet the competition of regular schools. The child of average intelligence who has a hearing handicap usually has a slower learning rate than his normal-hearing classmates. Learning problems will result in added hours of tutoring and special education. Such a situation, especially with an only child who is shy, may be seriously embarrassing to him when he compares his handicap with the advantages of normal hearing. This will result in his trying to withdraw from contact with his classmates, and eventually he can fall seriously behind. Those children who have great difficulty keeping up will undoubtedly do better in a specially structured learning situation, such as in a special class or in a special school where the environment is designed to promote communication. Some children with very little or no hearing who have exhibited very little aptitude for learning lip reading may learn to communicate better with a combination of lip reading and signing (total communication), but they should be given every opportunity to learn lip reading before this combination is tried.

Children suffering only a moderate permanent hearing loss present a different problem in education. They can communicate by ear as well as by eye, and their education should be planned for mainstreaming. If the hearing has been very poor before some of it has been recovered by means of surgery and/or amplification, the child will need some basic instruction in language as well as speech and lip reading, and this should be begun as early as possible. In this case, home instruction is necessary, as is an early start in a kindergarten prepared to teach the hearing-impaired child. After kindergarten, plans should be made to enter the child in a regular school that has the facilities for some special education. His schedule should be planned to include some time for special instruction in speech and lip reading.

The children with moderate to moderately severe conductive hearing loss need much less special instruction than those suffering sensorineural hearing loss because they hear undistorted speech: when they hear a word, it has all its normal components. If the children with conductive hearing loss are very young when fitted with an aid, they must be taught some language as well as speech and have some additional work on vocabulary. These children also do better if they get some instruction in lip reading.

The child with a moderate sensorineural loss has distorted hearing with a loss most marked in the high tones (above 250 Hz), which allows him to hear only the low-tone portions of a word. Such hearing results in his speech lacking sibilant sounds, which causes great difficulty in understanding for anyone trying to communicate with the child. A program for such a child should not only be designed for teaching lip reading, speech, and vocabulary, but some time must be devoted to instruction in correct pronunciation of words containing the high-tone sounds that the child does not hear so that he may be understood by those he communicates with. This is a tedious and frequently disappointing task for the child, teacher, and family and can be achieved only through careful instruction followed by practice and correction at home. The learning of a vocabulary is of necessity slow for such a child.

The best aids to provide vocabulary acquisition for all hearing-impaired children are reading and writing. Reading should be stressed in every program for them, and the permissive use of television should be discouraged.

The child with mild hearing loss usually gets along very well in a regular school setting provided a few concessions are made in the classroom and he receives some planned support in instruction. The child with conductive loss as well as one with a sensorineural loss needs preferential seating, and the teacher should make a special effort to face such a child when instructing the class. Children suffering conductive loss as well as those with sensorineural loss may need some help in homework and lip reading to keep them from dropping behind. The child with a mild sensorineural loss needs time set aside for special instruction as well. This help should be in speech to avoid distortion in speech production as much as possible. Like any child with a mild handicap, these children need understanding and support at home.

One factor must be emphasized: the importance for the family and the school-teachers to maintain rules of discipline for hearing-handicapped children. There is a tendency, especially for the family, to excuse breaches in discipline because the child is handicapped. This is one of the cruelest things that can happen to a child with such a handicap. He, more than the normal child, needs the security of knowing the rules of behavior in his family life as well as at school. He must realize that there are penalties to be paid for transgression of such rules. A permissive home environment for him may alienate his siblings, can cause him trouble in school, may weaken his determination, and, worst of all, may lower his morale. On the other hand, great care must be exercised by the family and the teacher not to discipline him for any breach resulting from his hearing loss, e.g., misunderstanding of instructions, failure to come from a distance when called, failure to understand when receiving instructions if the instructor's face is not visible. When a breach of discipline occurs under other circumstances, however, the child should be treated as a normal child, and if he has normal siblings, he should face the same type of discipline they do.

Much can be done today for the child with a hearing loss, but constant close cooperation is needed between the child, family, teacher, and pediatrician or general practitioner.

SELECTED READING

Brookhouser, P., and Bordley, J. E. (1980): Childhood communication disorders, present status and future priorities. *Ann. Otol. Rhinol. Laryngol.* [*Suppl.* 74], 80.

Hardy, W. G. (1970): *Communication and the Disadvantaged Child.* Williams & Wilkins, Baltimore.

Konigsmark, B. W., and Gorlin, J. G. (1976): *Genetic and Metabolic Deafness.* W. B. Saunders, Philadelphia.

Special issue (1979): Communication disorders in children. *Ear Nose Throat J.* 58(7).

Whetnall, E., and Fry, B. D. (1964): *The Deaf Child.* Whitefriars Press, London.

Chapter 4

Nose and Accessory Nasal Sinuses

Fetal Development 229
  Nose 229
  Accessory Nasal Sinuses 232
Anatomic Description 236
  Anatomy 236
  Blood Supply 237
  Innervation 239
Functions of the Nose 241
  Respiration 241
  Olfaction 242
  Role of the Nasal Sinuses 243
Examination of the Nose 243
Examination of the Sinuses 246
Nasal Disorders 247
  Congenital Disorders 247
  Infections 249
  Allergy 253
  Vasomotor Rhinitis 254
  Nasal Polyps 254
  Hypertrophied Turbinate 257
  Nasal Deformity 257
  Foreign Bodies 258
  Hypertrophied Adenoids: Role in Nasal Disorders 258
  Epistaxis 258
Obstructive and Destructive Conditions of the Nose and Sinuses ...265
  Polyps 265
  Granulomas 265
  Fungus Infections 270
  Tumors of Nonepithelial Origin 270
  Tumors of Epithelial Origin 270
  Tumors of Connective Tissue Origin 275

Osseous Tumors 279
Fibro-Osseous Disorders 280
Tumors of Neural Origin 282
Tumors of Vascular Origin 284
Mesodermal Tumors 285
Cysts 286
Atrophic Rhinitis/Ozena 288
Sinusitis 289
Signs and Symptoms of Acute Sinusitis 289
Causal Factors 290
Prevention 291
Examination and Nonsurgical Treatment of a Child with
    Suspected Sinusitis 291
Chronic Sinusitis 291
Complications 293
        Cellulitis/Osteomyelitis/Cavernous Sinus Thrombosis/
        Meningitis/Epidural Abscess/Brain Abscess/
        Mucocele and Pyocele
Facial Trauma 303
General Measures 303
Fractures of the Nose 304
Fractures Involving Nasal Sinuses 307
        Fractures of the Zygoma/"Blow-Out" Fractures/Frontal
        Sinus Fractures/Fractures of the Maxillary Sinus
Facial Fractures 310
        Le Forte I/Le Forte II/ Le Forte III
Fractures of the Mandible 314

FETAL DEVELOPMENT

Nose

The nose is one of the first organs to develop in the embryo. Paired epithelial thickenings, the olfactory placodes, appear during the third week on the wall of the forebrain. During the fourth week, these placodes develop into crescent shapes, and the centers gradually sink in to form the olfactory pits. As the pits grow down and backward, they approach the roof of the developing oral cavity until only two layers of epithelium separate them (Fig. 4-1). The pits now divide the caudal end of the nasofrontal process into medial and lateral sections. The medial portions, which have the more rapid growth rate, lie lateral to the frontonasal process. They extend and fuse in the midline to form the columella and premaxillary process.

OROFACIAL REGION

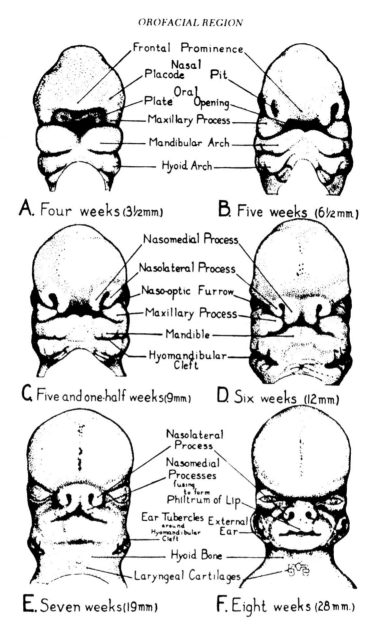

A. Four weeks (3½mm.)

B. Five weeks (6½mm.)

C. Five and one-half weeks (9mm.)

D. Six weeks (12mm.)

E. Seven weeks (19mm)

F. Eight weeks (28mm.)

FIG. 4-1. Development of the face. (Adapted from an original figure by W. Patten. From Patten, B.: *Human Embryology.* Blakiston, Philadelphia, 1946. With permission.)

During the third week, the first branchial arch splits to form the maxillary and mandibular processes. The maxillary process lies just lateral to the nasofrontal process and gradually fuses with the medial nasal process to form the inferior portion of the nasal vestibule and the ala nasi.

Compression of the tissue between the olfactory pits forms the primary nasal septum. The pits grow upward toward the brain and backward toward the oral cavity as separate pouches. They finally rupture the two-layered bucconasal membrane and merge with the oral cavity, forming the primitive choanae. The portion of the roof of the oral cavity that extends from the choanae to the nasal apertures forms the primitive palate (Fig. 4-1).

After the primitive palate is formed, the primitive nasal fossae increase in size, sink into the head between the eyes, and approach close to the brain. As they grow, the nasal fossae become oval and are separated from the remainder of the oral cavity by the true palate. The true palate is formed by the palatal ridges which appear on the maxillary process around the 45th day. These ridges grow caudally and medially as the primitive tongue descends, finally rotating medially and fusing with the primitive palate (Fig. 4-1).

Nasal Septum

During the sixth fetal week, the primary nasal septum (the medial nasal process) grows posteriorly, coincident with the lengthening of the nasal cavity anteroposteriorly. This transforms the primitive choanae into oval slits and facilitates their posterior migration. They lie on each side of the frontal process, which now becomes the posterior portion of the nasal septum.

The structures derived from the median nasal process by the time differentiation ceases are, from anterior to posterior, the columella, premaxilla, quadrilateral cartilage, perpendicular plate of the ethmoids, vomer, and crest of the palatine bone.

At birth the septum, unless fractured or dislocated during delivery (Fig. 4-2), lies in the midline and is straight. As the child grows to adulthood, the nose and cartilaginous septum may become curved or buckled into an "S" deformity as the result of growth stresses. These same stresses may cause dislocation of the cartilage from its inferior attachment to the maxillary crest. As the septum grows, a projection or spur may develop at the junction with the palatine crest. It usually is composed of cartilage and bone and may project from the midline into one or both nostrils; it can be obstructive (Fig. 4-3).

Lateral Nasal Wall

The lateral nasal wall in man differs from that in other mammals because of the reduction of the olfactory apparatus. This differentiation is associated with the formation of the turbinates or conchae and the recesses that lie between them, the meatuses. Killian stated that the conchal development is from three primary slit-

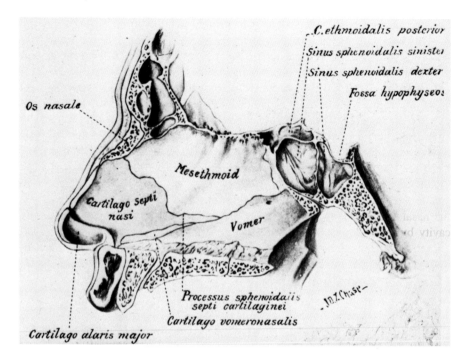

FIG. 4-2. Anatomy of the nasal septum. (From Onodi.)

like outpouchings from the lateral wall. These elevations are the maxilloturbinal, the ethmoturbinal, and the nasoturbinal. The maxilloturbinal in man becomes the inferior turbinate. The ethmoturbinal, which appears after and above the maxillo-turbinal, develops a second scroll just before birth and forms the middle and superior turbinates. The nasoturbinal remains rather rudimentary as a small ridge in front of the ethmoturbinal and becomes the agger nasi. Subsequent modification of the turbinates and the meatuses lying between them is associated with the first ap-pearance of the sinuses.

Accessory Nasal Sinuses

The nasal sinuses are irregular air-filled cavities adjacent to and communicating with the nose. In man there are an average of 13 ciliated mucous-membrane-lined cavities communicating with each nostril. They form the accessory nasal sinuses. These are divided into the maxillary sinus, the ethmoid complex (composed of 7 to 10 small air cells), the frontal sinus, and the sphenoid sinus.

The maxillary and frontal sinuses develop from direct extrusions (buds) from the nasal fossae, whereas the ethmoid cells and the sphenoid sinuses are primarily constrictions from the nasal fossae.

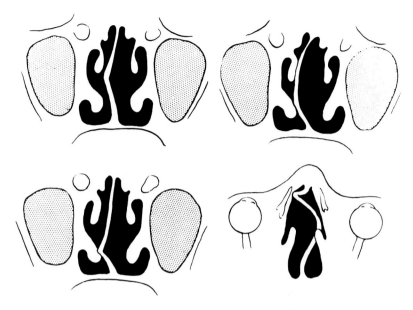

FIG. 4-3. Common deflections of the nasal septum. (From Deweese and Saunders: *Textbook of Otolaryngology*, p. 219. Mosby, St. Louis, 1968. With permission.)

The maxillary sinus, which at maturity has a capacity of 8 to 12 cc of air and occupies most of the space inferior to the orbit lateral to the nose and superior to the hard palate, first appears in the embryo during the middle of the third month as a small epithelium-lined sac at the side of the nasal fossae from which it has originated. By the sixth month, it measures about 5 mm across, and at birth it is 7 to 8 mm (Fig. 4-4). Until the eruption of the milk teeth, its growth is inhibited, and after the eruption of the first permanent teeth at six years, growth is further accelerated, and the sinus begins to assume its irregular adult shape. The first and second molar teeth and the second biscuspid remain in close approximation to the floor of the sinus. Infection around the teeth can affect the health of the maxillary sinus.

The ethmoid bone consists of two plates and two lateral masses. The median plate forms a portion of the nasal septum, and the cribriform plate attached to it at the top forms the roof of the nasal cavity and the cribriform process on each side. The lateral masses are attached to the lateral borders of the two plates. The masses lie on each side between the nasal cavity and the orbit. Within these masses the ethmoid cells develop, and they communicate with the nostril. Those cells draining into the middle meatus are designated the anterior cells. Those emptying above the posterior portion of the middle turbinate are the posterior ethmoid cells. The ethmoid cells are present at birth.

The frontal sinus (Fig. 4-5), which lies above the orbital roof and varies greatly in size and shape, is formed by extrusion of the nasal fossa during the third fetal

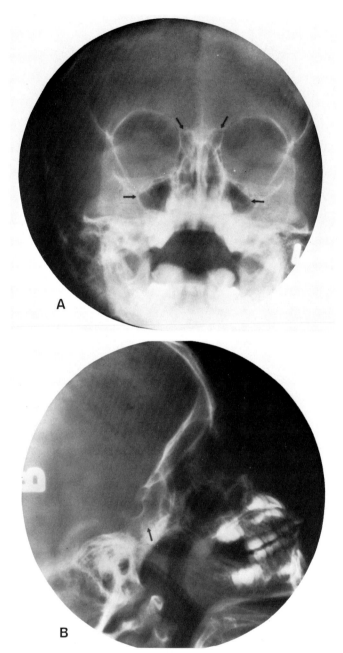

FIG. 4-4. Anteroposterior **(A)** and lateral **(B)** X-ray films showing normal sinus development in a 4-year-old girl. Note early development of the frontal sinus (*arrow*) and early growth of the maxillary antra (*arrow*). Lateral view shows unaerated sphenoid sinus (*arrow*).

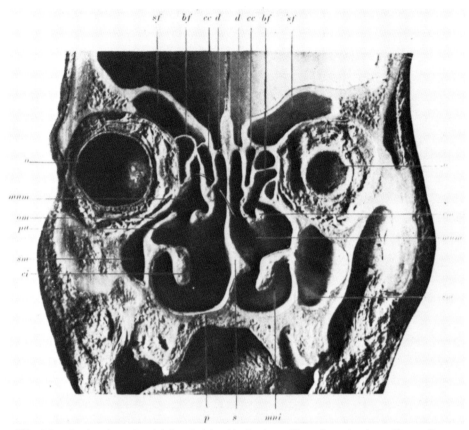

FIG. 4-5. Section through adult head. (*o*) orbit. (*sm*) maxillary sinus. (*om*) maxillary orifice. (*ci*) inferior turbinate. (*cm*) middle turbinate. (*s*) septum. (*mni*) inferior meatus. (*mnm*) middle meatus. (*bf*) (*cc*) ethmoid sinuses. (*sf*) frontal sinus. (*d*) cribriform plate. (From Onodi.)

month. It is so small that it is not recognized as a sinus until 6 or 7 years of age and remains small until puberty. It lies between the inner and outer tables of the frontal bone. In 4% of adults, only one frontal sinus develops.

The sphenoid sinus, which is the last to reach maturity, is formed by partial isolation of the posterior portion of the primitive nasal fossa during the third month. It remains rudimentary until the sixth or seventh year, when rapid absorption of the surrounding cancellous bone takes place, opening up the sinus, which continues to increase in size for another 7 to 8 years.

All the accessory sinuses are lined with ciliated, columnar, respiratory mucous membrane. All drain into the nose through ostia toward which the cilia of the lining membrane sweep the surface mucous blanket formed by the underlying goblet cells and the mucous and serous glands.

ANATOMIC DESCRIPTION

Anatomy

The child's nose has all the essential anatomic features of the adult nose, but in a number of areas, ossification is still proceeding. The nasal pyramid continues to grow for many years after birth. It consists of the paired nasal bones, the frontal processes of the maxillae (which form the ridged support of the upper nose), and the paired upper lateral cartilages (which are attached above to the under edge of the nasal bone and below to the underside of the upper edge of the lower lateral cartilage) (Fig. 4-6). The lower lateral cartilages form the flare and curve of the ala and most of the tip of the nose. They are divided into a lateral and medial crus. Molding of the nasal contours is additionally influenced by the lesser alar cartilages just lateral to the lower lateral cartilages and the fibroadipose tissue attached to the lower edge of the lower lateral cartilages. Additional support for the cartilaginous portion of the nasal pyramid is supplied by the anterior portion of the nasal septum and columella.

The internal nose is formed by the nasal septum medially and the medial wall of the maxilla and the ethmoid complex laterally. The turbinate bones (conchae) are attached to the lateral wall of each nostril and direct the air flow through the nostril. They consist of the superior, middle, and inferior turbinates and are attached to the lateral wall through the long axis running anteriorly and posteriorly from the vestibule to the nasopharynx. The superior and middle turbinates are outgrowths of the ethmoid complex. The inferior turbinate, the largest, is a separate bone that is attached to both the ethmoid complex and the maxilla. The longitudinal spaces between the turbinates and bounded by the medial wall of the maxilla are the superior, middle, and inferior meatuses (Fig. 4-7). The frontal sinus, anterior and middle ethmoid cells, and maxillary sinus all drain into the middle meatus, whereas the posterior ethmoid cells discharge into the superior meatus. The nasolacrimal duct empties into the anterior end of the inferior meatus. A rudimentary turbinate called the supreme turbinate is above and anterior to the superior turbinate and eventually becomes the agger nasi.

The development of the turbinates is somewhat governed by the shape of the septum. When there is a significant deflection of the septum to one side, compensatory hypertrophy of the turbinate takes place on the open side of the nose, thus tending to equalize the size of the air passages on the two sides. The turbinates, which are bulbous at their anterior ends, are rather streamlined, gradually tapering in size as they approach the nasopharynx. They divide the passage of air into narrow streams and deflect them up and back toward the olfactory mucous membrane. Olfactory mucous membrane covers the superior turbinate as well as the upper portion of the septum and extends up through the olfactory cribriform plate. This mucous membrane is slightly yellowish and differs from respiratory mucous membrane in that it lacks cilia. The mucous membrane covering the middle and inferior turbinates contains cavernous venous spaces that can expand or contract, thus

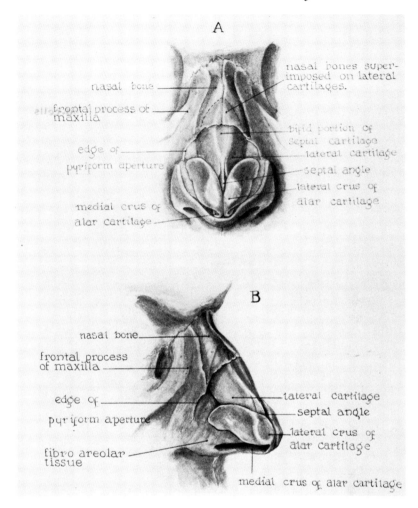

FIG. 4-6. Anatomy of the nasal pyramid: frontal **(A)** and lateral **(B)** aspects. (From Kazanjian, V. H., and Converse, J. M.: *Surgical Treatment of Facial Fractures,* p. 222. Williams & Wilkins, Baltimore, 1959.)

changing the size of the turbinates in order to regulate airflow and the temperature of inspired air and to modify the moisture content of the air.

Blood Supply

The blood supply to the nose is very rich and arises from a number of sources. The sphenopalatine branch of the internal maxillary artery supplies the nasal septum, turbinates, and meatuses (Fig. 4-8). The other principal source is the ophthalmic

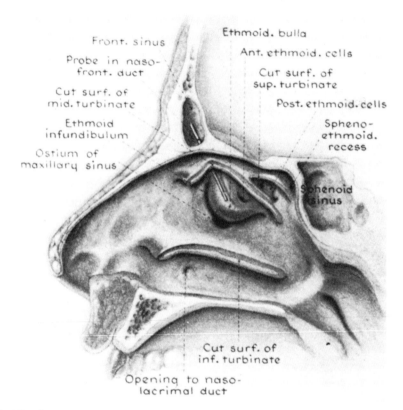

Front. sinus

Probe in naso-
front. duct

Cut surf. of
mid. turbinate

Ethmoid
infundibulum

Ostium of
maxillary sinus

Ethmoid. bulla

Ant. ethmoid. cells

Cut surf. of
sup. turbinate

Post. ethmoid. cells

Spheno-
ethmoid.
recess

Sphenoid
sinus

Cut surf. of
inf. turbinate

Opening to naso-
lacrimal duct

FIG. 4-7. Right lateral nasal wall, showing the relationships of the turbinates. (From Boies, L. R.: *Fundamentals of Otolaryngology*, p. 162. W. B. Saunders Co., Philadelphia, 1959. With permission.)

artery, which through its anterior, middle, and posterior ethmoid branches supplies the vault of the internal nose, the frontal sinus, and the ethmoid sinuses. The maxillary sinus is supplied by branches of the infraorbital, superior labial, and internal maxillary artery, and the sphenoid sinus receives its arterial blood from the pharyngeal branch of the internal maxillary arteries. The maxillary crest and inferior septum receive blood from a branch of the greater palatine artery. The venous system, which forms the cavernous spaces over the turbinates, lies beneath the mucous membrane and drains through the ophthalmic and sphenopalatine veins. There is a very rich plexus of veins on each side of the anterior septum [Kiesselbach's (Little's) plexus], which is very vulnerable to trauma from outside (see Fig. 4-21, below). Trauma of this area results in the majority of man's epistaxis. Veins draining the blood from this plexus and from the cavernous tissue of the turbinates drain in three directions: forward to the facial vein, backward to the sphenopalatine vein, and upward into the ethmoid veins. The venous drainage of the frontal sinus is separately described in the section on osteomyelitis of the frontal sinus.

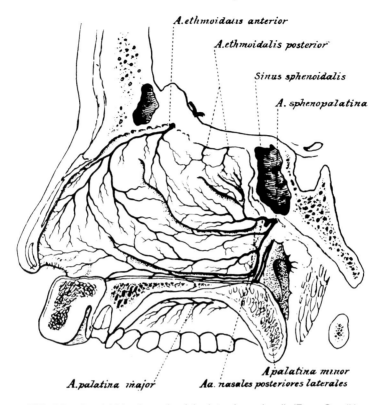

A.ethmoidalis anterior

A.ethmoidalis posterior

Sinus sphenoidalis

A. sphenopalatina

A.palatina major   *Aa. nasales posteriores laterales*   *A palatina minor*

FIG. 4-8. Arterial blood supply of the lateral nasal wall. (From Onodi.)

Innervation

The muscles of the external nose are innervated by branches of the seventh cranial nerve. The nasal spaces and the accessory sinuses are supplied principally by sensory fibers from the ophthalmic and maxillary branches of the fifth cranial nerve. The septum receives fibers from the anterior and posterior branches of the ophthalmic division and from the nasopalatine nerve out of the sphenopalatine ganglion (Fig. 4-9A). The latter crosses downward over the septum, anastomosing with the opposite side after passing through the anterior palatine canal. The nasociliary branch of the ophthalmic division supplies branches to the anterior portion of the nasal cavity and the anterior ends of the turbinates. The sphenopalatine nerve, which supplies branches to the bodies of the turbinates (Fig. 4-9B), enters the nasal space through the sphenopalatine foramen, which is located just behind and above the posterior end of the middle turbinate. The sphenopalatine ganglion, in which these fibers arise, is important because it receives and gives off parasympathetic fibers from the greater superficial petrosal nerve and sympathetic fibers from the deep petrosal nerve. The sphenoid sinus is innervated by fibers from the sphenopalatine ganglion.

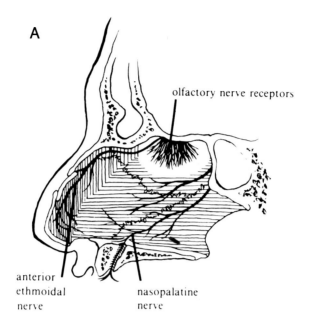

olfactory nerve receptors

anterior
ethmoidal
nerve

nasopalatine
nerve

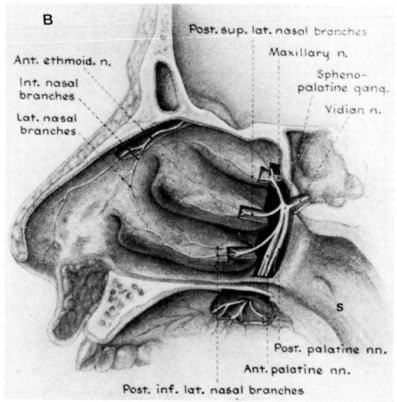

B

Post. sup. lat. nasal branches

Ant. ethmoid. n.

Maxillary n.

Int. nasal
branches

Spheno-
palatine gang.

Lat. nasal
branches

Vidian n.

S

Post. palatine nn.

Ant. palatine nn.

Post. inf. lat. nasal branches

FIG. 4-9. Nerve supply of the nasal septum **(A)** and the lateral nasal wall **(B)**. (A: From English, G.: *Anatomy of the Nose and Nasopharynx*, Vol. 2, Chapter 1.N, p. 14. Harper & Row, Philadelphia, 1984. With permission. B: From Boies, L. R.: *Fundamentals of Otolaryngology*, p. 167. Saunders, Philadelphia, 1959. With permission.)

The maxillary sinus receives filaments from the infraorbital nerve through its superior dental branches. The frontal sinus receives its nerve supply from branches of the supraorbital and nasal nerves, whereas the ethmoid cells receive fibers from the ethmoid branches of the nasociliary nerve.

FUNCTIONS OF THE NOSE

Respiration

Inspired air does not move in a flat anteroposterior direction between the vestibule of the nose and nasopharynx; rather, most of it moves in an arc, passing above the inferior turbinate and through the middle and superior meatus, where it is broken into narrow streams (Figs. 4-10, 4-11), exposing it to greater contact with the mucous membrane of the turbinates, the olfactory mucous membrane, and the septum.

In man, the chief function of the nose is in the support of respiration. The vibrissae in the vestibule of each nostril act as screens to filter out lightweight foreign bodies in the incoming air. The mucous blanket, secreted by the mucous glands and goblet cells in the mucous membrane, is propelled by the cilia toward the nasopharynx (Fig. 1-11) (see Chapter 1). The mucous blanket performs two functions: it is an air cleaner and a humidifier. It transports minute particles deposited from the air on its sticky surface to the nasopharynx and from there into the mouth to be swallowed. The enzyme lysozyme contained in the mucus has a bacteriostatic action. The mucous blanket provides the source of moisture that is added to dry, inspired

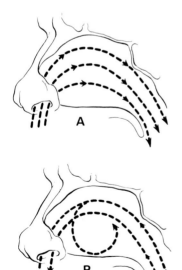

FIG. 4-10. Direction of air flow in the nose. **A:** Inspiratory current. **B:** Expiratory current. (From Ballinger, H. C., and Ballinger, B. S.: *Otology, Rhinology and Laryngology,* 4th edition. Lea & Fibiger, 1954.) (After Proetz.)

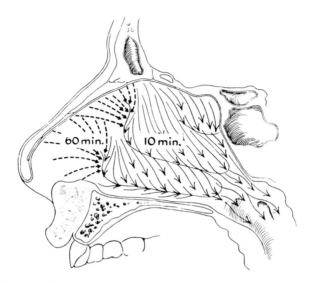

FIG. 4-11.   Direction and rate of flow of mucus in the nose. (From Boies, L. R.: *Fundamentals of Otolaryngology,* p. 167. W. B. Saunders, Philadelphia, 1959. With permission.)

air as it begins its final moisture saturation on its passage down the trachea and bronchi to the alveoli. The mucous membrane recovers a large amount of fluid (30%) given off during inspiration from that same air on expiration. The fluid exchange is facilitated by two mechanisms: (a) mucus can absorb and release fluid in proportion to the fluid content of the air in contact with it; and (b) air is warmed by the surrounding mucous membrane of the nose and turbinates as it passes toward the nasopharynx, thereby increasing its ability to carry a higher humidity, and is cooled on expiration, thereby lowering its humidity. The heat exchange in the nose is carried out largely by the turbinates, which provide a mucous membrane surface that can be expanded or contracted to regulate the internal dimension of the nasal passages and in which the temperature can be controlled by regulating the rate of blood flow through the venous spaces. In short, it is the nose that first cleans the air, heats and humidifies it, and prepares for its passage down the trachea and bronchi and into the alveoli (see Chapter 1).

Olfaction

Inspired or expired air passing through the vault of the nose contacts the olfactory mucous membrane where the branches of the olfactory nerve and olfactory end-organs lie. Nerve fibers from these end-organs pass upward through the cribriform plate, forming the first cranial nerve. The olfactory mucous membrane, which lacks cilia and has more cuboidal cells than the respiratory mucous membrane, covers the nasal vault and extends down over the upper portion of the superior turbinate

and to about the same level on the superior septum. Any alteration of the configuration of the upper nose that prevents air passage over this membrane can inhibit
the sense of smell (anosmia). The most common cause of anosmia is swollen nasal
mucous membrane resulting from the common cold or allergic rhinitis. Polyps,
scarring of the mucous membrane following trauma or surgery to the nose, or
tumors (nasal or intercranial) may also cause anosmia. Permanent anosmia of unknown origin is encountered in a number of patients without evidence of a causative
factor, although a number of authorities think it may be the result of a mild virus
infection.

The limited distribution of olfactory mucous membrane in man compared to that
in most other mammals suggests its decreasing importance as a warning signal and
its gradual denegration to the minor role of an aid to taste. The olfactory process
combines with the responses of the taste buds of the tongue to round out the gustatory
experience. In many animals, especially the carnivores, the olfactory mucous membrane covers a large percentage of the roof of the accessory nasal sinuses and
extends over the multiple turbinates found in the noses of such animals, resulting
in a much greater percentage of inspired and expired air coming into contact with
the olfactory surfaces than in man (see Chapter 1).

ROLE OF THE NASAL SINUSES

Much has been written about the function of the accessory nasal sinuses in man.
Negus believed that their original function was olfaction because in many animals
olfactory membrane is found in the sinuses. In man, however, the air exchange is
so small between the nose and the sinus that if olfactory mucous membrane were
present in the sinuses, it could not act very effectively. The ostia are so small in
man that the sinuses contribute little to the air-conditioning functions of the nose.
Air pressure in the sinuses drops during inspiration and increases on expiration—
opposite to the pressure in the lung. Today it is recognized that these sinuses are
capable of absorbing the force of blows directed toward the face with very little
damage resulting to the important structures lying behind them.

EXAMINATION OF THE NOSE

Determination of the nature of the disorders and diseases of the nose and sinuses
in an infant or young child can best be carried out by the attending physician
employing a number of simple examinations to establish the basic problems, after
which he can obtain further information from laboratory techniques such as cultures
and X-ray studies. The following steps are recommended.

1. *Inspection.* The child's face should be exposed in a good light and the following
   characteristics determined: swelling around the nose, over the cheeks, around
   the orbit, or of the eyelids; discoloration or inflammation of the skin over the

nose or sinuses; nasal discharges, unilateral or bilateral, and their character (clear, purulent, watery, or viscous). Note also if the child can breathe through one or both nostrils.

2. *Passage of catheter.* In infants, nasal patency can be determined by the passage of a soft catheter through the nose into the pharynx.

3. *Anterior rhinoscopy.* A light is projected into the nostril and directed along the floor of the nostril rather than into the nasal vault. Illumination can be obtained from a flashlight, a head light, or a head mirror (the latter two are much more effective and leave the examiner a free hand). The nasal tip should be elevated and the nostrils dilated in order to better expose the interior and permit better vision. Exposing the nasal passage can best be done with a nasal speculum. If the nostril is filled with discharge, it should be removed by having the patient blow the nose, by swabbing, or by applying gentle suction through a small suction tip attached to a rubber bulb or suction apparatus. When the nose is clear of discharge, the mucous membrane is examined for color and swelling, and the anterior ends of the inferior and middle turbinates are inspected to determine if they are swollen and obstructive (Fig. 4-12). Note if the septum is straight or if it deviates to one side enough to be obstructive. Note any nasal discharge and try to determine if it is coming from a specific meatus. Look for nasal polyps and foreign bodies. If the turbinates and nasal mucous membranes are so swollen as to obstruct examination, a drop of dilute phenylephrine solution (Neo-Synephrine®) can be placed in the nostril with the child in the prone position; within 4 to 5 min, the swelling should be reduced. Rhinoscopy seldom permits examination of a nostril beyond the anterior one-half but does give considerable information concerning nasal conditions. The child should be examined while in an upright position.

The following studies can be employed during nasal examination but require experience and training and are best done by otolaryngologists. They are described briefly to permit better understanding of consultation reports.

4. *Posterior rhinoscopy.* This can be accomplished by the use of a small laryngeal-type mirror inserted into the open mouth held just anterior to the posterior pharyngeal wall and directed upward toward the nasopharynx behind the soft palate. Here again, illumination is important and can best be obtained from a head light or a head mirror. A satisfactory examination can reveal the vault of the nasopharynx with the arch and posterior insertion of the septum, the eustachian tube orifices, the posterior openings of the nostrils (choanae), the posterior wall of the nasopharynx, and the adenoids.

5. *Nasopharyngoscopy.* This technique should not be attempted without careful training. It consists of passing a small periscope or fiberoptic flexible laryngoscope (2–3 mm) that provides its own illumination along the floor of the nose or through the middle meatus. With the angled vision obtained, it is possible to visualize the maxillary sinus orifice, the region of the anterior ethmoid orifices, bony growths on the septum, the sphenoid sinus orifice, the eustachian tube

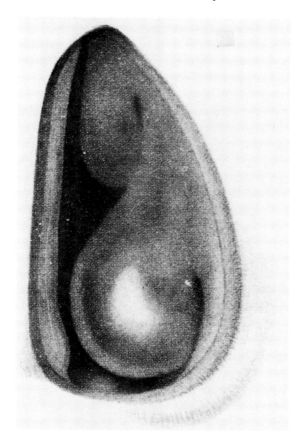

FIG. 4-12. Anterior rhinoscopy of the normal nose, showing the septum and middle and inferior turbinates. (From Hall, I. S., and Colman, B. H.: *Diseases of the Nose, Throat, and Ear,* p. 24. E & S Livingstone, Edinburgh, 1969. With permission.)

orifices, and the adenoids. Nasopharyngoscopy is also excellent for visualizing nasal polyps, foreign bodies that lie above the nasal floor, and some nasal and nasopharyngeal tumors. Only repeated use of the nasopharyngoscope will make it an effective diagnostic instrument.

6. *Rhinomanometry.* Like nasopharyngoscopy, rhinomanometry can give pertinent information. Its purpose is to measure the patency of the nostril for the passage of air and to determine nasal resistance to airflow. The instrumentation employed measures the amount of air passing through a nostril in a given time, during both inspiration and expiration. The conditions can be varied by the use of drugs that shrink the nasal mucous membrane and by variations in temperature and humidity.

7. *Ciliary transport.* Ciliary transport can be studied by placing various types of particles on the surface of the mucous blanket in the anterior portion of the

nostril and timing their appearance on the posterior pharyngeal wall. In the normal nose, the blanket is moved by ciliary action at a rate of up to 6 to 9 mm/min. Dry air, cold air, virus infections, and a number of drugs can alter the flow rate a great deal (see Chapter 1).

EXAMINATION OF THE SINUSES

1. *Inspection*. The child should be upright and placed in a good light as in the nasal examination. Swelling over the cheeks and around the orbit should be noted, and it should be determined if the swelling is inflammatory or cystic in character. Swelling of the eyelids and eye movement should also be checked, as well as equality of size of the pupils and pupillary response to light. Tenderness should be noted as well as crepitus over the brows and cheeks.
2. *Rhinoscopy*. For anterior rhinoscopy, nasal examination should be carried out as described in the section on the nose. Discharge and its location should be noted, and polyps should be identified. Posterior rhinoscopy should be carried out as described in the previous section.
3. *Nasopharyngoscopy*. This procedure is done as described above with emphasis on observation of discharge in the middle and superior meatuses.
4. *Transillumination of the maxillary sinus*. Maxillary sinus transillumination can be carried out by the pediatrician. The room should be completely dark, and a small flashlight placed on the tongue with the mouth closed around it. The maxillary sinuses will be illuminated. Any inequality of the illumination of the cheeks may indicate mucous membrane swelling, fluid, or polyp formation in the maxillary sinus on the less bright side. At times, such inequality of illu- mination results from one sinus being anatomically smaller than the other (Fig. 4-13).
5. *Transillumination of the frontal sinus*. Frontal sinus transillumination can be accomplished by placing a pencil light against the roof of each orbit on the medial side, directing the light upward, and comparing the illumination of the two sides. In children under 10 years of age, this is not a satisfactory examination because of the late pneumatization of the frontal sinuses (Fig. 4-13).
6. *X-ray examination*. X-ray examination of the sinuses has a distinct advantage over transillumination in that it visualizes the development and size of the child's sinuses. It can also give much information about the condition of the ethmoid and sphenoid sinuses as well as the maxillary and frontal sinuses. Polytomog- raphy and computed tomography (CT) scans can outline tumors and accurately define their position in the sinuses. Polytomography up to the present time seems best for the identification of sinus fractures. Note that all sinus X-ray films should be obtained in the erect position in order to identify fluid in the sinuses. A prone X-ray film does not show a fluid level, which is very important for identifying sinusitis (Fig. 4-14).

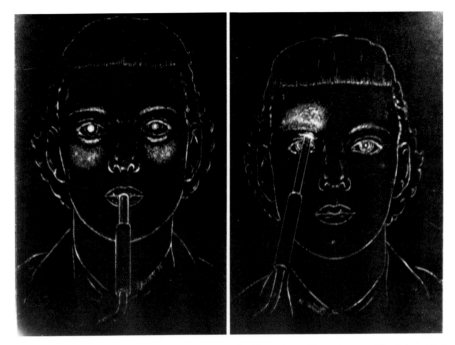

FIG. 4-13.   Transillumination of the sinuses. **Left:** Normal maxillary sinuses. The infraorbital areas light up with equal intensity. **Right:** Normal right frontal sinus. Frontal sinuses vary a great deal in their size and shape. They are frequently unequal in size, or one may even be undeveloped in an individual. (From Deweese and Saunders: *Textbook of Otolaryngology,* p. 27. Mosby, St. Louis, 1968. With permission.)

NASAL DISORDERS

Congenital Disorders

Atresia of the Nasal Passage

Unilateral or bilateral nasal obstruction in the newborn may result from choanal atresia. This is a development defect that arises from failure of the nasal–buccal membrane to rupture and the resulting retention of the posterior portion of the fetal nasal floor. The exact cause of this failure has not been fully explained. Estimates of its occurrence range from one in 60,000 births to a considerably higher incidence. This lack of consistency in medical statistics arises from the failure in many cases to make the diagnosis of unilateral atresia at birth. The obstruction may be bony or membranous, and it may be complete or partial with small perforations through the obstructing membrane (Fig. 4-15). It consists of a partition attached superiorly to the wall of the sphenoid sinus, laterally to the medial pterygoid process, medially

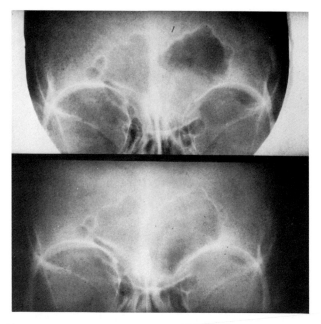

FIG. 4-14. X-rays of a boy with frontal sinusitis. These were taken at the same time, but the **upper view** was obtained when the patient was in the erect position and shows a fluid level in the left sinus. The **lower view** was taken when the patient was in a prone position and gives a very different impression of the condition of the sinus.

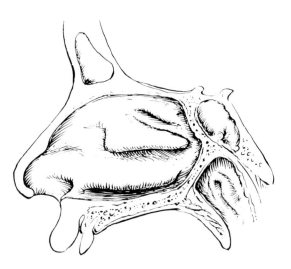

FIG. 4-15. Bony choanal artresia. This extreme form of artresia is caused by a bony partition extending from the posterior end of the hard palate to the basisphenoid. (From Benson, C. D. et al.: *Pedatric Surgery,* Vol. 1, p. 141. Year Book, Chicago, 1962. With permission.)

to the posterior edge of the vomer, and inferiorly to the horizontal process of the palatine bone. In some cases, partial obstruction results from an increased width of the posterior portion of the vomer and pterygoid process.

Unilateral atresia results in a chronic mucoid discharge from the obstructed nostril, which will be lined with smooth, swollen mucous membrane. Otherwise, it causes too few problems to warrant investigation of the infant's airway, so it may not be recognized until years later. Bilateral atresia in the newborn can be a serious emergency because it may result in asphyxiation in a suckling infant. Many newborns cannot adjust to mouth breathing while feeding. A nasal airway must be established if the infant is to be nourished. An indwelling airway may be required between feedings, and feeding by dropper, spoon, or gavage is usually necessary until the infant develops a rhythm of mouth breathing while sucking. Such infants require constant nursing care. A few infants adapt almost immediately after birth and are not critically endangered, but many do not. The time for surgery to relieve this obstruction depends greatly on the child's ability to adapt to its handicap and on its condition and nourishment. There is a general preference to postpone surgery and to allow growth and development of the nose and mouth. Diagnosis of complete unilateral or bilateral atresia should be made at the time of delivery by attempting to pass a small rubber catheter through each nostril into the pharynx. This examination should be a routine procedure at every delivery.

Syphilis

Acquired syphilis is rare in children, and congenital syphilis is also seldom seen in areas where adequate medical care is available. In congenital syphilis of the infant, the infection may come from passage through the birth canal, or it may be transplacental. The infant presents with "snuffles," an excoriating blood-tinged mucopurulent rhinitis, and nasal obstruction. Later there may be saddling of the nose secondary to destruction of the vomer, scarring around the mouth, and a prominent frontal bone. Pegged teeth appear later.

Histologically, biopsies show that obliterative endarteritis is very prominent, accompanied by epithelioid cells and fibroblasts. Small granulomas are present and are necrotic and avascular. Nontreponemal serologic tests can be used as a screening method followed by confirmatory treponemal serologic tests. For treatment of congenital syphilis, penicillin is presently the drug of choice.

Infections

Viral Infections

The common cold, which occurs three or four times a year in a normal child, can cause acute sinusitis. Sinusitis can result from the marked swelling of the nasal mucous membrane, especially over the turbinates and around the sinus orifices, which causes nasal obstruction and interference with normal drainage from the sinus through its orifice. The common cold is accompanied by marked watery nasal discharge, sneezing, and some coughing. After the third day the discharge becomes thicker, more tenacious, and more difficult to clear. If the discharge from one or both nostrils develops a purulent appearance on the fourth or fifth day, one should suspect that a secondary infection of bacterial origin is beginning to take over, which can involve the ethmoid sinuses and/or the maxillary sinuses. The average common cold is not ordinarily associated with fever and persists only 4 to 6 days, so the occurrence of fever is suggestive of some secondary infection in the sinuses or in the lower respiratory tract.

Children suffering from a cold show much variation in their responses to such a virus infection. These variations depend on the differences in bodily resistance to the infecting virus and on variation in the morbidity of the virus. A good rule to follow is to keep the child in bed at least 48 hr, force fluids, see that the room is well humidified, and except in the summer keep all windows of the bedroom closed at night. The child may be made more comfortable by raising his head on several pillows. For marked nasal obstruction, a mild nasal drop such as phenyleph-rine (Neo-Synephrine®) 0.25% may be used, or a mild vasoconstrictor can be administered by mouth. The average cold without fever should not be treated with antibiotics.

Influenza, which may be caused by a number of viral strains, presents as a febrile illness with generalized malaise and some cough. The upper respiratory tract in many instances is not involved, but when it is, the treatment should be the same as that outlined for the common cold. Influenza involving the upper respiratory tract is more likely to be followed by sinusitis than is the common cold.

Bacterial Infections

Acute or chronic bacterial infection of the nose or nasal sinuses usually follows viral infections and results from nasal and sinus swelling that interferes with proper drainage. The obstruction can be either unilateral or bilateral. Obstruction is more likely to occur when there is anatomic narrowing of a nostril, as by a septal deflection. In both acute and chronic sinusitis of bacterial origin, the nasal obstruc-tion is accompanied by a purulent nasal and/or postnasal discharge. The acute form usually runs a febrile course, and both may be associated with cough and/or tracheitis (see "Sinusitis," below).

Abscess of the nasal septum causes bilateral or unilateral nasal obstruction. It may result from trauma to the septum, excessive nose-picking, or septal surgery (Fig. 4-16). The abscess presents as a rather smooth swelling in the anterior portion of the septum in one or both nostrils. It is fluctuant and may be painful. It may or may not be accompanied by fever. The usual treatment is incision and drainage (one side only), local heat, and an appropriate antibiotic. Untreated septal abscesses may result in destruction of the septal cartilage and some of the bony septum,

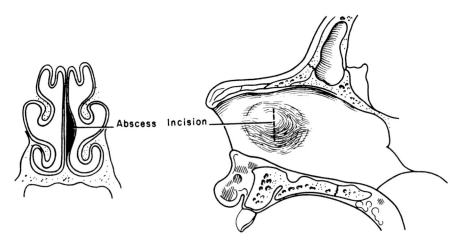

Abscess   Incision

FIG. 4-16. Septal abscess. **Left:** Note the elevated perichondrium over the septum as a result of pus formation. **Right:** Location of most septal abscesses in the anterior third of the septum. (From Montgomery, W. W.: *Surgery of the Upper Respiratory System,* Vol. 1, p. 298. Lea & Febiger, Philadelphia, 1971. With permission.)

producing deformity of the pyramid. It may also extend through the cribriform area, causing meningitis or brain abscess.

Furunculosis usually develops in the vestibule of the nose, the sebaceous glands, or hair follicles of the vibrissae. Single furuncles are the common type of infection, but multiple boils can occur. Pain and swelling are usually marked, and although nasal obstruction is not complete, a great deal of crusting occurs, which can occlude the nostril (Fig. 4-17). Furuncles in the nose are potentially dangerous because the venous drainage of this area empties into the cavernous sinus, and such infection can result in a cavernous sinus thrombosis. The treatment of choice is local application of wet heat to the nose, specific antibiotic therapy, and careful removal of crusts that occlude the nostril employing a clean technique. It is preferable to allow the furuncle to rupture and drain, rather than to open it surgically. Under no circumstances should the "head" be picked off with a finger, nor should it be squeezed. Repeated furunculosis in some children results from a chronic *Staphylococcus* infection in the vestibule. In such cases, specimens for cultures should be carefully obtained to identify the infecting agent at a time when no furuncles are present. A specific vaccine made from the infecting agent may be helpful.

Erysipelas is an acute inflammation of the skin secondary to the invasion of the skin lymphatics by a specific form of group A *Streptococcus*. It seldom occludes the nostrils because it primarily affects the skin. It frequently occurs in the skin of the nose, spreading across the skin of the cheek and extending to and sometimes involving the ear (Fig. 4-18). It occurs with raised, red margins. When both sides of the nasal pyramid and cheeks are involved, it has a typical butterfly appearance. It is more common in children and is usually accompanied by a high fever. Unless

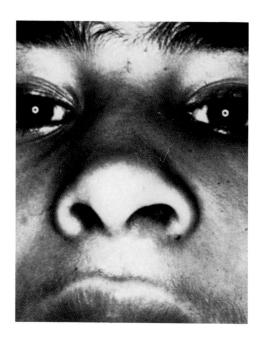

FIG. 4-17. Nasal furunculosis. Note the elevation of the floor of the left nostril in this boy. (From El Sarafy, S.: *Atlas of Ear, Nose and Throat Diseases,* p. 80. Ali Bin Ali, Doho, Qatar, Egypt, 1977. With permission.)

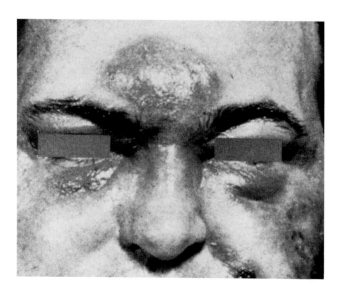

FIG. 4-18. Erysipelas. Note the raised edges and the clear demarcation of the infection. (From Deweese and Saunders: *Textbook of Otolaryngology,* p. 220. Mosby, St. Louis, 1968. With permission.)

treated, it can be very dangerous to young children. It can be transmitted through contact, and it can be identified by demonstration of large numbers of hemolytic streptococci in the nasopharynx. It should be treated promptly with a specific antibiotic.

Nasal diphtheria still occurs occasionally in children. It can cause marked nasal obstruction, either unilateral or bilateral. Obstruction is caused by the pseudomembrane that may appear in the vault of the nasopharynx or in the nostril itself. The child presents the same symptoms as those associated with pharyngeal diphtheria (see Chapter 5). Treatment is by administration of diphtheria antitoxin.

Allergy

Allergic rhinitis may be seasonal or perennial. It is thought by many clinicians that inheritance may predispose an individual to allergic reactions. It presents the picture of obstructive swelling of the nasal mucosa, which usually is pale or bluish and has a shiny, smooth appearance as opposed to the fiery red appearance seen in rhinitis from infection. Eosinophils are present in scrapings of the mucous membrane and in nasal secretions. The turbinates are very swollen, and there is a profuse watery discharge from both nostrils. Itching of the nose may be a presenting symptom. Sneezing is common, and frequently the eyes are irritated and water constantly. In some severe cases, especially in young children, the patient suffers attacks of bronchial asthma. Patients with perennial allergic rhinitis frequently complain of frequent colds or symptoms that they attribute to chronic sinusitis. Nasal discharges in such cases, however, contain a significant number of eosinophils as compared to the lymphocytes and polymorphonuclear cells found in the common cold and bacterial infections.

The diagnosis of allergy and the differential diagnosis of the seasonal or perennial types can usually be made by taking a careful history. A family history of allergy can be significant in reaching the diagnosis of allergic rhinitis.

Seasonal allergy is usually the result of exposure to pollens of trees, grasses, and flowers. It appears usually in the spring and fall, producing acute symptoms that last 6 to 8 weeks. In some instances, especially sensitive individuals have symptoms all summer, probably associated with grasses. Those patients who spend winter months in warm subtropical climates where flowers bloom throughout the year may confuse the examining physician by describing allergic symptoms during the winter, which could lead to the classification of a perennial allergy.

True perennial allergic rhinitis is usually associated with substances with which the patient is in daily contact throughout the year, e.g., house dust, molds, tobacco smoke, wool in clothes, dander of dogs or cats, or feather pillows. Sometimes children suffer from food allergies that result in perennial symptoms. Perennial rhinitis can result in marked hypertrophy of the turbinates, which may remain obstructive even after the child has shown marked improvement following removal of the allergens or after hyposensitization. Surgical or chemical reduction of the hypertrophied mucous membrane may be necessary but should be avoided if possible. Removal of contact with the sensitizing agents and hyposensitization are the preferred methods of treatment. Temporary relief of symptoms can frequently be obtained by the use of antihistamines. Cortisone, which relieves the symptoms of allergy, should be used only with great caution in children. Chronic use of nasal drops should be avoided, as this may induce a severe rebound swelling of the mucous membrane and cause chronic nasal obstruction.

Complications of allergic rhinitis are serous sinusitis secondary to closure of the sinus ostia by swollen mucous membrane and nasal polyps, which can cause either unilateral or bilateral sinus symptoms as well as marked nasal obstruction. Bacterial infection of the sinus may follow this obstruction. Control of the allergy and removal of the polyps either by a short course of cortisone or by surgery clears this condition.

Vasomotor Rhinitis

Recurrent nasal obstruction without evidence of the common cold and without the laboratory findings associated with allergic rhinitis is referred to as vasomotor rhinitis. This is thought to be the result of an imbalance between the sympathetic and the parasympathetic systems, resulting in swelling of the nasal mucous membrane with general engorgement of the turbinate mucosa. It is aggravated by tension states in older children or by thyroid deficiency. In pregnant women such symptoms are attributed to ovarian deficiency or hypometabolism. Such a condition can also result from the overuse of vasoconstrictors contained in "nose drops." The patient finds that eventually the use of nose drops gives a shorter and shorter period of relief until there is little improvement in airway. Withdrawal of the drops is not easy but offers the only lasting relief. Many patients must learn to live with vasomotor rhinitis knowing that they will experience occasional periods of remissions.

Nasal Polyps

Nasal polyps are translucent pedunculated tumors covered with thin mucous membrane containing a few lymphocytes and eosinophils in a gelatinous matrix. They are associated with chronic nasal infection, sinusitis, or allergies. They are sessile and fluctuant and may vary in size from 1 to 2 mm to 1 to 4 cm. They are freely movable except at the base, and they arise from the mucous membrane of the nasal sinuses or the turbinates. They may obstruct one or both nostrils completely or partially, and they cause increased nasal secretions (Fig. 4-19). Polyps developed in the sinuses can extrude into the nostril and as they grow can extend into and fill the nasopharynx. These are known as choanal polyps. Polyps can occur very rapidly at times and when surgically removed may recur very quickly. The best treatment is to determine the cause—allergy or infection—and take measures to correct the causative factor. Sometimes polyps cause secondary sinusitis as a result of obstruc-

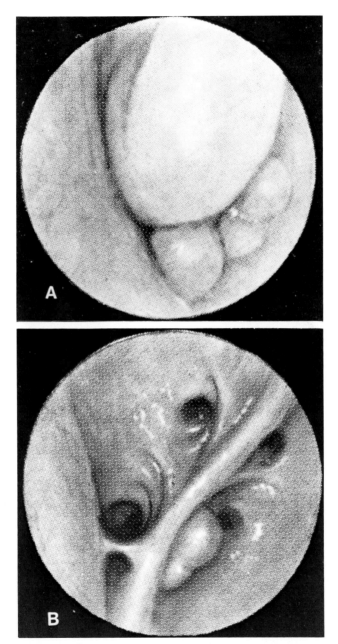

FIG. 4-19. Observations made through a nasopharyngescope showing the reduction of polyps in the ethmoid region of patient under steroid therapy. **A:** Before therapy. **B:** After 3 weeks of steroid therapy. (From Bordley, J. E.: Observations on changes taking place in the upper respiratory tract of patients under A.C.T.H. and cortisone therapy. *Bull. Johns Hopkins Hosp.,* 87(5):419, 1950. With permission.)

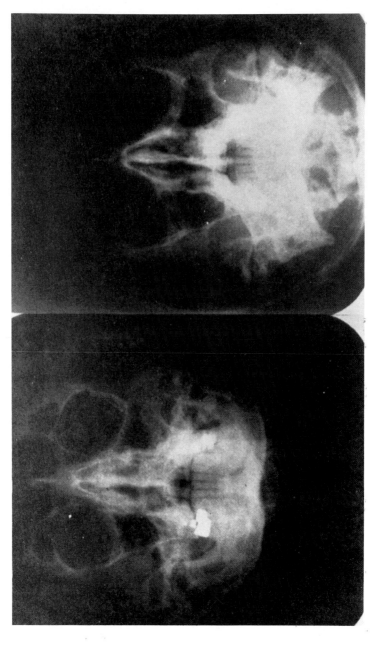

FIG. 4-20. X-rays of an allergic male showing a polyp on the floor of the left maxillary sinus **(left)** and after 11 days of treatment with cortisone, showing nearly complete resolution of the polyp **(right)**. (From Bordley, J. E.: Observations on changes taking place in the upper respiratory tract of patients under A.C.T.H. and cortisone therapy. *Bull. Johns Hopkins Hosp.,* 87(5):421, 1950. With permission.)

tion of the sinus ostium. The employment of a course of cortisone with covering doses of a specific antibiotic is usually very effective in reducing or eliminating polyps, but care must be taken to remove the basic cause for their formation (Fig. 4-20). Sometimes medical therapy is ineffective, especially if there is chronic sinusitis present, and it is then necessary to surgically remove the polyps to cure the sinusitis. Choanal polyps rarely respond to medical measures and for the most part require surgical removal. Where possible, any nasal obstruction such as that caused by septal deviation or fracture should be surgically corrected in those individuals suffering from polyps in order to improve nasal ventilation. Any sinus infection must be cleared up after a polypectomy to avoid a recurrence of polyps.

Hypertrophied Turbinate

Occasionally, nasal obstruction or partial obstruction can result from a hypertrophied turbinate. This most frequently occurs in one nostril. Two careful nasal examinations spaced several days apart when the patient is free from nasal or sinus infection can identify this. Care must be taken, however, to rule out an allergy, and the physician must be sure that nasal drops have not been used for several days before examination. Turbinates can be reduced by submucous resection of some of the turbinate bone, but surgical removal of the turbinate should be avoided because it frequently results in the development of atrophic rhinitis.

Nasal Deformity

Nasal deformity can cause nasal airway obstruction in one or both nostrils. Such deformities may be congenital (see p. 247, Atresia) or may result from trauma at the time of birth, a blow to the nose, or unequal growth rates in the nasal skeleton. Anterior septal deformities are more likely the result of trauma, whereas posterior deformities are the result of unequal growth rates resulting in the posterior septum being twisted against the skull base. Birth injuries and developmental deformities of the nose, if severe, should be referred to an otolaryngologist for correction. Saddle nose deformity from congenital syphilis results primarily from destruction of the vomer, which causes "saddling." Fractures from a blow on the nose require immediate attention while the bony and cartilagenous fragments are still freely mobile. Fractures can usually be easily detected because of external deformity, either deviation from the midline or depression of the nasal dorsum. Fractures are usually accompanied by epistaxis. In most instances crepitus can be elicited over the nasal bones when the fracture is "fresh." Such fractures may involve the septum, resulting in its deviation, or may cause a hemorrhage under the perichondrium, causing a septal hematoma that increases the width of the septum. Ecchymosis developing in one or both orbits is commonly associated with nasal fractures (see "Facial Trauma," below).

Foreign Bodies

Foreign bodies in the nose can result in nasal infection and obstruction. They may be small objects that a child can insert into his nose, and as a result of his efforts to dislodge them they are pushed well into the nostril. Such objects become lodged in the anterior part of the nose on the floor, wedged against the inferior turbinate. They may remain for some time before they cause observable symptoms. The first sign of a foreign body in the nose is frequently unilateral nasal discharge followed in some cases by nasal obstruction of varying degrees. As time passes, the discharge becomes thicker and more purulent and develops a fetid odor. Rhinoliths impacted in the nostril can give the same picture. In some instances the rhinoliths become embedded in the posterior portion of the nostril. Treatment in both instances is to identify the object and have it removed by a specialist. In cases of foreign bodies, it is well to try to find a matching object in order to determine if it can better be delivered anteriorly through the nostril or pushed into the nasopharynx for delivery.

Hypertrophied Adenoids: Role in Nasal Disorders

Adenoids can be the cause of nasal obstruction, either unilateral or bilateral. The obstruction is, of course, postnasal. A large adenoidal mass in the nasopharynx is the usual cause of the obstruction, but in a few children the adenoids not only fill the vault of the nasopharynx but extend into the posterior nares. In some allergic children, when conventional adenoidectomy does not relieve nasal obstruction and obstruction is thought to be secondary to allergy, it has been found that there is residual adenoidal tissue in the choanae. Such tissue when present must be delivered into the nasopharynx in order to remove it at the time of operation. (Obstruction secondary to neoplasms and cysts is described later in the chapter).

Epistaxis

Next to nasal obstruction, epistaxis is the most common nasal disorder of childhood, and it requires immediate attention. It is the number-one nasal emergency. Bleeding can begin in many places in the nose and can result from many conditions.

The blood supply of the nose is through two arterial systems. The ethmoid arteries arise from the internal carotid system, and the sphenopalatine artery is supplied by the external carotid system through the internal maxillary artery. When bleeding is from the anterior and superior portion of the lateral nasal wall or from the posterior portion of the nose, it is usually from the internal carotid system through the ophthalmic artery, which supplies the ethmoid arteries.

The most common site of bleeding is Kiesselbach's (Little's) plexus, which lies near the surface of the mucous membrane covering the anterior third of the nasal septum and its anteriorly located septal spurs (Fig. 4-21). This plexus is formed

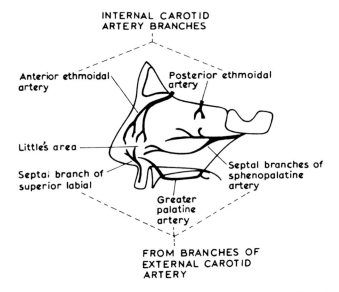

INTERNAL CAROTID
ARTERY BRANCHES

Anterior ethmoidal
artery

Posterior ethmoidal
artery

Little's area

Septal branch of
superior labial

Septal branches of
sphenopalatine
artery

Greater
palatine
artery

FROM BRANCHES OF
EXTERNAL CAROTID
ARTERY

FIG. 4-21. Blood supply of the nasal septum, showing the two branches of the ethmoid artery, the septal branches of the sphenopalatine artery, and branches from the superior labial artery and the greater palatine artery, all of which supply the highly vascular Little's (Kiesselbach's) area. The septum is supplied by both the internal and external carotid arteries. (From Dyal, V. S.: *Clinical Otolaryngology*, p. 117. Lippincott, Philadelphia, 1981. With permission.)

by the anastomosis of the septal branches of the sphenopalatine artery with the septal branches from the ethmoid arteries. It is in a position to be exposed to the drying effect of domestic low-humidity heating. It crusts easily. It can be reached easily by the finger for picking, and it is also injured by trauma to the nasal pyramid. Other areas of hemorrhage are found around the anterior end of the inferior turbinate and posteriorly at the posterior end of the inferior meatus.

The common causes of epistaxis are trauma (external and internal), environmental conditions, perforation of the septum, blood dyscrasias, growths, genetic factors, and debilitating illness. Epistaxis associated with hypertension is rare during childhood.

Trauma

External trauma may be from a blow on the nose resulting in fracture of the septal cartilage and/or nasal bones. In this instance, the bleeding results from a tear in the mucous membrane covering the septum, the turbinates, or the vault of the nose. Fractures may cause bleeding almost any place in the nose (see "Facial Trauma," below).

Internal trauma may result from picking off of crusts, excessive cleaning of the nose, or the pushing of foreign bodies such as sticks into the nostril. This usually results in bleeding from Kiesselbach's plexus. Ulceration of the septum can also result from nose picking and cause bleeding.

Environmental Conditions

Ulceration of the septum with epistaxis may also be the result of extreme environmental conditions. Epistaxis occurs most frequently during the winter in those climates where homes must be heated and dry air causes drying and cracking of the mucous membrane or in working conditions where there is excessive dust or chemical fumes.

Perforation of the Septum

Perforation of the septum causes excessive crusting around the margins, which when dislodged causes epistaxis. In children such perforations can also be caused by nose picking, septal abscesses, fractures of the septum, syphilis, and debilitating diseases, particularly enteric diseases such as typhoid fever and dysentery.

Growths

Bleeding is commonly seen in children when granulomas, hemangiomas, and papillomas grow in the exposed anterior third of the nostril. These tumors ulcerate and bleed very easily. They should be removed as soon as discovered in order to prevent repeated epistaxis. The first evidence of nasal malignancy is spontaneous bleeding.

Blood Dyscrasias

Epistaxis is a common complication in children suffering from blood dyscrasias. The most commonly associated conditions are purpura and leukemia. In these conditions, there is a general failure of normal circulation in the mucous membrane, resulting in crusting and ulceration over the septum and turbinates. Bleeding occurs frequently, and although it is usually from the exposed surfaces in the anterior nose, it may originate almost any place.

Genetic Factors

Hemophilia is the most common hereditary bleeding disorder and is associated with failure of normal coagulation. It is sex linked and is caused by a recessive mutant gene; it is limited almost exclusively to males. Coagulation is defective at birth. Therefore, epistaxis may occur at any time after birth. Bruising and hematomas occur after the mildest trauma. Epistaxis more frequently occurs from the anterior nose but may occur from any place in the nose that has been traumatized. Bleeding may also occur from the membranes of the nasopharynx and the mouth, so it is important to locate the bleeding site if bleeding is to be completely controlled.

Purpura may be hereditary or acquired. The hereditary form is transmitted to both sexes. In this condition, the blood vessels are thought to be incapable of response to the body's vasoconstrictors. It can be diagnosed by increased capillary fragility and prolonged bleeding time. As in hemophilia, bleeding is commonly seen around the anterior third of the nose, especially in Kiesselbach's plexus, but can occur from almost any place in the nose.

Hereditary hemorrhagic telangiectasia (Osler–Weber–Rendu disease) is transmitted as a simple dominant trait to both sexes. Bleeding results from vessel wall defects that form small hemangiomas or spider telangiectases. They occur in the mucous membrane and the skin. They are very sensitive to trauma, and the nasal mucous membrane around them ulcerates easily when they are treated. They occur very frequently on the septum and may also be seen in the nasopharynx and mouth. Epistaxis occurs in these cases more frequently in adults than in children but can occur at any age. The lesions may occur at any place in the body, so if one is identified in the nose or mouth, a thorough search should be made to identify other lesions. Some articles have reported successful destruction of telangiectases by use of a laser beam.

In all these hereditary conditions, nasal bleeding is difficult to control. It is important to call in a specialist as soon as possible. Only emergency measures should be undertaken to control bleeding at home. Transfusions are frequently required when bleeding starts in individuals suffering from these conditions.

Debilitating Diseases

Epistaxis can occur during prolonged and debilitating diseases. Nasal hemorrhage occurs with acute rheumatic fever when a child has had a long and severe febrile course, as well as with typhoid fever and other enteric diseases such as severe prolonged diarrhea and dysentery. The bleeding usually occurs as a result of crusting and ulceration around Kiesselbach's plexus. Such bleeding is usually easily controlled with an anterior nasal pack or cotton pledget. In these cases, it is important to keep the nostril clean and eliminate crusting by the periodic application of some mild ointment.

Control of Epistaxis

Epistaxis is an emergency, and it is important for the pediatrician and the general practitioner to know the basic steps to be taken to control nasal bleeding before the patient loses much blood. In the normal child, nasal bleeding is rarely terminal, although mild shock can occur. It is more serious in debilitated children. Shock results in some natural control of the bleeding but may be of short duration. Healthy children usually bleed from sites in the anterior nose as a result of local trauma, but repeated nosebleeds should be considered a serious symptom and the child should be thoroughly studied.

The following steps are helpful when treating epistaxis. These basic steps can be carried out in an emergency by the pediatrician or general practitioner in the home:

1. Raise the head. Where possible place the child in a sitting position. This lowers the blood pressure in the head.

2. Keep the head level or tilted slightly forward. If the bleeding is in the anterior half of the nose and the anterior blood clots are removed by blowing the nose or by suction, this position keeps the blood from dropping into the pharynx and being swallowed, which may cause vomiting. If the bleeding is posterior, this position does not prevent blood from entering the pharynx; thus, it aids in localization of the site of the bleeding.

3. Have good illumination for examining the nose.

4. When clots have been removed by having the patient blow his nose or with suction, examine Kiesselbach's plexus on the septum. If a septal spur is present, examine its anterior tip; then look under the spur. The anterior end of the inferior turbinate should be inspected next, followed by examination of the posterior septum when possible and the inferior and middle meatus. Bleeding from the middle meatus may be caused by hemorrhage in one of the nasal sinuses with blood passing into the nose through the sinus orifice.

5. If the bleeding is from the anterior septum or the anterior end of the turbinate, obtain some temporary control of bleeding while preparations are being made to treat the bleeding area by having the patient or a parent compress the ala against the septum between finger and thumb. In cases of simple bleeding from the anterior septum or turbinate, place a cotton pledget soaked with 1:1,000 epinephrine, 1% ephedrine solution, or 0.5% phenylephrine (Neo-Synephrine®) solution in the nose to cover the bleeding area and apply external compression for 5 to 6 min. Carefully remove the pledget, and if the bleeding is controlled, apply a local anesthetic to the area and gently touch the bleeding area with a silver-nitrate-tipped applicator. If there is continued oozing, insert another pledget and take the child to the hospital emergency room or to an otolaryngologist.

6. If the bleeding is profuse and cannot be controlled by the above method, it may be necessary to pack the nose. The mode of packing should be adapted to the area of bleeding, anterior or posterior. Many times attempts to control hemorrhage by packing fail because the pack is placed anteriorly or posteriorly to the bleeding area and does not compress it. The posterior end of the pack (0.5 inch selvaged gauze) should be laid along the floor of the nose posterior to the bleeding area and two or three folds of packing placed on top of this to form a buttress. The first folds should be fluffed. The pack is then placed against the barrier in accordian

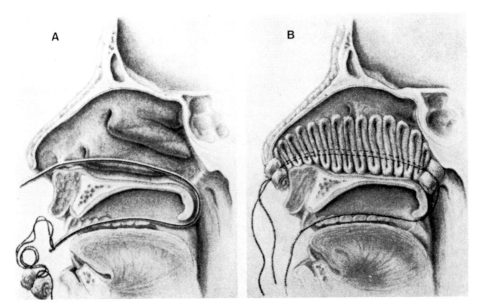

FIG. 4-22. **A:** Method for inserting a postnasal pack. **B:** Placement of the anterior nasal pack against the posterior pack. (From Boies, L. R.: *Fundamentals of Otolaryngology*, p. 277. W. B. Saunders, Philadelphia, 1959. With permission.)

pleats and extended anterior to the bleeding area. Pressure should then be exerted against the anterior end of the pack in order to tighten it within the nose (Fig. 4-22).

7. In those cases in which the bleeding is very posterior, it may first be necessary to insert a postnasal pack or a Foley catheter and then pack through the nostril against this. Posterior packs can be made from gauze squares, bunched and tied gauze strips, or a folded strip of linen torn from a handkerchief. The posterior pack should be large enough to completely fill the choana when it is drawn into place. It should be made up with two strings attached—one to control insertion of the pack and a second to facilitate its withdrawal. The strings should be long enough to extend out of the front of the nose and out of the mouth at least 6 inches. To insert, pass a rubber catheter through the nose into the pharynx on the side of the bleeding and retrieve it through the mouth. Attach the insertion string of the pact to it and draw it out through the nostril. Guiding the pack with a finger in the mouth, pull it up behind the soft palate and into the choana. Anchor the insertion string firmly to the face or to a small roll of gauze to keep the pack from slipping out of the choana, and tape the mouth string to the cheek to facilitate later removal of the postnasal pack. Place the nasal pack in the nostril, pushing it firmly against the postnasal pack. Such packs should remain in place at least 16 to 24 hr. The

nasal packing should be removed first; then the postnasal pack should be withdrawn with the string that has been brought out through the mouth.

Comments on Epistaxis

Children with repeated epistaxis, except those in known good condition who have experienced repeated mild bleeding from easily identified areas that has been controlled without difficulty, should be put on a suspect list and referred to an otolaryngologist. Such children should also undergo a pediatric hematology study.

It is very difficult to estimate blood loss in children without laboratory tests to measure it. Such measurements should be made in children experiencing serious bleeding (enough to require full packing). This is especially important in children who vomit large amounts of blood following epistaxis. Transfusions should be considered in any child with much blood loss and should always be available for children suffering from leukemia, purpura, and genetic conditions associated with hemorrhage.

The time-honored method of packing has been described in detail to help the attending physician who frequently must cope with epistaxis as an emergency at home. A number of substitutes for nasal packing in epistaxis are available to the pediatrician for the control of epistaxis, and all work under optimum conditions.

Balloons have been much improved in recent years, but often they do not tamponade the bleeding area, especially areas in the meatus or under a spur. They can be very easily inserted in the nostril and inflated. Overinflation should be carefully avoided because it can destroy nasal mucous membrane. When a balloon fails, repeated attempts to use it should not be continued, and a pack should be placed in the nostril.

Expandable packs have been developed that swell after insertion into the nostril. They may fail for the same reasons that defeat the balloon, so caution should be exercised not to continue to readjust them in the presence of continued bleeding, but withdraw them and pack the nose.

A Foley catheter can be inserted through the nose into the posterior nares or the nasopharynx and inflated gently as a substitute for a postnasal pack.

Control of the Patient

One of the greatest problems a physician faces when called to attend a bleeding child is the state of panic in the house or fear that is apparent in the parents who bring the child to the emergency room. This is usually caused by what appears to be a great blood loss during epistaxis because of the piles of blood-soaked tissues and clothes. Panic usually starts among the adults and is quickly communicated to the bleeding child. Such children are very difficult to treat. It sometimes is very helpful if the parents can be calmly reassured while preparations to control the bleeding are under way. A calm parent can do wonders in helping control a child during such procedures.

OBSTRUCTIVE AND DESTRUCTIVE CONDITIONS OF THE NOSE AND SINUSES

Tumors in the nose commonly result in increasing nasal obstruction that is usually unilateral and are frequently associated with chronic nasal discharges. When the tumors are benign, this discharge is usually mucoid or mucopurulent, whereas malignant tumors occasionally bleed.

Polyps

Polyps are the most common tumors found in the nose and sinuses (see p. 254, Nasal Polyps).

Granulomas

Foreign Bodies

Granulomas caused by foreign bodies consist of chronic inflammatory exudative fibrosis of the nasal mucosa with masses of giant cells and mononuclear cells. These obstructive masses can be associated with thick nasal discharge and an unpleasant odor. Removal of the granuloma and the related foreign body usually results in a rapid cure.

Sarcoidosis

Sarcoidosis occurs in the nose as noncaseating tubercles composed of epithelioid cells, giant cells, and lymphocytes. Large areas of nasal mucous membrane can be involved by these lesions, with resultant nasal obstruction. Treatment for this condition is not specific. Cortisone has been administered with only questionable success.

Tubercular Infection

Tubercular infection may involve the nose, causing granulomas that are more destructive than those previously described. This is usually secondary to a primary infection in the lungs or throat. In the nasal infection, there is marked thickening of the mucous membrane, especially over the inferior and middle turbinates, which

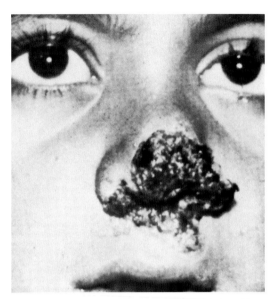

FIG. 4-23. Tuberculous granuloma of the nose in a 10-year-old boy. It involves not only the nostril but also the skin of the nasal tip. (From El Sarafy, S.: *Atlas of Ear, Nose and Throat Diseases,* p. 81. Ali Bin Ali, Doho, Qatar, Egypt, 1977. With permission.)

are covered by tubercles composed of masses of epithelioid cells and lymphocytes and show some central necrosis surrounded by squamous metaplasia. These lesions can extend forward, involving the nasal vestibule, and are locally destructive (Fig. 4-23). Local removal should be attempted only if the lesion is very slow in resolving and while the patient is under general medical treatment for the infection.

Wegener's Granulomatosis

This is a nonneoplastic granulomatous condition originating in the midline of the nose or hard palate; it is associated with periarteritis. It occurs in older children and young adults. It has been theorized that it may be caused by some abnormality in the immune system. In the later stages it becomes a generalized disease, involving the kidneys and respiratory tract, and in some cases there is interstitial keratitis and rheumatoid-type arthritis.

Stewart in 1933 described it as progressive through three stages. The initial stage usually begins with nasal obstruction and a watery nasal discharge, often mistaken for rhinitis or sinusitis. The septum may develop some thickening, followed by an ulcer on the septum, the floor of the nostril, or the midline of the hard palate (Fig. 4-24). As the disease progresses, the septum and/or the hard palate perforates. The nasal discharge increases and develops a disagreeable odor. The structures of the midface become involved, the septum is destroyed, and necrosis spreads to the ethmoid labyrinth, the maxilla, and the orbit and begins to destroy the palatal bone. During this destructive process there is very little change in the white blood cell

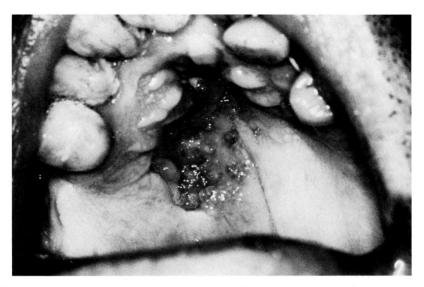

FIG. 4-24. Early lesion in the hard palate of boy suffering from Wegener's granulomatosis.

picture, although X-ray films frequently show a "snowball" appearance in the lungs. The patient becomes severely debilitated. In the advanced stage of the disease, granulomas develop in the nasopharynx, pharynx, larynx, and trachea, renal failure begins, and the lungs become involved with periarteritis. The histologic picture is one of angiocentric infiltration, occasional immature lymphocytes, and periarteritis.

Treatment is a course of cytotoxic drugs combined with steroids; however, prolonged high doses of steroids should be monitored very carefully. Two of the patients observed by the author to whom steroids were administered developed osteoporosis.

Lethal Midline Granuloma (Polymorphic Reticulosis)

This condition is closely related to Wegener's granulomatosis, but a number of investigators consider it to be a separate entity. It may begin as a unilateral lesion in the nose but attacks the midline structures in much the same manner as Wegener's disease; however, it is not as extensive in its involvement. The kidney is not attacked, there is no rheumatoid arthritis, and there is less involvement of lower respiratory tract. The sedimentation rate is quite elevated, and the histologic picture is much the same as in Wegener's granulomatosis with a chronic inflammatory condition accompanied by marked necrosis and necrotizing vasculitis. Except for symptoms of glomerular nephritis and arthritis, clinical symptoms are the same in the two conditions. Suggested treatment is a combination of repeated small doses of irradiation combined with corticosteroids. However, the prognosis is poor.

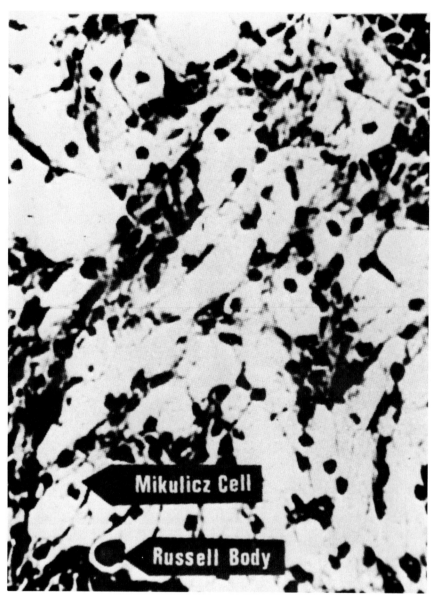

FIG. 4-25. Histologic section through the nasal mucous membrane in a case of rhinoscleroma showing the typical vacuolated macrophage (Mikulicz cell) and a Russell body, which are found in this disease. (From El Sarafy, S.: *Atlas of Ear, Nose and Throat Diseases*, p. 87. Ali Bin Ali, Doho, Qatar, Egypt, 1977. With permission.)

Rhinoscleroma

This is a granulomatous disease involving the nose, sinuses, pharynx, and trachea. It is endemic in the Middle East and southern Europe and has been reported in Mexico and southern California. It begins as a foul rhinorrhea, and shortly after onset a small flat nodule appears on the septum followed by the development of nodules in the nose that rapidly become heavily scarred. The disease is confined to the soft tissues. The bacillus *Klebsiella rhinoscleromatis* has been identified as the infecting agent, although some investigators think that a virus may also be involved. The infection is characterized by granuloma formation involving the nose, sinuses, pharynx, larynx, and trachea. These granulomas contain vacuolated macrophages and Russell bodies (Fig. 4-25). The resultant scar formation causes stenosis of the nostrils and occasionally of the nasopharynx and larynx (Fig. 4-26). Treatment of this infection with specific antibiotics and small doses of X-ray has proved moderately successful.

Leprosy

In tropical countries leprosy may result in development of nasal masses causing nasal obstruction in children and young adults. These nodular masses come from heavy infiltration of the nasal mucous membrane by the infecting organism *Mycobacterium leprae* surrounded by masses of vacuolated histiocytes. At present there is no satisfactory treatment for this problem.

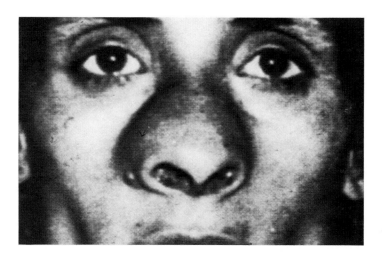

FIG. 4-26. Rhinoscleroma in the proliferative stage of the disease, with the nose distended by nodular masses that have developed in the nasal mucosa. This stage will be followed by contractures of the nose and upper lip from the formation of heavy scar tissue. (From El Sarafy, S.: *Atlas of Ear, Nose and Throat Diseases,* p. 87. Ali Bin Ali, Doho, Qatar, Egypt, 1977. With permission.)

Fungus Infections

Mucormycosis is caused by *Mucor*, a phycomycete with nonseptate hyphae that is generally considered a saprophyte. It is found frequently under the fingernails. The nasal and sinus infection caused by *Mucor* has usually been associated with severe diabetes. (The author, however, examined a young pregnant girl with confirmed mucormycosis of the ethmoid sinuses in India who had no trace of diabetes.) The infection may be transferred into the nostril from the finger. It grows into the turbinates, which turn black; it spreads through the mucous membrane of the sinuses causing dry necrosis and, if untreated, extends into the orbit and the cranium. Histologically, the mycelium with cross septa are easily recognized in extensive areas of necrosis: they appear to grow into the lumen of the blood vessels, causing advancing thrombosis and necrosis (Fig. 4-27). Treatment consists of massive surgical debridement and administration of amphotericin or griseofulvin.

Rhinosporidiosis is a fungus infection caused by *Rhinosporidium seeberi* (Fig. 4-28). It is quite common in southern India and the Middle East, affecting children and adults. It also occurs in Argentina, and a few cases have been reported in the United States. It causes a granulomatous lesion having the appearance of a reddish polyp composed of thick layers of granulomatous material rich in spores. This is usually attached to the septum and protrudes from the nostril (Fig. 4-29). The spores can easily be identified. As it grows it can completely obstruct the nostril. Treatment is removal with a rather wide margin. Failure to remove the entire infected area results in recurrence.

Tumors of Nonepithelial Origin

Melanoma in children is a pigmented tumor that can occur in the vestibule of the nose or on the septum. Its first symptom is unilateral nasal obstruction frequently accompanied by epistaxis. It is a dangerous tumor, as it metastasizes very early. Diagnostic biopsies should not be performed because they may cause spread of the tumor; therefore, an excisional biopsy should be carried out that includes a wide margin of normal tissue.

Tumors of Epithelial Origin

Although common (65% of all neoplasms of the nose and sinuses), carcinoma occurs only rarely in children. It most commonly is seen in the nose but also occurs in the maxillary, ethmoid, frontal, and sphenoid sinuses, in that order. The most common location in the nose is the anterior septum, where it results in nasal obstruction and epistaxis. It may also develop on the anterior portion of the turbinates. These anterior nasal tumors are most often classified as squamous cell carcinomas. The transitional cell variety is seen in the sinuses and the posterior portion of the nose and represents the nonkeratinizing form of squamous cell car-

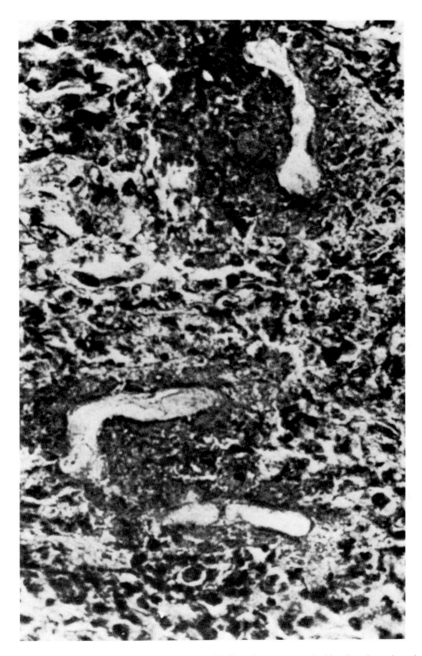

FIG. 4-27.   Nasal mucormycosis in a 17-year-old. Broad nonsegmented hyphae have invaded small vessels and have stimulated inflammatory eosinophilic granular areas. (From Ash, J. E., and Raum, M.: *An Atlas of Otolaryngic Pathology,* p. 179. Armed Forces Institute of Pathology, Washington, D. C., 1949. With permission.)

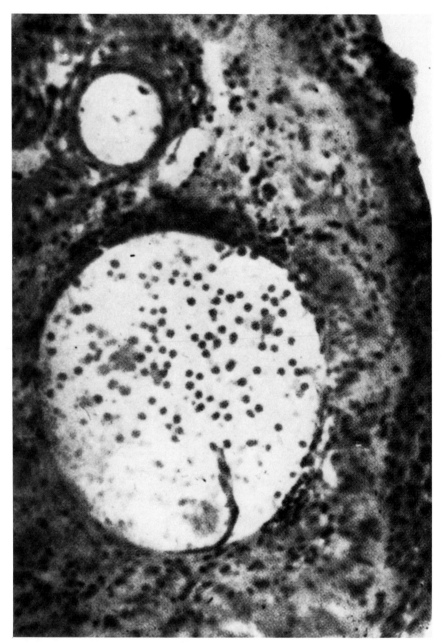

FIG. 4-28. Histologic section of a nasal mucous membrane infected by *Rhinosporidium see-beri*, showing the loose myxedematous tissue and the sporangia-containing spores. (From El Sarafy, S.: *Atlas of Ear, Nose and Throat Diseases,* p. 89. Ali Bin Ali, Doho, Qatar, Egypt, 1977. With permission.)

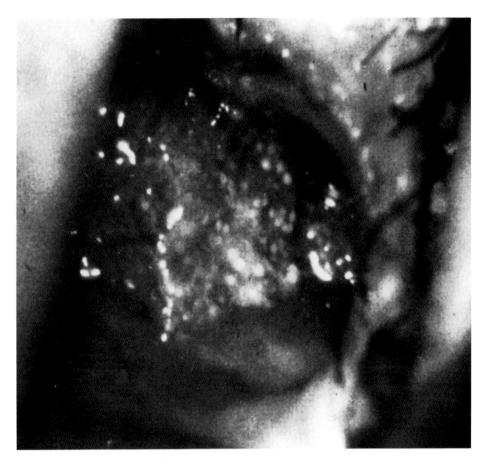

FIG. 4-29. Rhinosporidiosis, showing the obstruction of the nostril by a granulomatous mass covered by a chronic discharge. Nasal polyps are also seen in this mycotic infection. (From El Sarafy, S.: *Atlas of Ear, Nose and Throat Diseases,* p. 89. Ali Bin Ali, Doho, Qatar, Egypt, 1977. With permission.)

cinoma. These tumors can cause external swelling, occasional nasal obstruction, pain, and severe epistaxis. X-ray studies are helpful in establishing a presumptive diagnosis, which must be confirmed by biopsy. After staging, a practical program for therapy can be planned. Excisional surgery, combined with X-ray therapy, is providing an increasingly improved cure rate.

Papilloma is a benign epithelial tumor that most commonly occurs as a pedunculated tan mass on the skin of the nose or on the mucous membrane of the nose, usually around the vestibule. If traumatized it bleeds. It is benign and can be easily removed surgically. It occurs rather commonly in children (Fig. 4-30). Histologic

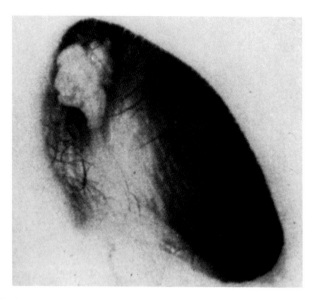

FIG. 4-30. Pedunculated papilloma of the nose growing at the mucocutaneous border. (From El Sarafy, S.: *Atlas of Ear, Nose and Throat Diseases,* p. 99. Ali Bin Ali, Doho, Qatar, Egypt, 1977. With permission.)

sections show neoplastic proliferation of benign epithelium. It may be verrucous or a fibroepithelial polyp. The outer layers are hyperkeratotic and contain large vacuolated cells.

Inside the nose and sinuses papilloma develops different characteristics. It arises from the respiratory mucous membrane of the septum as a benign neoplastic proliferation or as a sessile growth with a lobular surface and at first is asymptomatic. The nasal wall and sinus tumors are more bulky than those developing on the septum, and they have a grayish-pink appearance, often extending along the wall as squamous metaplasia. They can erode neighboring bone but do not invade it. This type is known as inverting papilloma and may become very extensive. Histologically, the tumor appears to be inverting on itself, pushing into the stroma. The epithelial element has a uniform epidermoid appearance in the basal portion with cylindrical cells near the surface. Microcysts are present throughout the tumor. The surface is covered with respiratory epithelium. This tumor occurs most frequently in middle-aged white males but can occur in adolescents. Malignant degeneration has been reported in about 14% of these tumors. Differential diagnosis must rule out inflammatory polyps. Treatment is surgical removal with a large normal margin. X-ray treatment is not effective. Recurrences must be watched for.

Tumors of Connective Tissue Origin

Chondroma

The chondroma associated with nasal involvement arises from the perichondrium and is less aggressive than the enchondroma that arises from cartilage rests in bone. This chondroma develops early during the time of active bony and cartilaginous growth but may not be detected until adult life. It commonly originates from the septum but can arise in the ethmoid cells. It grows slowly and becomes obstructive, and the mucous membrane covering it can become ulcerated and bleed. Surgical removal offers the best chance to restore the breathing space, but recurrence has been reported a number of times, which may have resulted from incomplete removal. This tumor is considered benign.

Chondrosarcoma

This tumor usually occurs in children (Fig. 4-31). It begins frequently in the ethmoid cells or the septum and is aggressive, destroying surrounding structures (Fig. 4-32) and often deforming the nasal pyramid (Fig. 4-33). It seldom metastasizes. Treatment is surgical removal. X-ray therapy is reported to slow the progress of the tumor. The prognosis is guarded.

Lymphosarcoma (Malignant Lymphoma)

This tumor frequently occurs in the long bones. It can occur in children around the face, involving the nose and the sinuses, or it can arise primarily in the sinuses, the maxillary sinus being most often involved. It is composed of undifferentiated cells with hyperchromatic nuclei. The cells are atypical lymphocytes, and mytotic figures are plentiful. Some authors believe that this tumor is related to leukemia.

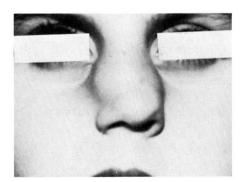

FIG. 4-31. Chondrosarcoma in an 11-year-old girl. It originated in the right ethmoid region, causing nasal pyramid deformity.

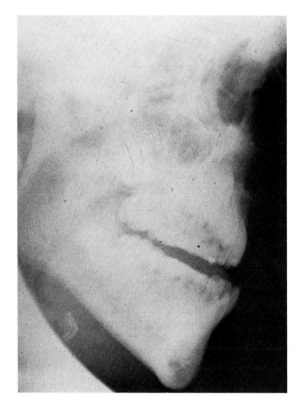

FIG. 4-32. Lateral X-ray showing the destruction of the nasal bones by a chondrosarcoma.

The tumor is highly infiltrative, and the usual treatment is X-ray therapy. Such treatment appears to retard the growth but is not considered curative. X-ray combined with chemotherapy appears to be slightly more effective.

Burkett's Lymphoma (African Lymphoma)

This is the most common tumor during childhood in the Sub-Sahara region of Africa; it is also endemic in New Guinea and appears in South America and the southern United States. It appears most commonly in young children around the age of 7 and 8. It is twice as common in male children as females. It can be primary in the maxilla or orbit as well as the mandible, invading the nose and orbital contents. Swelling of the jaw is a common presenting symptom. It may also invade the central nervous system. When it is in the sinuses, there may be marked facial swelling. The lymphoid system is not necessarily involved in this disease, which may attack the thyroid gland, retroperitoneal area, and viscera. Histologically, there is diffuse

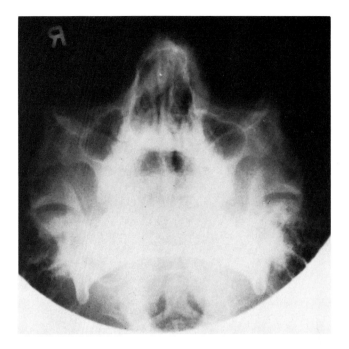

FIG. 4-33. Anteroposterior X-ray demonstrates the nasal deformity and the perforation in the septum by a chondrosarcoma.

lymphoblastic cell infiltration with numerous macrophages throughout the tumor. The etiology of the tumor is thought to be viral, and the Epstein–Barr virus is considered a likely cause, although this has not been definitely proved. A differential diagnosis must rule out retinoblastoma and neuroblastoma, which also produce osteolytic lesions in the mandible and maxilla. The most effective therapy up to the present time has been obtained from chemotherapy employing nitrogen mustard or cyclophosphamide. X-ray therapy has not been successful.

Ewing's Sarcoma

This tumor appears predominantly in children and adolescents. It is very malignant, most frequently involving the long bones, but does occur as a primary lesion in the maxilla and mandible. When in the maxilla, it involves the sinus. It is very destructive in the sinus and surrounding tissue, causing external swelling and great pain. The tumor is composed of densely packed sheets of small, round or oval spindle cells, which are poorly differentiated; necrosis is seen throughout the tumor. It is only moderately sensitive to X-ray therapy, and where possible, such therapy is combined with radical surgical removal.

Osteosarcoma

This very malignant bone tumor may arise in the ethmoid cells and extend into the nose. It can occur at any age, but the average age of appearance is 10 years; it is found three times more often in males than females. It can first be detected as an external swelling and histologically consists of immature osteoid cells; malignant bone production is present, and there are cartilage rests in the tumor. Treatment of any kind has proved ineffectual, and the survival rate is about 3 years.

Fibrosarcoma

This usually originates in the nasal cavity but occurs occasionally in the sinuses. It appears most frequently in adults but can occur in children. Nasal obstruction, external swelling, and pain may be the first signs of this tumor (Fig. 4-34). It is slow-growing and does not metastasize. Its cells are irregular in size and shape;

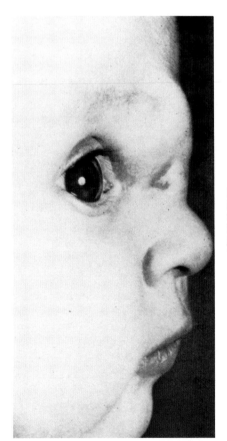

FIG. 4-34. Fibrosarcoma of the face originating in the region of the glabella and involving the inner canthus of the right eye. (From Benson, C. D. et al.: *Pediatric Surgery,* Vol. 1, p. 101. Year Book, Chicago, 1962. With permission.)

nuclei are flat and oval; and there are atypical spindle cells and giant cells containing multiple nuclei. This tumor is one of the most frequently occurring sarcomas in the nose and sinuses, and treatments of all kinds have been unsuccessful for its eradication.

Osseous Tumors

Osteoma is a bone tumor; when it appears in the nasal region, it is found most commonly in the frontal sinus, but it also can occur in the ethmoid and sphenoid sinuses. It begins early when osteogenesis is very active, and it arises from osteogenic periosteum. Ordinarily its growth is slow, and it is discovered by accident during X-ray studies. Although it is benign, it can become obstructive and can cause pressure damage to neighboring structures (Fig. 4-35). Headaches are reported in a few cases, and sinusitis can result from its obstructive growth. The rate of growth of these tumors may vary greatly, so it is wise to check them regularly by X-ray films. Surgical removal can be accomplished if its position and growth become a menace to nasal airway or sinus drainage.

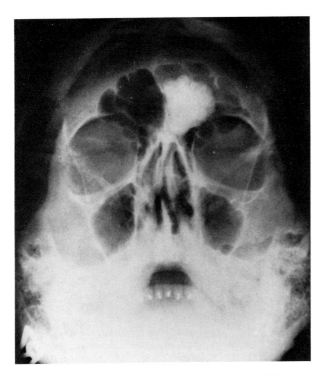

FIG. 4-35. Osteoma of the frontal sinus in a 13-year-old boy.

Fibro-Osseous Disorders

Ossifying Fibroma

These tumors occur most often in the maxilla and may occur in children and young adults following puberty. They are closely associated with fibrous dysplasia. Early in their development, they tend to invade the maxillary sinus. The tumor is destructive because of its expansion and is not considered malignant. It begins with replacement of fatty marrow by fibrous tissue but also appears to be slightly osteogenic. The etiology is unknown, but the origin of some lesions has been associated with trauma.

The first symptom of the tumor is swelling, which may be accompanied by pain (Fig. 4-36). It is slow-growing, and the growth rate seems to diminish with age. X-ray films describe a dense mass with osseous fragments distributed throughout. Total surgical removal is the treatment of choice, but in advanced cases, surgical debulking may be done because of the morbidity of exenteration. X-ray therapy should be avoided because of the danger of malignant degeneration of the tumor.

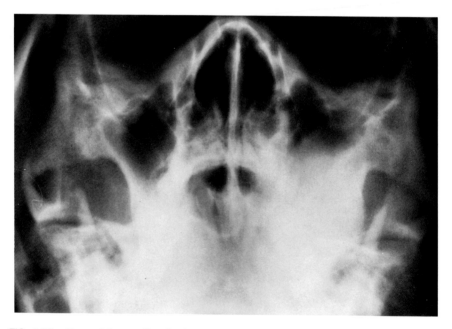

FIG. 4-36. X-ray of the maxilla of a 6-year-old girl showing a dense mass involving the left maxilla and alveolus. She developed pain and swelling of the right upper jaw 10 months earlier and underwent extraction of her right upper molar teeth. Diagnosis: ossifying fibroma.

Fibrous Dysplasia

Monostotic fibrous dysplasia is the most common form of such dysplasias. This is closely related to the polyostotic fibrous dysplasia (Albright's syndrome) that includes multiple bone lesions involving bones throughout the body, endocrine dysfunction manifested by precocious puberty in females, and *café-au-lait* spots on the skin. Monostotic and polystotic dysplasia are thought not to have the same etiology. Monostotic fibrous dysplasia frequently involves the bones of the jaws, and it has been identified as an ossifying fibroma, a fibrous osteoma, and by some pathologists as a neoplastic process rather than dysplasia.

Jaw lesions appear to be more aggressive than those that involve the maxillary sinus and the nose. Fibrous dysplasia is most often seen after puberty, the first symptoms being swelling over the affected area, in most cases accompanied by pain (Fig. 4-37). In general, growth is rather slow, but in some patients the process is very rapid and painful. There is no redness or inflammation over the swelling, and blood chemistries are normal. X-ray studies show a circumscribed osteolytic lesion. Biopsy is necessary for a diagnosis. Histologically, the lesion is covered by a thin layer of cortical bone. There is a stroma of fibrous tissue that is vascularized

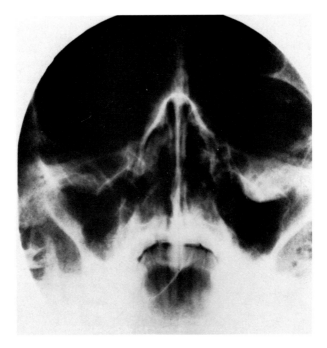

FIG. 4-37. Fibrous dysplasia of the left maxilla in a young girl that caused moderate swelling and severe local pain.

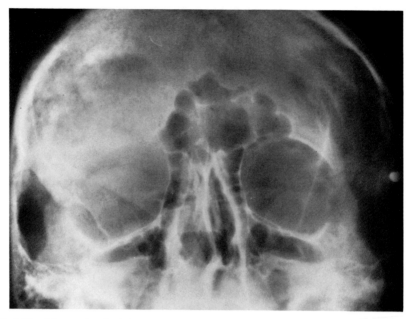

FIG. 4-38. Fibrous dysplasia in a 19-year-old male. A small mass on the right forehead had been present since 5 years of age. It gradually increased in size, and in recent years several temporal headaches had developed. Note erosion of the supraorbital rim and, above this, destruction of the frontal bone.

in its periphery and contains many osteoclastic giant cells; tiny spicules of bone can be seen throughout the specimen. This mixture of fibrous tissue and cancellous bone spicules may vary greatly in different lesions.

This lesion may involve the facial bones (Fig. 4-38) to the point of causing marked facial deformities. The treatment is total surgical removal. X-ray therapy should be avoided.

Tumors of Neural Origin

Tumors of neurogenic origin that present in the nose during childhood are relatively rare, and few of them originate within the nasal spaces.

Neuroblastoma

This usually originates in the vault of the nostril. Although they are rare during childhood, the author has seen two in older children. The tumors develop from either peripheral neural elements or the neural crest. They are invasive and are rather vascular and cause early nasal obstruction. Obstruction and bleeding from the nose are the usual symptoms. The treatment is irradiation.

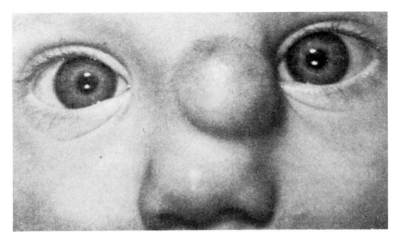

FIG. 4-39. Frontonasal glioma (encephalocele) in a 7-month-old child. (From Whitaker, S. R. et al.: Nasal glioma. *Arch. Otolaryngol.*, 107:551, 1981. With permission.)

Encephalocele

This results from herniation of brain tissue and meninges and their growth downward into the nose. The most common routes are through a defect in the cribriform plate or through an open suture line in the ethmoid region. Encephaloceles present in the anterior vault of the nose and above the inner canthus of the eye, are soft and slightly fluctuant, and intranasally have the appearance of a polyp. Some appear as fluctuant swellings of the external lateral nasal wall (Fig. 4-39). They are submucosal so that in the nose they are covered with respiratory or olfactory mucous membrane. They can become partially or completely obstructive. They are present at birth, grow slowly, and are frequently mistaken for nasal polyps, which are rarely seen in babies. When an external nasal swelling is seen in a newborn or a very young child, an encephalocele should be suspected. Diagnosis is usually confirmed by X-ray studies, which show the bony defect through which the tumor has descended. The usual treatment is surgery. The stalk is severed within the cranium, and the skull defect is closed with bone or some other material that affords a permanent closure; the nasal portion is allowed to remain. Following this, the nasal tumor usually shrinks, although it may remain large enough to require eventual surgical removal from the nose. A rhinotomy approach has proved satisfactory.

Meningioma

These tumors, which originate in the anterior cranial fossa around the olfactory groove, may descend through the cribriform plate and invade the nose. They present as a firm mass covered by mucous membrane with its base in the vault of the nose.

They are very firm to the touch, and X-ray studies should reveal the cranial defect. They are seldom totally obstructive, and they present a surgical problem for both the neurosurgeon and the otolaryngologist, who usually work together to remove them. The tumors are occasionally associated with von Recklinghausen's disease, so the child should be checked for multiple neurofibromas and *café-au-lait* spots.

Neurofibroma

These tumors are relatively rare in the nose and sinuses and are usually associated with multiple tumors elsewhere in the body. In most cases they are considered to be a manifestation of von Recklinghausen's syndrome, which is also accompanied by *café-au-lait* spots on the skin. They occur along the pathways of cranial nerves and are reported in the nose and the sphenoethmoid area. When such a tumor is identified in the nose or sinuses, a thorough neurologic examination should be arranged.

Schwannoma (Neurilemmoma)

This tumor is very closely related to the neurofibroma; they are both neurogenic tumors. The schwannoma tends to occur as a single tumor along a peripheral, cranial, or autonomic nerve. It is most commonly seen along the auditory nerve but may occur in the sinuses. It is rare before puberty. It is somewhat infiltrative and slow-growing, and it does not metastasize. Diagnostic signs are usually neurologic, and if it has enlarged considerably, it can be identified by X-ray studies. Biopsy is necessary for final diagnosis. The tumor is of neuroectodermal origin, whereas the neurofibroma is of connective tissue origin. Histologically, Schwann cells are prominent. There are a thin fibrous capsule and masses of bipolar spindle cells with oval nuclei in palisades. The eosinophilic stroma contains myxomatous elements. Surgical removal is the treatment of choice.

Tumors of Vascular Origin

Hemangiomas

These can occur in the nose and nasal sinuses at almost any age. They consist of masses of blood vessels embedded in loose connective tissue (Fig. 4-40). They are usually sessile, and their surfaces become ulcerated. They most frequently develop on the anterior nasal septum, where they are exposed to trauma; in children they stimulate nose picking. They can become partially obstructive to the airway. Their structure is very delicate, and their vessels are easily ruptured; epistaxis then is usually the first indication of these tumors, and such epistaxis can be very severe. After control of the bleeding, these tumors should be removed surgically with wide

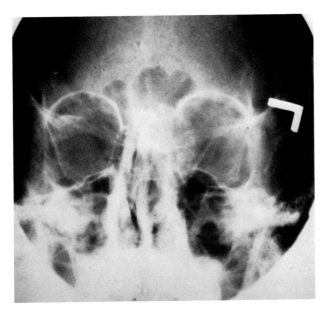

FIG. 4-40. Hemangioma of the left ethmoid and left frontal sinus with invasion of the left orbit. The growth was removed from a 14-year-old boy who complained of diplopia on right lateral gaze.

margins of normal mucous membrane. Local cauterization, either chemical or thermal, cannot be considered a satisfactory form of therapy.

Angiofibromas

These tumors develop in the upper nasopharynx. They may grow forward through the choanae into one or both nostrils, resulting in nasal obstruction and epistaxis (see Chapter 5).

Mesodermal Tumors

Myxomas are closely associated with the fibromas. They are thought to be the result of early disruption of the development of a tooth. The myxoma occurs in the sinuses, most often in the maxillary sinus. It is aggressive, eroding neighboring structures, invading the orbit, and frequently presenting in the nose. Eye symptoms may develop early, and invasion of the alveolar process has been reported. It can erode into the intercranial spaces. This tumor is considered unlikely to metastasize and appears to be much less active after puberty. It is soft and contains a large

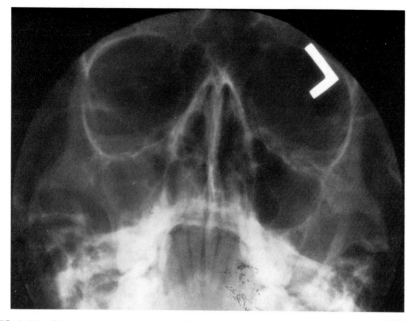

FIG. 4-41. Fibromyxoma in the right maxilla of an 11-year-old boy who had a history of swelling of the right upper jaw for 6 months. Note the soft tissue mass involving the right maxilla eroding the lateral and anterior walls.

proportion of mucoid material resembling mesenchyme. The cells are stellate, and delicate fibrils are seen throughout its structure (Fig. 4-41).

The treatment is surgical removal, and usually by the time this tumor is identified such removal requires extensive and radical surgery. In one case—a 12-year-old boy under the author's care who had undergone surgery three times—the growth rate of the tumor was greatly inhibited by inducing puberty, and the tumor subsequently was removed successfully.

Cysts

Mucous Retention Cyst

The most common cyst associated with the nose is the mucous retention cyst arising from a mucous gland in the nasal mucous membrane. The most common sites for these cysts are the nasal septum and nasal floor. They appear as smooth, round, slightly fluctuant masses that are covered with normal-appearing mucous membranes. Surgical saucerization of the larger cysts or removal of both small and large cysts is usually successful. Saucerization occasionally results in recurrence.

Mucocele

Cystic tumors such as mucoceles (see "Sinusitis," below) that arise in the sinuses and expand into the nostril through the middle meatus can rapidly become obstructive. They present as thick-walled, smooth tumors that are slightly fluctuant. If tapped, they are filled with turgid mucus or a mucopurulent, rather viscid material as a result of low-grade infection in the mucocele. They slowly erode surrounding structures. When studied by X-ray, an occasional mucocele demonstrates a snowstorm appearance as a result of small collections of calcium in the cyst's contents. Mucoceles are very rarely found before puberty. Treatment consists of total removal of the cyst from the sinus where it originated.

Dermoid Cyst of the Nose

These usually present as a flattening and widening of the nasal bridge. They may be slightly fluctuant, and occasionally a small pore is seen in the midline of the nasal pyramid. Hairs have been reported growing out of this pore. Sometimes they are associated with a small midline fistula (Fig. 4-42). The cyst forms because of the pinching off of a small piece of epithelium at the time of midline fusion of the structures. The cysts contain elements of skin and hair and have a stalk that penetrates the region of the septum. If they become infected, they can expand rapidly. They seldom cause any nasal obstruction. Treatment is surgical, and complete removal of the cyst and stalk is necessary because otherwise it may recur.

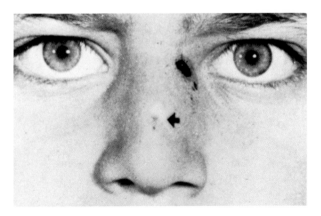

FIG. 4-42. Dermoid cyst of the nose. The dimpled area on the bridge has the appearance of a large pore. The discolored area opposite the left inner canthus is a draining sinus, communicating with the cyst. (From Benson, C. D. et al.: *Pediatric Surgery,* Vol. 1, p. 101. Year Book, Chicago, 1962. With permission.)

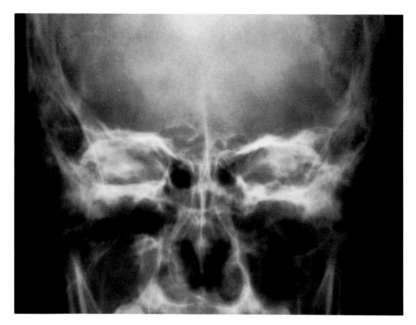

FIG. 4-43. Anteroposterior view of a benign bone cyst of the right maxilla of a 15-year-old male. There was a history of swelling of the right maxilla and upper lip which rapidly increased until it destroyed the lateral wall and caused a bulging of the right hard palate. The swelling was painless.

Benign Bone Cyst

This may occur in the sinuses of children and is usually asymptomatic until it causes facial swelling. Occasionally there is some nasal obstruction. Because of slow growth the cyst causes little discomfort unless it becomes infected. Surgical removal is recommended (Fig. 4-43).

Atrophic Rhinitis/Ozena

A number of authors consider atrophic rhinitis and ozena to be separate entities. They believe atrophic rhinitis to represent atrophy of the mucous membrane of the nose and replacement of ciliated membrane in the anterior portion of the nose by squamous epithelium. There is marked loss of glandular elements as the result of damage to the parasympathetic postganglionic fibers of the nose. Other authors believe that ozena is an advanced phase of atrophic rhinitis. Both groups believe that virus infections play some part as causative factors in the two disorders.

Both disorders include atrophy of the nasal mucous membrane, loss of cilia and mucous glands, loss of cavernous venous spaces over the turbinates, and increased nasal air space; later in ozena there is formation of large crusts on the floor of the nose, which have a very fetid odor.

Symptoms are paradoxical in that despite the increasing air space the patient complains of marked nasal obstruction. He is very much aware of the odor present and much disturbed by the nasal crusts.

These disorders, which usually begin during puberty, present a therapeutic problem. The use of nasal douches of warm saline to remove the crusts often gives much relief. Nasal sprays of sugar solution or insufflation of confectioner's sugar has been reported as helpful if used after the crusts have been removed. Surgical procedures designed to decrease the nasal air space are also successful in some cases not relieved by simple medical treatment.

SINUSITIS

All normal accessory nasal sinuses have certain characteristics in common. They are noncollapsible, nonexpandable bony cavities filled with air, and they are lined with ciliated mucous membrane, which moves a mucous blanket formed by its mucous glands toward a small exit, the ostium, where it is discharged into the nose. Their blood and nerve supply is usually remotely located in relation to the ostium. Obstruction of the ostium, destruction of the cilia, which occurs in viral infections, or destruction of the lining mucous membrane drastically interferes with drainage and alters normal physiological function. Therefore, we find that edema of the mucous membrane, masses of thickened untransported mucus, destruction of the cilia, the formation of polyps, tumors, and granulations, or trauma can obstruct the ostium and result in retained material. The presence of infection in this retained material results in inflammation, increased intersinus pressure, interference with normal blood flow within the sinus, pain, tenderness, fever, and unless relieved, eventual destruction of the sinus walls.

Signs and Symptoms of Acute Sinusitis

The signs and symptoms of acute sinusitis result from inflammation of the lining mucous membrane and the failure of adequate drainage of the sinus. The first sign of sinusitis is usually purulent or mucopurulent nasal and/or postnasal discharge and nasal obstruction. Such drainage may cease rather suddenly if the ostium becomes occluded, and the symptoms will increase in intensity. As sinusitis progresses and internal sinus pressure increases, pain, tenderness, and fever can occur. X-ray studies show a fluid level in the sinus and thickened mucous membrane (Fig. 4-44). Such increased pressure can also interfere with circulation of the sinus, resulting in thrombosis and local osteomyelitis. As the infection proceeds, swelling and erythema and tenderness may develop around the face. When the infection penetrates the sinus wall, severe facial cellulitis and/or orbital cellulitis and abscess

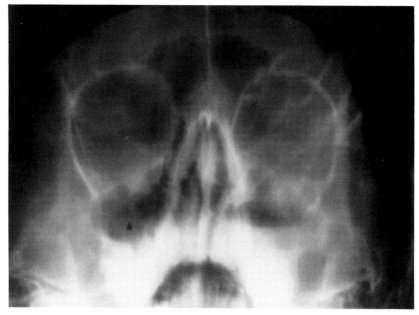

FIG. 4-44. Acute orbital cellulitis right in 10-year-old boy. Note the fluid level in the frontal sinus and antrum with clouding of the ethmoid cells on the same side. The X-ray diagnosis was pan-sinusitis right.

formation can result. In older children, when the frontal sinus and sphenoid sinus have developed, infection can result in intercranial extension of the disease, causing meningitis or intercranial abscess formation.

Causal Factors

Sinusitis in children may result from a number of causes. The predisposing cause is usually a virus infection often associated with an upper respiratory infection. The virus invasion causes increased serous and mucous discharge, mucous membrane swelling, and damage to the cilia, which interferes with drainage. Such a condition invites a secondary bacterial invasion of the sinus. Sinusitis may also develop as a complication of debilitating respiratory conditions (e.g., bronchiectasis or cystic fibrosis) or blood diseases such as leukemia. The actual acute sinusitis associated with such illnesses is the result of bacterial secondary invasion and local thrombotic processes in the lining mucous membrane of the sinus. Obstructive conditions within the nose itself, e.g., septal deviations, septal spurs, hypertrophied turbinates, certain tumors, and polyps, markedly increase the incidence of sinusitis. Children who swim and dive a great deal in unclean water are subject to sinusitis, and allergic states that cause nasal edema appear to predispose a child to sinus disease.

TABLE 4-1. *Treatment of a cold*

Total bed rest for 2 to 3 days.
Humidify the room.
Avoid marked temperature changes; keep the window closed at night except in summer.
Force fluids.
For severe nasal obstruction, use steam inhalations morning and evening or expose the face for 6 min three times a day to an infrared light from 30 inches with the patient sitting up with eyes closed.
If severe nasal obstruction persists after inhalations or infrared treatments, consider the use of mild nasal drops such as phenylephrine (Neo-Synephrine®), 0.5% solution twice a day for a restricted period. In older children, oral nasal decongestants may be preferable.
Children known to be allergic appear to handle a cold better if they are put on antihistamines.

Prevention

Because the most common predisposing factor to sinusitis is the common cold, it is recommended that families adopt a routine for the care of their children when they develop colds in order to avoid complications in the upper or lower respiratory systems. The regimen shown in Table 4-1 is suggested.

Examination and Nonsurgical Treatment of a Child with Suspected Sinusitis

Examination cannot be carried out in the home by the pediatrician as thoroughly as in a well-equipped otolaryngologist's office. However, the face can be examined for local erythema and swelling; the nostrils can be examined to determine the type and amount of discharge present and which nostril contains the larger amount of discharge. The pharynx can be examined for postnasal discharge, and simple transillumination can be carried out with a small flashlight to get an idea of involvement of the maxillary and/or frontal sinuses. The area over the sinuses should be palpated to determine tenderness. At the time of examination, a specimen of the discharge should be taken for culture.

If the above examination suggests sinusitis and the child is running a fever, the routine shown in Table 4-2 can be adopted.

Chronic Sinusitis

Children may develop chronic sinus infections especially if (a) they have had a number of attacks of acute sinusitis, (b) they have internal nasal deformity or polyps obstructing drainage of the sinuses (Fig. 4-45), (c) they are allergic, (d) they are debilitated, and/or (e) they have chronic lung disease (cystic fibrosis or bronchiectasis).

TABLE 4-2. *Treatment of acute sinusitis*

Penicillin according to weight until culture studies indicate a specific antibiotic sensitivity.
Bed rest with head elevated.
Humidify room.
Force fluids.
Keep windows closed except in summer.
Vasoconstrictors (for no longer than 1 week): drops twice a day or oral vasoconstrictors.
Infrared heat to face from 30 inches for 6 min with eyes closed two or three times a day.
When findings of culture are reported, adjust to optimum antibiotic. Antibiotics should be
  continued for 3 or 4 days after disappearance of symptoms. This is very important in
  order to avoid recurrence of sinusitis.
If after 5 or 6 days of therapy there is no relief of symptoms, child should be referred to
  an otolaryngologist for complete nasal and sinus examination, X-rays, and more
  specific therapy, which may include surgical drainage.

Symptoms

The symptoms of chronic sinusitis are not constant. They may disappear for long periods, especially during the summer, only to reappear during bad weather. This condition is characterized by nasal congestion, slightly increased nasal discharge, and chronic postnasal discharge. During an exacerbation, the symptoms are much the same as, but milder than, those of acute sinusitis. Purulent nasal and postnasal

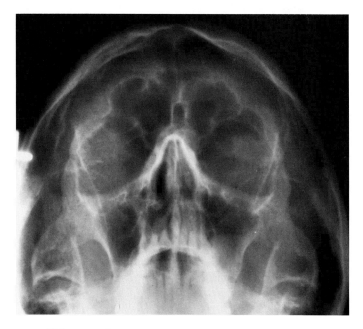

FIG. 4-45. Polyp on the floor of the right maxillary sinus.

discharge and nasal obstruction are the three most common symptoms, but pain, tenderness, and fever can also accompany flare-ups. Care must be taken to differentiate chronic sinusitis from an allergic condition. It is well to have X-ray studies made. Thickening of the mucous membrane of the affected sinus with or without fluid level or polyp formation is the usual X-ray finding.

Postsinusitis Precautions

After any acute attack of sinusitis or if there is evidence of chronic sinusitis, care should be taken to determine any factors contributing to the development of sinusitis; an attempt should then be made to eliminate them. An otolaryngologic consultation should be obtained in order to identify nasal conditions that might interfere with proper sinus drainage and for advice as to the best method of eliminating or controlling such conditions. Allergic surveys should be made if a hypersensitivity state is suspected.

Complications

Because of the location and the thin-walled structure of the sinuses and their rich venous drainage, sinusitis can be complicated by the spread of the infection to the adjacent structures and to more remote areas. The spread may be (a) through rupture of the sinus wall with local cellulitis, (b) secondary to local osteomyelitis, or (c) via thrombotic spread by way of the rich vascular bed associated with the sinuses.

Cellulitis

The most common complication of acute infection of the frontal, ethmoid, or maxillary sinus in young children is cellulitis of the orbit. This is secondary to the spread of infection through (a) the very thin bony wall between the ethmoid sinuses and the orbit, (b) the roof of the orbit in frontal sinusitis, and (c) the floor of the orbit in maxillary sinusitis (Fig. 4-44). This spread can be the result of local osteomyelitis, thrombosis, or rupture. Such a spread results in swelling and redness of the skin and eyelids and marked chemosis of the eye. Later proptosis may develop with outward displacement of the globe and then loss of movement of the eye. Finally, as the interorbital pressure increases, vision may be endangered.

When the infection does not penetrate the periorbita, it dissects under the periosteum and forms an orbital abscess (which usually spreads posteriorly and can involve the optic foramen) (Fig. 4-46). It causes proptosis and limits eye movement. In some cases the abscess points in one of the lids. When orbital cellulitis or an orbital abscess is not controlled, it can result in total loss of vision in the affected eye. Such cellulitis is accompanied by fever, occasionally a chill, and severe pain. This orbital spread of infection is a serious emergency, and the child should be

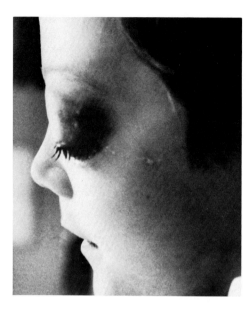

FIG. 4-46. Orbital abscess in a 7-year-old girl showing proptosis of the left eye with ecchymosis of the lid following an acute ethmoid infection. She had marked diplopia. (Photo courtesy of P. Brookhouser.)

started at once on antibiotics and hot compresses. Consultations should be sought immediately with an ophthalmologist and otolaryngologist. The eye grounds should be studied frequently because any evidence of retinal hemorrhage, increasing pallor of the disk, or visual failure makes surgical decompression mandatory. Routine X-ray examination is of limited help in such cases, but CT scans will demonstrate the extent of the cellulitis (Fig. 4-47). The usual surgical approach by the otolaryngologist is through an incision medial to the inner canthus and extending superiorly and inferiorly around the orbital rim. The periosteum is elevated over the lamina papyracea and posteriorly until the abscess is reached and drained. After drainage is established, the ethmoid cells should be exenterated and a large opening made between the orbit and the nose. The frontal or maxillary sinus, when involved, should be drained, and any areas of osteomyelitis of the orbital floor or roof should be removed (see next section).

Osteomyelitis

Osteomyelitis can occur locally in the ethmoid complex with local destruction of cell walls, but it occurs more frequently in the frontal and maxillary sinuses. It is rare in the sphenoid sinus.

The most common and most serious osteomyelitis is that which occurs in the frontal bone secondary to a frontal sinus infection or to trauma to the sinus in the presence of infection. It occurs in children any time after the development of the frontal sinus is nearly complete but with greater frequency in young adolescents than in mature adults, and it is more common in males. It results from the spread of thrombophlebitis originating in vessels of the submucosa of the sinus through

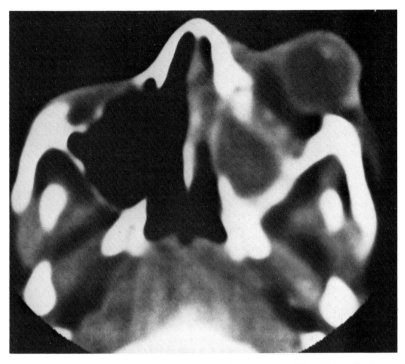

FIG. 4-47. CT scan showing marked anterolateral displacement of the globe of a 7-year-old secondary to intraorbital pressure. (Photo courtesy of P. Brookhouser.)

the penetrating vessels (canals of Breschet) into the veins of the diploic systems of the anterior and posterior bony walls of the sinus or upward into the frontal bone. This spread can result in local subperiosteal abscess formation over the anterior wall (Pott's puffy tumor) or can penetrate inward, causing meningitis or forming an epidural, subdural, or frontal lobe abscess. When the frontal bone becomes involved, there is marked necrosis of the bone with focal areas quickly coalescing into larger areas of decalcified decomposing bone (Fig. 4-48). True sequestration does not take place in the frontal bone. In those cases in which there is downward extension of infection, the superior ethmoid cells and the roof of the orbit may become involved. Such spread can result in a periorbital abscess or a chronically draining fistula around the eye. The close communication of the frontal bone diploic system with the intercranial veins can result in an infected thrombotic process penetrating the cavernous sinus by way of the superior sagittal sinus or the ophthalmic veins. Osteomyelitis is usually caused by frontal sinus infection, but it may also be secondary to external trauma to the frontal bone or to surgical manipulation in an infected frontal sinus without proper measures to control the infection.

Symptoms are pain and tenderness over the sinus. Involvement of the anterior table often results in swelling over the sinus with pitting edema (Pott's puffy tumor)

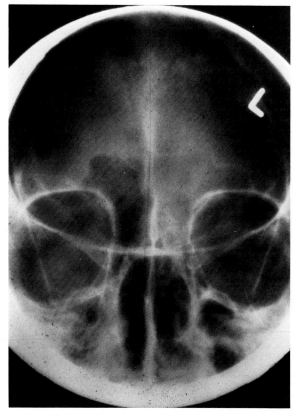

FIG. 4-48. Frontoethmoid osteomyelitis in a young male. Note loss of the bony margin of the frontal sinus and clouding of frontal bone above and ethmoid cells below.

and swelling of the upper eyelid. There may be purulent nasal discharge. X-rays show a blurring of the sinus bony margins, loss of fine bony structure with areas of decalcification, and thickened mucous membrane lining. In cases in which the infection has spread through the inner table of the diploic bone, signs of meningismus, meningitis, and later headaches with personality changes may warn of the development of a frontal lobe abscess. (The symptoms of cavernous sinus thrombosis are discussed separately.)

Osteomyelitis of the frontal bone is primarily a surgical problem and is best treated by antibiotic therapy and radical resection of the infected bone including in the resection a safe margin of normal bone (Fig. 4-49).

FIG. 4-49. Anteroposterior **(A)** and lateral **(B)** projections of the skull of a 12-year-old boy 6 months after surgery. He had developed extensive osteomyelitis of the frontal sinuses and frontal bone following a fall on his face while suffering from an acute cold. He had a small fracture through the anterior wall of the sinus which was untreated. Note the areas of bone regeneration in the posterior table.

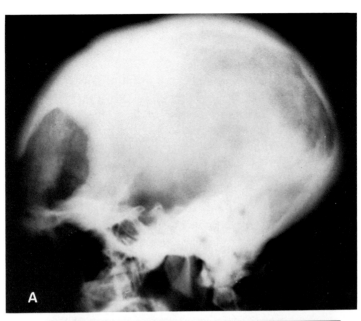

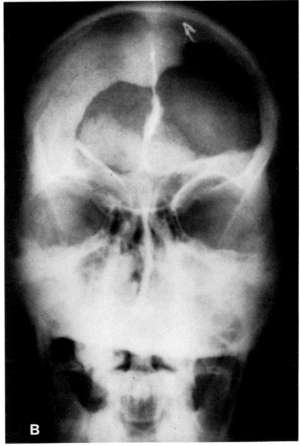

Osteomyelitis of the maxilla is much less common than that of the frontal bone. It is a different type of disease because the maxilla is composed of a different type of bone and contains no diploic system. The disease usually originates from a dental infection or external trauma in the presence of sinus infection but can also result from a surgical attack on the nose or sinuses in the presence of acute infection. Usually the process develops as thrombophlebitis involving the mucoperiosteum of the maxillary sinus and extends into the infraorbital vascular system and ascends from the alveolar region of the maxilla to the infraorbital foramen; from the foramen it may involve the orbital floor. The thrombotic process can progress into the ophthalmic venous system and from there into the cavernous sinus. Usually before there is involvement of the cavernous sinus, sequestration takes place in the anterior wall of the maxilla extending up to and including the orbital floor. Other complications of osteomyelitis of the maxilla are antral–oral fistulas and orbital cellulitis and/or abscess.

Symptoms include marked swelling, erythema, and tenderness over the cheek, swelling of the lower lid, supraorbital headache, and fever. X-ray studies usually outline the involved area of bone and show thickened mucous membrane in the

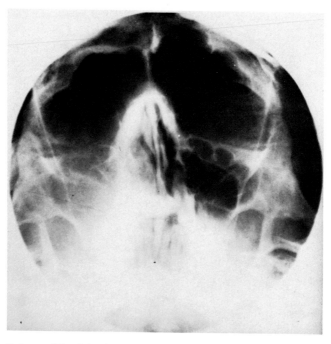

FIG. 4-50. Osteomyelitis of the right maxilla. Note opacification of the medial portion of the maxilla and the nasal bones, and the loss of bony outline of the inferior orbital rim. (From Bordley, J. E.: Modern indications for sinus surgery. *Transactions of the Pacific Coast Oto-Ophthalmological Society,* 50:294, 1969. With permission.)

maxillary sinus (Fig. 4-50). Treatment should be undertaken quickly and consists of high-dose antibiotic therapy and hot compresses. Otolaryngologic consultation should be obtained. When X-ray reveals bone destruction, the sequestrum should be removed and with it any dead bone in the orbital floor; a margin of normal bone should be established.

Cavernous Sinus Thrombosis

Cavernous sinus thrombosis usually occurs secondary to an infected thrombotic spread from the accessory nasal sinuses or to spread of infections in the soft tissues of the nostrils (furunculosis) or following extraction of infected upper teeth. From the nasal sinuses, infection spreads by way of the angular vein and the ophthalmic venous return and/or the sagittal sinus. If not recognized and treated vigorously, cavernous sinus thrombosis is associated with an extremely high mortality rate. Symptoms usually begin with a chill, fever, and headache with pain behind the eyes. The usual course is selective ocular palsy followed by bilateral proptosis (Fig. 4-51), complete bilateral ophthalmoplegia, and meningitis. There are swelling of the lids and marked chemosis. The patient is extremely ill. Consultation should be mandatory. Treatment consists of heavy antibiotic therapy (intravenous) and the administration of anticoagulants. Drainage should be established in any nasal sinus contributing to this condition, and osteomyelitic bone should be removed.

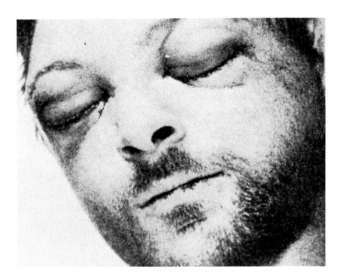

FIG. 4-51. Bilateral cavernous sinus thrombosis following nasal polypectomy and extraction of molar tooth. There is left exophthalmos and bilateral orbital edema. (From Ash, J. E., and Raum, M.: *An Atlas of Otolaryngic Pathology*, p. 538. Armed Forces Institute of Pathology, Washington, D. C., 1949. With permission.)

Meningitis

Extension of an infection from the frontal, ethmoid, or sphenoid sinus can cause penetration of the posterior bony table, reaching the dura, meninges, and frontal lobe of the brain. This extension can result from the development of an infected thrombotic process in a vessel in the mucoperiosteum of a sinus during an acute infection, and in a few instances it is secondary to erosion of the posterior table by longstanding chronic infection. When the infection is the result of such direct communication between sinus and intercranial spaces, there can be recurrent attacks of meningitis until this source has been identified and corrected. Meningitis of sinus origin presents the same clinical picture as any acute bacterial meningitis. A chill is usually followed by a high fever, and the patient develops a severe headache followed by nuchal rigidity, vomiting, convulsions, and coma. Spinal fluid examination will show increased fluid pressure and cloudy fluid with many white blood cells; a culture of the fluid will confirm and identify the infecting agent.

Treatment includes massive doses of antibiotics intravenously and general supportive measures. X-ray studies of the sinuses should be carried out on the child after the meningitis has been resolved to determine the status of the sinuses. If there is evidence of chronic sinusitis, the child should have a thorough investigation of his sinuses. In cases in which meningitis recurs and there is evidence of some relationship between an attack of acute sinusitis and the onset of meningitis, the sinuses should be explored.

Epidural Abscess

Epidural abscess can occur as the result of infection spreading from the sinuses through the penetrating veins of the posterior table to the dura. This presents a slowly developing, ill-defined condition, sometimes very difficult to diagnose. When the infection reaches the dura, there may be a fever preceded by a mild chill. The patient complains of a headache. He does not improve while receiving antibiotic therapy or when there is evidence that the sinusitis has cleared. The white blood cell count, which is usually only slightly elevated, shows a relative increase of lymphocytes. Headache and fever persist, and occasionally tenderness can be elicited by percussion over the frontal bone. An untreated epidural abscess can progress to a brain abscess or can rupture into the arachnoid space. A neurosurgical consultation is advisable for early identification and surgical drainage.

Brain Abscess

Nearly all brain abscesses of sinus origin are located in the frontal lobe. Some authors believe that they are the result of infected thrombi in the terminal portion of the penetrating vessels from the mucoperiosteum of a sinus. A sudden rise of fever accompanied by a chill during acute sinusitis must be considered by the physician as possibly associated with encephalitis and as a precursor to brain abscess. Abscesses in the frontal lobe may be very slow to produce symptoms. Early symptoms are afternoon fever despite clearing of the sinusitis, persistent headache, occasional unexplained nausea, and vomiting. The patient seems unwell, and as the condition progresses personality changes can occur; combativeness and short temper are the most common changes. Facial weakness can also develop in advanced frontal lobe abscesses. Repeated examination of the eyes may show progressive papilledema. Computed tomographic scans and a neurologic consultation can usually establish the diagnosis. Surgical drainage or excision is the usual treatment for such abscesses. The attending physician should make certain that children who have suffered from recurrent meningitis or from an epidural or brain abscess have an otolaryngologic consultation for a complete evaluation of the status of their sinuses.

Mucocele and Pyocele

Mucoceles and pyoceles, which have been briefly described in the section of nasal obstruction, occur very rarely in young children, but they do occur at puberty and in early adult life after maturation of the sinuses. They occur most frequently in the frontal sinuses but can occur in any sinus. The most common causes of mucocele formation are (a) total obstruction to the sinus ostium or drainage duct as the result of previous sinusitis, (b) external trauma including surgery causing damage to or closure of the sinus outlet, and (c) obstruction from growths that impinge on and close the outlet.

A mucocele is a respiratory mucous-membrane-lined cyst containing an accumulation of mucoid secretion resulting from an obstruction to the sinus outlet or trapping of mucous membrane in some defect in the sinus wall (see "Fractures Involving Nasal Sinuses," below). It gradually expands because of the continued production of mucus by the mucous membrane. This results in thinning of and, in some cases, extension through the sinus walls. By its expansion it may erode into and fill a neighboring sinus, appear as a fluctuant mass in the forehead, cheek, or hard palate, expand into the orbit displacing and limiting the movement of the eye, or extend intercranially.

These benign cysts can expand so slowly that the cause of their formation may have occurred years before onset of symptoms. Unless mucoceles become infected, they usually cause no symptoms such as pain, fever, nasal obstruction, or nasal discharge; occasionally a patient complains of a persistent dull headache. If mucoceles expand externally, they can erode through the covering bone, forming a smooth mass that is fluctuant and painless and may be associated with palpable crepitus (egg shell). If they expand into the orbit, they cause a very slow-growing,

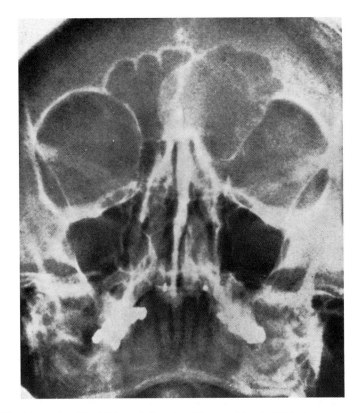

FIG. 4-52. Mucocele of the left frontal sinus in a 13-year-old male. Patient presented with mild left proptoses and diplopia on right lateral and upward gaze. Note destruction of the upper medial portion of the left orbit and the cyst outlined by the calcification. (From Bordley, J. E., and Bosley, W. R.: Mucoceles of the frontal sinus: Causes and treatment. *Ann. Otol. Rhinol. Laryngol.,* 82(5):696–702, 1973. With permission.)

rounded, palpable, fluctuant, painless tumor in the orbital wall 1 to 2 cm posterior to the orbital rim; mucoceles in the frontal or ethmoid sinus as they grow may cause proptosis and/or diplopia because of the limitation of eye movement (Fig. 4-52). Mucoceles in the sphenoid sinus can destroy the sella turcica and involve the third, fourth, and sixth cranial nerves; the earliest symptom of a mucocele in that sinus may be an ophthalmoplegia.

When mucoceles become infected, they are called pyoceles. These can cause fever and because of rapid expansion may cause pain. They also accelerate expansion into the neighboring sinuses, the face, the orbit, or intercranially. Sinus X-ray is of little help in the diagnosis of early mucoceles but may reveal some results of their expansion; CT scans are far more helpful but are not infallible. Antibiotics are not successful in the treatment of pyoceles but should be employed to control an inflammatory flare-up before surgery is undertaken. These cysts should be removed entirely and not treated medically or surgically drained.

FACIAL TRAUMA

Facial fractures can occur as early as at the time of birth, and they increase in frequency and severity as full growth is attained. The frequency of fractures in older children and young adults depends very much on their environment and their occupation.

General Measures

When called to attend a child suffering a possible facial fracture, the physician's first examination should include the evaluation of a number of possibilities before any course of action is planned concerning the fracture. This is particularly important in the event that the patient has suffered a severe blow to the head and/or neck in an automobile accident or in a contact sport. These are listed in order of their importance: (a) Ascertain that there is no airway obstruction; (b) determine the level of consciousness and rule out head injuries; (c) determine any injury to the eye; (d) ascertain that any lacerations have not injured the facial nerve or punctured the parotid duct or gland; and (e) estimate the blood loss and the patient's degree of shock.

Airway obstruction can be determined by observing the patient's color and by listening for the gurgling sounds caused by blood or mucus in the hypopharynx or trachea. Check for backward displacement of the tongue, marked respiratory stridor, and superclavicular retraction during respiratory effort. When repositioning the tongue and cleaning out the hypopharynx fail to relieve respiratory embarrassment, auscultation over the larynx and trachea should be done to determine if the level of obstruction is in the larynx or the upper trachea (see Chapter 7). Such injury may require tracheotomy or insertion of an endotracheal tube.

The level of consciousness should be evaluated. If there is evidence of loss of alertness, the patient should be examined to determine the presence of specific head injury.

The physician should examine the orbital rim and orbital contents and determine any gross loss of visual acuity, limitation of eye movement, and periorbital hemorrhage or proptosis. He should check for facial lacerations to determine if these have injured the facial nerve or penetrated the parotid gland or parotid duct.

It is imperative to check the child's general condition to determine the degree of shock, and in the presence of obvious bleeding try to estimate the blood loss. As a general rule, the physician(s) should control bleeding and suture lacerations before attending to the fracture.

Fractures of the Nose

The most common facial fracture is that of the nose (Fig. 4-53). In man, the prominence and fragility of the nasal structure expose it to frequent injury. If a child's nose bleeds after being struck, it is a presumptive sign of a fracture of the nasal bones or the septum. Common findings in nasal fractures are as follows.

1. *Fracture of the nasal bones.* This may result in a slight or severe depression of the nose at the site of the fracture, ecchymosis, swelling over the pyramid, and deflection of the pyramid. Crepitus may be elicited over the site of the fracture (Figs. 4-54 and 4-55). Discoloration around the eyes is common.

2. *Nasal deformity.* This can be classified as (a) deviation of the nasal pyramid, (b) saddling of the nose from the crushing of the dorsum, and (c) widening as the result of lateral displacement of the nasal bones.

3. *Fracture or dislocation of the nasal septum.* The most frequent fracture of the septum is in the quadrilateral cartilage, with dislocation of its columellar end. Fractures of this cartilage can be associated with a tear in the covering mucous membrane resulting in serious nasal hemorrhage; when the mucous membrane is not torn, bleeding within the septum can result in a septal hematoma (Fig. 4-56).

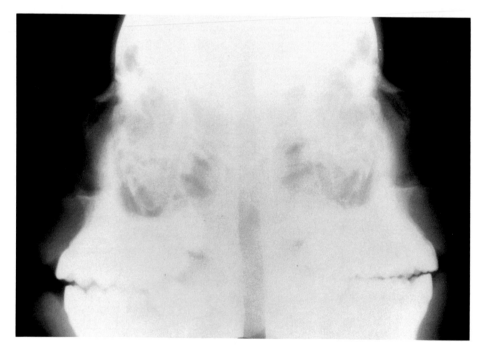

FIG. 4-53.   Normal nasal bones in a 14-year-old boy.

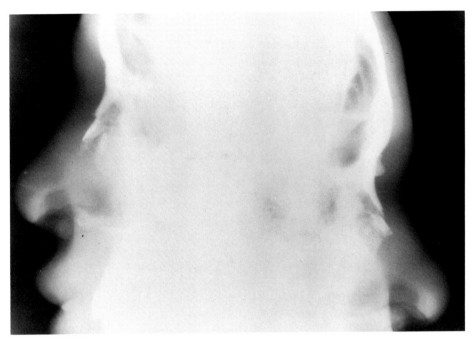

FIG. 4-54. Fracture and displacement of nasal bones in an 18-year-old male.

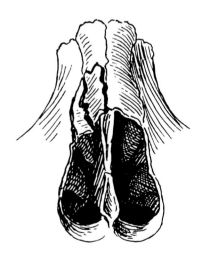

FIG. 4-55. Simple fracture of the right nasal bone with slight depression of fragments. (From Kazanjian, V. H., and Converse, J. M.: *The Surgical Treatment of Facial Injuries,* p. 229. Williams & Wilkins, Baltimore, 1959. With permission.)

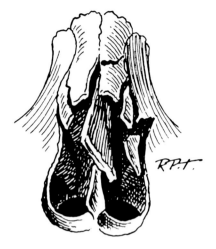

FIG. 4-56. Fracture of the nose involving both nasal bones and a fracture dislocation of the septum. (From Kazanjian, V. H., and Converse, J. M.: *The Surgical Treatment of Facial Injuries,* p. 229. Williams & Wilkins, Baltimore, 1959. With permission.)

With crushing injuries of the vault of the nose, the perpendicular plate of the ethmoid bone may be shattered and the cribriform plate fractured. Such fractures usually result in cerebrospinal fluid (CSF) rhinorrhea.

4. *Nasal obstruction.* This can occur as the result of dislocation of fractured fragments, severe nasal deflection, or intranasal hematomas. However, organized clots in the nostril are the most frequent cause of obstruction.

5. *Nasal bleeding.* In most instances when there is a fracture of a nasal bone or cartilage, there is a tear in the nasal mucosa resulting in some bleeding. Usually the greater the damage to the nose, the greater is the blood loss. In some crushing injuries to the nose, the cribriform plate may be fractured. This causes serious bleeding that is extremely difficult to control. Fractures through the cribriform plate also result in CSF rhinorrhea. In the presence of CSF rhinorrhea, nasal packing should be avoided if possible.

Simple measures should be undertaken to control bleeding before a complete examination is undertaken. When bleeding is controlled, the physician may wish to have an X-ray study, if available, before examination. If possible, before any physical examination is done a careful history should be obtained. This should include a careful description of the accident and of the shape of the nose before the accident, any previous trauma to the nose, and any bleeding tendencies of the child or his family. Recent photographs are helpful.

External examination should include observation of the shape of the nasal pyramid, the presence of ecchymosis, orbital swelling, proptosis, limitation of eye movement, nasal obstruction (if the obstruction is unilateral or bilateral), and if the bleeding and/or rhinorrhea are unilateral or bilateral. The nose should be bimanually palpated to see if the pyramid is mobile and to note crepitus resulting from the movement of bone fragments. The orbital rim should be palpated to determine if there is a "step" deformity suggesting a possible fracture extending into the orbit.

Anterior rhinoscopy reveals any anterior dislocation of the septal cartilage. It also gives information about the nasal airway. A septal hematoma appears as a smooth expansion on one or both sides of the septum. A fracture of the septum with laceration of the mucous membrane is frequently seen, and care must be taken not to insert an instrument or a pack into the septum through the tear. X-ray films will show a fracture line or displacement of fragments of the nasal bones but are not very helpful for septal fractures.

Treatment

Many simple nasal fractures involving only the nasal bones with free mobility of the fragments can be corrected by elevating the bridge of the nose with a thin instrument placed in the nostril and manually realigning the fragments of the nasal bones. A small pack and external stent may be needed to hold the fragments in alignment. Such cases should be referred to an otolaryngologist.

Fractures of the nose involving the septum, the orbit, or saddling of the nose from a crushing blow, or when there has been serious hemorrhage and/or rhinorrhea following an accident, should always be referred to an otolaryngologist for examination and reduction because such fractures may involve the orbit and/or the cribriform plate. If not treated with great expertise, a fractured septum may result in permanent nasal obstruction or septal perforation. Nasal packing should be avoided in the presence of CSF rhinorrhea.

Fractures Involving Nasal Sinuses

Fracture of the Zygoma

The zygomatic arch, through which the coronoid process of the mandible slides, is composed of a temporal portion arising from the temporal bone and a malar portion from the malar process of the maxilla. Fractures may cause simple collapse of the thinnest portion of the arch or may include fractures of the malar root.

When the force of the blow is directed to the side of the head against the arch, the temporal portion of the arch is most likely to break because it is the weakest portion of the arch. Such fractures result in flattening of the temporal prominence of the cheek and limitation of motion of the mandible.

Fractures involving the malar process as well as the temporal portion of the arch are much more serious because they frequently involve the root of the malar process and may result in a fracture known as "trimalar" fracture, involving the inferior and lateral portion of the orbit and the maxillary sinus. They can also involve the infraorbital foramen (Fig. 4-57). Such fractures result in flattening of the zygomatic arch, limitation of motion of the mandible, a step deformity of the inferior orbital rim, and the loss of sensation over the cheek. Ecchymosis can occur in the orbit, resulting in a "black eye" and diplopia. In a few such fractures the malar eminence is freely movable.

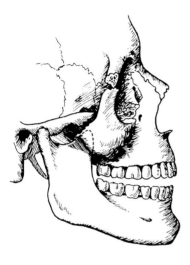

FIG. 4-57. Trimalar fracture right showing the fracture of the zygoma with inward and downward displacement of the detached fragment. This causes a step-down fracture of the orbital floor and flattening of the cheek. (From Kazanjian, V. H., and Converse, J. M.: *The Surgical Treatment of Facial Injuries,* p. 246. Williams & Wilkins, Baltimore, 1959. With permission.)

Simple fractures involving only collapse of the zygomatic arch can be reduced by slipping a flat elevator through a small incision in the skin just above the arch, passing it under the arch, and elevating it. The "trimalar" fracture is considerably more complicated, frequently requiring wiring of the fracture at the orbital rim and/or the arch itself. All fractures of the zygoma should be referred to the otolaryngologist for X-ray examination and reduction.

"Blow-Out" Fractures

"Blow-out" fractures involve the floor of the orbit, which is also the roof of the maxillary sinus. The bone here is extremely thin, and when the force of a blow directed against the orbit suddenly increases the intraorbital pressure, the floor is blown out, forcing some of the orbital contents into the maxillary sinus (Fig. 4-58). In many instances the orbital rim is not fractured, so there is no step deformity. A common complication of such fractures is the incarceration (trap door effect) of the inferior rectus muscle. This causes limitation of motion of the eye, resulting in diplopia on upward gaze. Such accidents also cause ecchymosis in the orbit and a resulting "black eye" and conjunctival hemorrhage. Enophthalmos and limited upward gaze may develop if the condition is not corrected.

Blow-out fractures are corrected by exposing the floor of the orbit (the roof of the maxillary sinus) in order to elevate the displaced contents and free the entrapped muscle. When the displaced tissues and muscle have been returned to the orbit, the defect in the floor is closed, employing a bone graft from the anterior wall of the maxillary sinus or a sheet of some plastic substance that will be tolerated by the recipient's tissues. Occasionally a pack is placed in the antrum to support the repaired orbital floor.

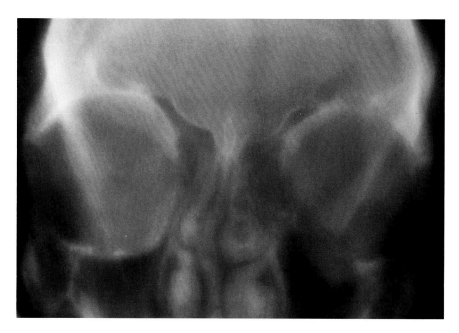

FIG. 4-58. Tomogram showing fracture of the nasal bones and the orbital floor, with a small blow-out fracture in the left maxillary sinus.

Frontal Sinus Fractures

Frontal sinus fractures occur very rarely in children before 10 to 12 years of age because of the late development of this sinus. After the sinus is developed, the fractures that occur can be classified as follows: (a) simple fracture of the anterior table without displacement of fragments; (b) fracture of the anterior table with displacement posteriorly of fragments; (c) fracture of the anterior table and the posterior table, with or without CSF rhinorrhea; and (d) fractures that involve the nasofrontal duct.

Frequently frontal sinus fractures are missed because they may not cause noticeable external deformity and because there is no demonstrable palpable crepitus. However, when a child has received a severe blow over the frontal sinus, a fracture should be carefully ruled out. In all cases in which nasal bleeding or watery nasal discharge occurs after a blow to the forehead, the physician should assume that a fracture has occurred. Bleeding suggests a fracture that has torn the mucous membrane of the sinus, and CSF rhinorrhea indicates a fracture through the posterior table of the sinus that has caused a dural tear or a fracture through the cribriform plate. The best way to rule out a fracture or to determine the type of fracture that has occurred is by a careful X-ray study. Tomograms have proved most useful in identifying this fracture and are preferred here to CT scans. Whenever there is doubt about a possible frontal fracture, routine X-ray studies should be superseded by tomograms.

A simple fracture of the anterior table without displacement rarely needs any surgical treatment. A depressed fracture of the anterior table can frequently be treated by surgical elevation and alignment of the displaced fragments. Sometimes it is necessary to wire the fragments. It will probably require an open reduction.

Fractures involving the posterior table, the orbital roof, or the nasofrontal duct require exploration of the frontal sinus and so should be referred immediately to the otolaryngologist. When the mucous membrane of the sinus or duct has been lacerated, and when there is separation of the posterior table fragments or those of the orbital roof and/or a dural tear, the dural tear should be repaired, the mucous membrane lining of the sinus and duct carefully removed, and the sinus obliterated. Obliteration can be done with the use of a fat graft, or the sinus can be collapsed by removing the anterior table and allowing the cavity to be filled with the soft tissues of the forehead. Such fractures if untreated often result in later formation of mucoceles.

Fractures of the Maxillary Sinus

Fractures of the maxillary sinus are rare and usually come about because a small object such as a stone or a pellet or a small ball strikes the anterior wall. Such fractures cause nasal bleeding and result in crepitus over the cheek. They may also involve the anterior ethmoid sinuses (Fig. 4-59). If the fragments are displaced, the child should be referred to the otolaryngologist for X-ray study and for realignment of the fragments.

Precautions to be observed by the attending physician in all accessory nasal sinus fractures are as follows:

1. The patient should be advised not to blow his nose. Nose blowing can force infected secretions into the cranium in those patients with fractures extending into the intercranial spaces. It can cause soft tissue or orbital emphysema and proptosis where the fracture tears the mucous membrane of the anterior wall or orbital wall of the maxillary or ethmoid sinuses.
2. Care should be taken not to push instruments into the nose or to pack the nose in cases of suspected CSF rhinorrhea.
3. If there is a history of sinus infection or there is an acute upper respiratory infection at the time of the fracture, the patient should be placed on antibiotics.

Facial Fractures

Facial fractures in children include the same types of fractures that occur in adults, although they occur with less frequency than in adults for two reasons. A child's bones are more elastic than mature facial bones and therefore have less

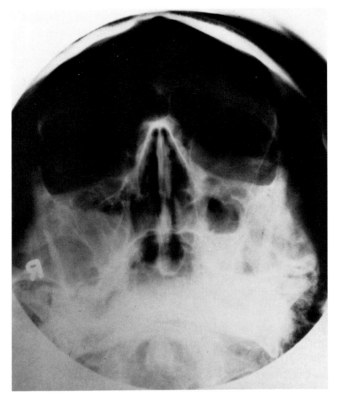

FIG. 4-59.   Fracture of the right maxilla of a young boy with depression of the orbital rim and a fluid level in the right maxillary sinus.

tendency to shatter from a blow. Moreover, the average child is exposed to less severe facial trauma than adults who compete in contact sports and drive automobiles.

Facial fractures occurring in children respond to the same corrective measures as those employed for adults. A complicating factor faced by the doctor treating such fractures in children is the presence of unerupted teeth. These can be injured by the trauma causing the fracture or by the methods employed to care for the fracture. In all facial fractures, one of the primary objectives is to obtain good dental occlusion because the patient suffering malocclusion after facial fracture will have difficulty until the occlusion can be restored.

Facial fractures in children are classified in the same manner as those in adults; they fall into three categories—the Le Forte I, II, and III fractures, which represent an increasing damage to the facial bony structures. They all should be managed by a specialist and require special X-ray studies before treatment.

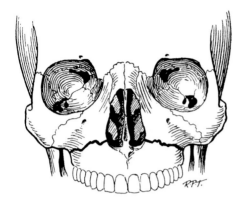

FIG. 4-60. Le Fort I fracture which separates the lower maxilla from the alveolar process, palate, and pterygoid process. (From Kazanjian, V. H., and Converse, J. M.: *The Surgical Treatment of Facial Injuries*, p. 193. Williams & Wilkins, Baltimore, 1959. With permission.)

Le Forte I

This fracture involves the lower midfacial structures, and the fracture line is a transverse one across the lower maxilla and into the bony nostril apertures (Fig. 4-60); it creates a floating segment of the lower maxilla that includes the alveolar process, the hard palate, and the teeth (both milk teeth and permanent teeth). Occasionally the fracture line lies below the nasal structures and results in a floating alveolus. Such floating structures may be complicated by a vertical fracture line that splits them into two.

These fractures can be reduced by wiring "arch bars" to the upper and lower teeth and then passing a stabilizing wire from the upper arch bar and attaching it to the zygoma. Proper occlusion can be maintained by the use of elastic traction between the arch bars.

Le Forte II

Here the fracture line is higher in the face. It extends through the pterygoid plate and passes forward through the orbital rim and the upper portion of the nasal bones (Fig. 4-61). This penetrates the upper portion of the maxillary sinus and the upper ethmoid cells, and it may include the cribriform plate. Fractures through the ethmoids and cribriform plate can result in a CSF leak.

Treatment here applies the same principles as those employed for Le Forte I fractures. Displaced segments are rocked into as correct a position as possible. Then arch bars and elastic traction are employed to stabilize the fragments and to bring the occlusion into the proper alignment.

Le Forte III

This fracture is sometimes known as a "midfacial dissociation." In this case, the midfacial bony structure is separated from its bony attachments to the skull (Fig.

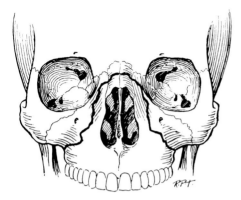

FIG. 4-61. Le Fort II, or pyramidal, fracture, which is a fracture line that runs transversely through the maxilla extending through the nasal bones. (From Kazanjian, V. H., and Converse, J. M.: *The Surgical Treatment of Facial Injuries,* p. 194. Williams & Wilkins, Baltimore, 1959. With permission.)

4-62). A transverse fracture line separates the nasal bones from the nasal process of the frontal bone, passes through the orbit, the frontomaxillary suture, and the zygomatic–maxillary suture line. The upper portion of the midface is usually displaced backward. This results in a "dished face" with the bite locked open anteriorly because the posterior teeth of the upper jaw are moved forward and downward by midfacial displacement. These fractures are usually accompanied by multiple fractures around the face, and often there is associated CSF rhinorrhea.

The treatment of such fractures usually depends on the wiring of arch bars to the upper and lower jaws and the application of elastic traction to realign the segments and restore the bite. All Le Forte-type fractures require very special care by a surgeon trained to handle such fractures. Most of them, when properly treated, have a very good prognosis.

FIG. 4-62. Le Fort III fracture showing craniofacial disjunction. (From Kazanjian, V. H., and Converse, J. M.: *The Surgical Treatment of Facial Injuries,* p. 194. Williams & Wilkins, Baltimore, 1959. With permission.)

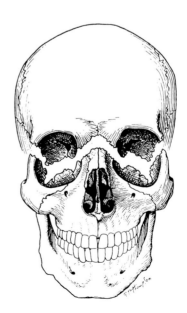

Fractures of the Mandible

Mandibular fractures rank second to nasal fractures as the most common of all facial fractures. The mandible is the largest of the facial bones and, next to the nose, the most exposed. Its main body is U-shaped, and its posterior portion has an upward curve, the ramus, which divides superiorly into an anterior coronoid process and a posterior condylar process. The upper end of the condyle forms the inferior articular surface of the temporomandibular joint. Fractures often occur simultaneously on the side of impact and on the opposite side (Fig. 4-63). The most common fracture is through the neck of the condyle (Fig. 4-64), and the second most frequent is at the angle of the ramus. Displacement upward of the ramus is common when fractures occur at the angle because of the upward pull of the powerful masseter, temporalis, and pterygoid muscles.

The diagnosis of mandibular fractures can be greatly facilitated if the type and direction of the blow can be ascertained. A blow from the front impacting the chin frequently causes bilateral fractures of the condyles, whereas one impacting from the side causes a fracture of the opposite condyle and a fracture of the body of the mandible at the site of impact. Displacement of the ramus occurs with angle fractures. Fractures of the mandible usually result in malocclusion because of upward displacement of the posterior fragment by the strong "grinding" muscles and downward displacement of the anterior fragment because of the action of the digastric, geniohyoid, and mylohyoid muscles. Point tenderness and local ecchymosis are usually present as well as restriction of jaw movement. Occasionally a fracture line is palpated on examination of the mandible.

The usual treatment of mandibular fractures is closed reduction, and proper occlusion is obtained by the use of elastic traction between upper and lower jaws. Open reduction may be necessary in the presence of a shattered jaw.

Fractures of the coronoid process are rare. They may lock the bite open if the upper fragment becomes engaged under the zygomatic arch; however, they seldom require treatment, as the coronoid is well splinted by its surrounding muscles.

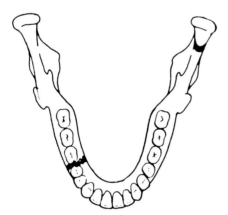

FIG. 4-63. Common sites of double fractures of the mandible. In this case a blow delivered from the right fractured the body of the jaw at the site of impact and the condyle on the opposite side. (From Paparella, M. M., and Shumrick, D. A.: *Otolaryngology, Vol. 3: Head and Neck,* p. 437. W. B. Saunders Co., Philadelphia, 1973.)

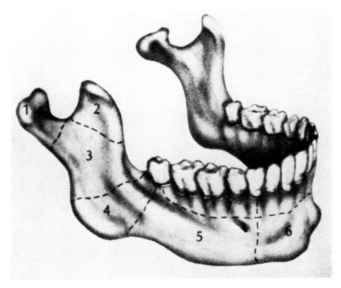

FIG. 4-64. Common sites of mandibular fractures: (*1*) condyle. (*2*) coronoid process. (*3*) ramus. (*4*) angle. (*5*) body. (*6*) symphysis. (*7*) alveolus. (From English, G. M.: *Otolaryngology,* Vol. 4, Chapter 33, p. 17. Harper & Row, New York, 1983. With permission.)

SELECTED READING

Ambrus, P. S., et al. (1981): Management of nasal septal abscess. *Laryngoscope,* 91:575–582.

Ash, J. E., and Raum, M. (1949): Chap. 3: Histology of the nose and sinuses. Chap. 18: Tumors of the nose and sinuses. In: *Atlas of Otolaryngic Pathology.* Armed Forces Institute of Pathology, Bethesda, Md.

Bordley, J. E. (1950): Observations on changes taking place in the upper respiratory tract under ACTH and cortisone therapy. *Bull. Johns Hopkins Hosp.,* 87(5):482–504.

Bordley, J. E. (1969): Modern indications for sinus surgery. *Transactions of the Pacific Coast Oto-Ophthalmological Society,* pp. 281–301.

Bordley, J. E., and Bosley, W. R. (1973): Mucoceles of the frontal sinus: Causes and treatment. *Arch. Otol. Rhinol. Laryngol.,* 82:696–702.

Bordley, J. E., and Farrior, J. (1982): Frontal fractures. In: *Otolaryngology Looseleaf Series,* Vol. IV. Harper & Row, Denver.

Dupin, C. L., and Le Jeune, F. E., Jr. (1978): Nasal masses in infants and children. *South. Med. J.,* 71(2):124–128.

Fairbanks, D. N. F., et al. (1974): Intercranial complications of sinusitis. In: *Otolaryngology Looseleaf Series,* Vol. III, Chap. 19. Harper & Row, Denver.

Flake, C. G., and Ferguson, C. (1964): Congenital choanal atresia in infants and children. *Ann. Otol. Rhinol. Laryngol.,* 73:458–573.

Friedman, I. (1973): Wegener's granulomatosis. In: *Otolaryngology,* Vol. 3, edited by M. M. Paparella and D. A. Shumrick, pp. 26–28. Saunders, Philadelphia.

Furstenburg, A. C. (1931): Osteomyelitis of the skull. *Ann. Otol. Laryngol. Rhinol.,* 40:996–1012.

Godel, V. G., et al. (1981): Maxillary meningioma appearing as exophthalmos. *Arch. Otolaryngol.,* 107:October.

Hinderer, K. H. (1971): Chap. 4: Developmental anatomy. Chap. 5: Adverse conditions affecting development of the nose. In: *Fundamentals of Anatomy and Surgery of the Nose.* Aesculopius, Birmingham, Alabama.

Hinderer, K. H. (1978): Nasal problems in children. *Ear Nose Throat J.,* 57:116–126.

Jones, H. M. (1981): Some orbital complications of nose and throat conditions. *J. R. Soc. Med.*, 74:409–414.

Kazanjian, V. H., and Converse, J. M. (1959): Fractures of the maxilla. In: *Surgical Treatment of Facial Injuries,* Chap. 7. Williams & Wilkins, Baltimore.

May, M., et al. (1970): Nasofrontal duct in frontal sinus fractures. *Arch. Otol.*, 92:534–538.

Negus, V. (1961): *Biology of Respiration.* Williams & Wilkins, Baltimore.

Parkin, J. L., and Dixon, J. A. (1981): Laser photocoagulation in hereditary hemorrhagic telangiectasia. *Otolaryngol. Head Neck Surg.*, 89:204–208.

Templer, J., and Davis, W. E. (1979): Congenital tumors of the nose. *Ear Nose Throat J.*, 58:481–487.

Chapter 5

Mouth and Pharynx

Embryology and Anatomy 318
   Oral Cavity 318
   Hard Palate and Alveolar Process 319
   Tongue 320
   Potential Spaces in the Floor of the Mouth 321
   Salivary Glands. 321
   Pharynx 322
   Parapharyngeal or Lateral Pharyngeal Space 323
   Tonsils and Adenoids 323
   Lymphatics 325
   Muscles of the Pharynx 325
   Teeth 326
Examination of the Mouth and Pharynx 326
Disorders and Diseases of the Mouth 332
   Dental Problems 332
   Congenital Deformities. 336
   Tumors of the Jaw 341
   Abnormalities of the Tongue 343
   Burns of the Mouth and Oropharynx 345
   Infections of the Oral Cavity 346
   Blood Dyscrasias 350
   Tumors in the Mouth 351
Tonsils and Adenoids 352
   Role in Immunity 352
   Hypertrophy of the Tonsils 353
   Infections of the Tonsils and Adenoids. 354
   Pseudotonsillitis 359
Infections Involving the Pharyngeal Spaces .359
   Submental Space Infection. 360
   Peritonsillar Space Infection 360
   Retropharyngeal Space Infection 361

Parapharyngeal Space Infection 361
Submaxillary Space—Ludwig's Angina 363
Tumors of the Tonsils 366
   Benign Tumors 366
   Malignant Tumors 367
Nasopharynx 367
   Disorders of the Nasopharynx 367
   Foreign Bodies in the Nasopharynx 369
   Tumors of the Nasopharynx. 369
Laryngopharynx (Hypopharynx) 376
   Benign Lesions 376
   Infections 377
   Cysts 377
Tonsillectomy and/or Adenoidectomy: Reasons For and Against 378
   Indications for Tonsillectomy 379
   Indications for Adenoidectomy 379
   Complications of Tonsillectomy and Adenoidectomy 380

This chapter discusses the embryologic development and clinical anatomy of (a) the mouth and its contents and (b) the pharynx (nasopharynx, oropharynx, and laryngopharynx). It also describes and discusses the congenital deformities, disorders, and diseases of these areas.

EMBRYOLOGY AND ANATOMY

Oral Cavity

Development and Anatomy

The primitive oral cavity begins as a depression (the oral pit) on the stomodeum of the embryo beneath the anterior cerebral vesicle. Its development commences on the 13th day. The oral pit is separated from the upper end of the head gut by the pharyngeal membrane. Rupture of the pharyngeal membrane composed of opposing surfaces of ectoblastic and entoblastic origins is followed by deepening of the oral pit, which opens into the head gut forming the primitive pharynx. On about the 20th day, the first visceral arch (mandibular arch) splits, differentiating the maxillary and mandibular processes. The mandibular processes grow ventrally and fuse in the midline; combined with the second visceral arches, they form the boundaries of the floor of the mouth. At 5 weeks, the nasomedial process descends and lies between the maxillary and mandibular processes, fusing with the maxillary

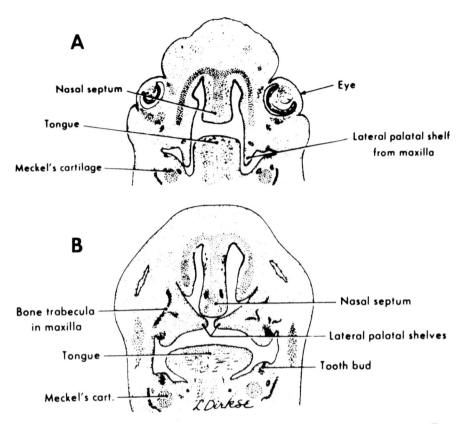

A

Nasal septum

Tongue

Meckel's cartilage

Eye

Lateral palatal shelf from maxilla

B

Bone trabecula in maxilla

Tongue

Meckel's cart.

Nasal septum

Lateral palatal shelves

Tooth bud

FIG. 5-1. Development of the palate. **A:** Seven-week embryo. **B:** Eight-week embryo. (From Patten, B.: *Human Embryology,* Blakiston, Philadelphia, 1946. After an original figure by W. Patten. With permission of McGraw-Hill.)

processes at 6 weeks and forming the midportion of the upper lip and the intermaxillary segment of the upper jaw (Fig. 5-1).

Hard Palate and Alveolar Process

The hard palate and alveolar process are formed by fusion of the lateral palatal shelves of the maxillary processes and the nasofrontal process at the time when the tongue flattens out, leaving space above it for the processes to move toward the midline. It becomes covered with firmly attached mucoperiosteum and mucous membrane.

The normal palate at birth consists of three portions: hard palate, soft palate, and uvula. These are covered with nonciliated mucous membrane continuous with that of the alveolus and meet as a raphe (ridge) in the midline. The mucous membrane forms rugae on the oral surface of the hard palate. The palatine bones are continuous with the alveolus laterally and are supported from above in the midline by the vomer. The soft palate is attached to the posterior border of the hard palate. The uvula is the small midline mass of muscle at the posterior margin of the soft palate.

The soft palate develops from a fold of mucous membrane arising from the posterior border of the hard palate. Its lower border is concave on each side with a medial elongation that later forms the uvula. The lateral borders of the soft palate extend downward in two folds, which form the anterior and posterior faucial pillars. With the mouth closed the soft palate rests on the tongue, and with the mouth open it hangs free. When the soft palate is raised, it separates the oropharynx from the nasopharynx.

The anterior faucial pillar is formed by the palatoglossus muscle, which attaches to the lateral border of the posterior tongue; the posterior pillar is formed by the palatopharyngeus muscle, which attaches to the superior cornu of the thyroid cartilage. The other muscles forming the body of the soft palate are the tensor palatini arising from the scaphoid fossa, which attaches along the eustachian tube, and the levator palatini, which arises from the apex of the petrous bone and attaches to the cartilagenous portion of the eustachian tube.

Tongue

The tongue is a muscular organ attached to the floor of the mouth and the hyoid bone. It has a double origin. The main body arises from paired anlagen in the anterior portion of the floor of the mouth, and the root of the tongue is derived from a median elevation of the floor of the mouth, the copula, and from portions of the second visceral arch. The thyroglossal duct opens at the junction of these two structures in the midline of the tongue just posterior to the circumvallate papillae. This opening is the foramen caecum. The tongue is covered with mucous membrane that is continuous with the floor of the mouth. Under its anterior tip a fold of mucous membrane forms the frenum, which attaches to the floor of the mouth. Medial to the insertion of the anterior pillars is a line of eight or nine large papillar masses— circumvallate papillae—which are surrounded by taste buds.

The tongue has two sets of muscles, intrinsic and extrinsic. The extrinsic muscles are the genioglossus, hyoglossus, styloglossus, palatoglossus, and geniohyoid. They are paired, and all except the palatoglossus receive their innervation from the n. hyoglossus. The nerve supply for the palatoglossus comes from the pharyngeal plexus, probably from the spinal accessory nerve.

The intrinsic muscles form the body of the tongue. They are the lingualis and the transversus. A few vertical fibers in the tongue are referred to by some anatomists as the muscle perpendicularis.

Motor innervation is supplied by the n. hyoglossus. Sensation of the anterior two-thirds of the tongue is supplied by the lingual branch of the fifth nerve, and the posterior one-third of the tongue by the glossopharyngeal nerve; taste over the anterior third of the tongue is mediated by the chorda tympani nerve, which descends from the geniculate ganglion of the facial nerve in the temporal bone. The bilateral blood supply is by the lingual arteries, which are branches of the external carotid arteries.

Between the floor of the mouth and the tongue is the sublingual space. The ducts from the submaxillary gland (Wharton's duct) and the sublingual salivary glands pass forward through the space and empty on each side of the attachment of the frenum to the floor of the mouth.

Potential Spaces in the Floor of the Mouth

There are three potential spaces on the floor of the mouth that can become involved in serious infection: (a) the submental space, (b) the submaxillary space, and (c) the sublingual space.

The submental space is the smallest of the three. Its side walls are the anterior bodies of the digastric muscles; the roof of the space is formed by the mylohyoid muscles; the posterior wall is bounded by the hyoid bone; and the floor is composed of the fascia of the skin.

The submaxillary space extends superiorly between the ramus of the mandible and the lower border of the temporal bone. The styloid muscles and the posterior digastric muscle form its posterior wall, and the mylohyoid and hyoglossal muscles form the roof. The anterior wall is formed by the anterior digastric muscle, and its floor is the deep fascia of the chin. The submaxillary gland lies in this space.

The sublingual space is bounded by the mandible anteriorly and laterally; the posterior wall is formed by the styloglossus muscles, the palatoglossus muscles, and the hyoid bone. The roof is formed by the mylohyoid muscles.

Infection in these spaces can compromise the child's airway and may require surgical drainage (see "Infections Involving the Pharyngeal Spaces," below).

Salivary Glands

The parotid gland, the largest salivary gland, lies behind the upper part of the ramus of the mandible with an extension overlapping the external side of the ramus. It extends foward over the masseter muscle. It is divided into lobules and is surrounded by a tough capsule of fibrous tissue. The gland extends forward from just anterior to the auditory meatus and styloid process and occupies a space bounded anteriorly by the ramus of the jaw, the masseter, and the internal pterygoid muscles. The external carotid artery enters the gland from the inner side and divides into the temporal and internal maxillary branches. The facial nerve enters the gland through its posterior surface, passes obliquely foward, lying external to the artery, and divides within the gland into its two main trunks. The parotid (Stenson's) duct emerges from the anterior surface of the gland, passing forward and downward across the external surface of the masseter muscle. It runs through the buccinator muscle and empties into the mouth opposite the first or second upper molar tooth.

The submaxillary gland lies within the submaxillary space just inside and slightly forward of the angle of the mandible, external to the mylohyoid and hyoglossus muscles. Its duct (Wharton's) runs forward along the floor of the mouth and opens at the base of the frenum.

Pharynx

The pharynx is described as a bag with musculomembranous walls that are lined with mucous membrane, and it opens anteriorly into the nose and mouth. It extends from the base of the skull to the lower border of the larynx at the level of the seventh cervical vertebra, and behind it lies the spinal column covered by the prevertebral muscles and fascia. The roof of the pharynx is the basilar process of the occiput and the base of the sphenoid bone.

The pharynx is enclosed by the loose mucopharyngeal fascia, which allows free movement of the pharynx on the prevertebral fascia. It can be divided into: (a) the nasopharynx, which is that portion lying above the lower edge of the soft palate extending upward behind the posterior aspect of the nasal chambers; (b) the oropharynx, which opens into the mouth and extends downward behind the tongue to the hyoid bone; and (c) the laryngopharynx, which extends below the hyoid bone, its posterial wall formed by the anterior surface of the larynx and its lower limits being the pyriform sinuses and the orifice of the esophagus. The posterior wall of the upper two divisions of the pharynx is anterior to the prevertebral structures of the cervical vertebrae and is covered by nonciliated mucous membrane up to the midportion of the adenoids. The lateral walls of the upper pharynx are formed by the eustachian tube orifices and the fossae of Rosenmüller, and below the faucial tonsils and lingual tonsils.

The upper two-thirds of the pharynx contains a number of important lymphoid structures that reach their greatest development during childhood: (a) the adenoids, which lie on the posterior superior wall of the nasopharynx, sometimes extending into the fossae of Rosenmüller; (b) the faucial tonsils, which lie on the lateral walls of the oropharynx between the anterior and posterior pillars; and (c) the lingual tonsils, which extend from the lower border of the faucial tonsils across the base of the tongue.

The posterior wall of the pharynx is important particularly in young children because of the glands in the retropharyngeal space. The posterior wall is separated from the anterior surfaces of the first five cervical vertebrae by the loose connective tissue covering the anterior wall of the prevertebral fascia. Tuberculous infection of the cervical vertebrae can perforate the prevertebral fascia and form an abscess in the retropharyngeal space. In the event of acute bacterial infection involving the retropharyngeal glands, abscesses can form between the prevertebral fascia and the posterior wall of the pharynx (see "Retropharyngeal Space Infection," below).

Parapharyngeal or Lateral Pharyngeal Space

The parapharyngeal or lateral pharyngeal space is a large triangular potential space that lies next to the tonsillar fossa at the lateral aspect of the pharynx. It is divided into anterior and posterior spaces by the styloid muscle. The posterior space extends from the base of the skull to the visceral cervical space and is contained within the carotid sheath. Important structures in this space are the internal carotid artery, the vagus nerve, and the internal jugular vein. The anterior space contains the ascending pharyngeal artery, loose connective tissue, and lymph glands. It extends from the base of the skull to the level of the angle of the jaw. Its posterior wall is formed by the carotid sheath and the fascia and muscles attached to the styloid. The medial wall is covered by the alar fascia; the anterior wall is formed by the buccopharyngeal fascia. This fascia-lined potential space communicates with the retropharyngeal peritonsillar spaces and extends down along the great vessels to the superior mediastinum; it can become a channel for the spread of infection originating in the retropharyngeal space, in the vicinity of the tonsils, and around the molar teeth or the base of the tongue. (See p. 361, Parapharyngeal Space Infection.)

Tonsils and Adenoids

The distribution of lymphoid (adenoid) tissue in the pharynx is referred to as Waldeyer's ring, a ring of lymphoid tissue that roughly encircles the pharynx. It is present in the fetus and grows rapidly during the last month *in utero* and less rapidly during the first 3 to 4 years of childhood. Atrophy of the lymphoid tissue begins at puberty, and by age 30, healthy adenoids and tonsils have become small. Waldeyer's ring lies in the region of the junction of the air and food passages. In the child this lymphoid tissue forms the adenoids, which grow on the upper posterior wall of the nasopharynx, the faucial tonsils that grow between the anterior and posterior faucial pillars, and the lingual tonsils, which grow from the base of the faucial tonsils on each side of the tongue anterior to the valleculae extending from the circumvallate papilla to the epiglottis. In addition, some submucosal plaques of lymphoid tissue form on each side of the posterior pharyngeal wall medial to the posterior tonsillar pillar, the lateral pharyngeal bands.

All of these structures are composed of lymphoid tissue, but their anatomic composition is not the same. The adenoids are formed by orderly masses or follicles of lymphoid tissue held together by a delicate reticulum of connective tissue. The lobules consist of germinal centers surrounded by maturing lymphoid cells and extend across the posterior wall of the nasopharynx between the eustachian tube orifices. The adenoids are grouped around a central depression, the pharyngeal bursa, and their upper two-thirds are covered by ciliated respiratory mucous membrane that is punctuated by numerous small depressions formed by epithelium-lined simple crypts. The lower third is covered by nonciliated mucous membrane.

The tonsils consist of more compact lymphoid follicles than the adenoids, also containing germinal centers; they are covered by nonciliated mucous membrane and are indented by numerous epithelium-lined compound crypts (Fig. 5-2), which extend to the capsule of the tonsil. The embedded portion of the tonsil is covered by an adherent fibrous sheath, the tonsillar capsule, separating it from the surrounding muscles. The vascular supply of the tonsil is derived from several sources, a branch of the ascending pharyngeal artery entering the midportion of the tonsil and a branch of the facial artery entering the base of the tonsil. Several small arteries may enter it at the upper pole. It is innervated by branches from the fifth nerve and the glossopharyngeal nerve.

The lingual tonsils are separated from the underlying muscles of the tongue by a layer of thick connective tissue. They are covered with adherent nonciliated mucous membrane and contain a few simple crypts, which are numerous crater-like irregularities that contain mucous glands.

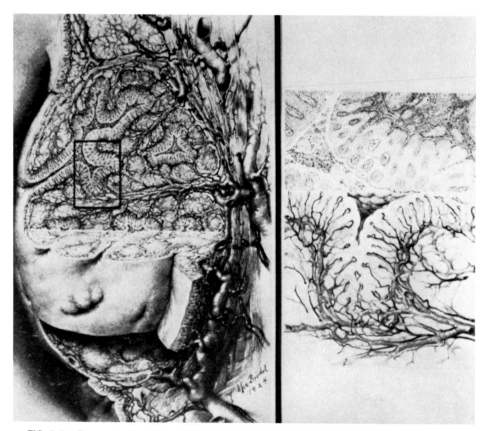

FIG. 5-2. Reconstruction of tonsil. The rich vascular network surrounds the crypts that extend to the tonsillar capsule. (From M. Brodel: The Johns Hopkins University. With permission.)

In children, great care should be taken not to confuse aberrant thyroid tissue growing on the base of the tongue with enlarged lingual tonsils. This mistake has been made many times, and removal of such tissue may result in cretinism.

Lymphatics

The posterior cervical chain of lymph glands drains the retropharyngeal region, the area of adenoid growth, and the region of the fossae of Rosenmüller. The anterior cervical chain drains the faucial and lingual tonsils as well as the main body of the tongue. The submental nodes receive lymph channels from the floor of the mouth and the tip of the tongue.

Muscles of the Pharynx

The muscles of the pharynx differ from the arrangement of muscles elsewhere in the digestive tract: those running longitudinally are placed internally, and the circular muscles are external. Three sets of muscles form the constrictors of deglutition. (a) The superior constrictor muscle arises from the hamular process of the internal pterygoid plate, the pterygomandibular ligament, the mylohyoid ridge, and the side of the tongue. The muscle passes posteriorly, meeting its twin in a median raphe. This extends most of the length of the posterior wall of the pharynx, attaching to the pharyngeal tubercle of the basilar process. (b) The middle constrictor muscle arises from the lower end of the stylohyoid ligament, the lesser horn of the hyoid bone, and the upper border of the greater horn. The fibers fan out, meeting their twins in a median raphe. (c) The inferior constrictor, heaviest of the constrictors, arises from the posterolateral portion of the cricoid cartilage, the triangular surface of the thyroid cartilage, and its anterior horn. It overlaps the middle constrictor; its lowest fibers join the circular fibers of the gullet.

The longitudinal stylopharyngeus muscle arises from the inner side of the styloid bone, descends between the middle and superior constrictors, and ends in an expansion on the side of the pharynx; some fibers insert on the posterior border of the thyroid cartilage, and the rest insert into the expanded portion of the palatopharyngeus. One bundle of fibers passes from the thyroid division to the side of the epiglottis, forming a fold on the side of the larynx, the plica pharyngoepiglottica; the salpingopharyngeus arises from the eustachian tube and extends to the back of the hard palate.

The action of the constrictors is to decrease the size of the pharynx. The longitudinal muscles raise the larynx and pharynx to promote the act of swallowing.

The nerve supply of the constrictors is from the pharyngeal plexus and the recurrent laryngeal nerve except the stylopharyngeus, which is innervated by the glossopharyngeal nerve.

The chief blood supply of the pharynx is the ascending pharyngeal artery. Some vascular support in the lower pharynx comes from the superior thyroid artery.

Lymphatic drainage of the pharynx is to the prevertebral nodes and the deep cervical nodes.

Teeth

Development of the teeth begins at the seventh week of fetal life with thickening along the margins of the oral cavity. This develops into the labiodental strand of epithelium, which grows into the mesoblast and divides into two plates. The inner plate (the dental ledge or bar) is the precursor of the teeth. During the third month, anlagen of the milk teeth (dental germs) develop, which in turn become tooth sacs in which the teeth take final form.

The permanent teeth develop from a second set of "dental germs," which are formed while the milk teeth are developing. They also arise from a dental bar. The dental germs of the first molar teeth appear during the 17th week, preceding the germs of the permanent incisors and canines, which appear during the 24th week. The first bicuspids are seen during the 29th week, and the second bicuspids appear a month later. The germs of the second and third molars are formed at 4 months and at 3 years after birth, respectively.

At birth there are 20 crowns of milk teeth in the jaws. Cusps of the permanent molars, except the first molar, are uncalcified at birth, as are the rudiments of the permanent incisors and canines. The rudiments of the permanent teeth lie behind and above the milk teeth in the upper jaw, and below and behind the milk teeth in the lower jaw (Fig. 5-3).

Milk teeth erupt in five groups separated by intervals, as shown in Table 5-1. Calcification of the permanent teeth is as follows: first molars just before birth, incisors and canines at 6 months, bicuspids and second upper molars during the third year, second lower molars at 6 years, and wisdom teeth at 12 years. The first permanent molars come into line with the milk teeth and begin to perforate the gums even before the milk teeth are lost.

EXAMINATION OF THE MOUTH AND PHARYNX

Every physical examination of this or any other area or system of the body should be preceded by a careful history. A simple model of history-taking in this area follows.

1. *Present illness.* This history should include the patient's major complaint, its onset, and course of the disease or disorder to date, including symptoms as they have developed. (a) Onset sudden or gradual? Preceded by other illness? (b) Pain location and duration? (c) Fever and/or chills. (d) Course—any additional symptoms that have developed during illness. (e) Duration and description of any treatment carried out before this examination and all medication.

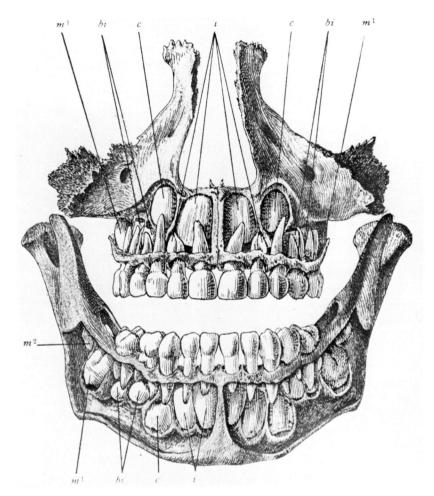

FIG. 5-3. Jaws of a child showing tooth development. (*bi*) biscuspids. (*c*) canines. (*i*) incisors. (*m*) molars. (Piersol Anatomy, 1923.)

TABLE 5-1. *Eruption of milk teeth*

Age (months)	Teeth (number)
6	Middle lower incisors (2)
8–10	Upper incisors (4)
12–14	Lower incisors (2)
18–20	Canines (4)
24–34	Second molars (4)

2. *History*. Describe any previous similar illness, number of occurrences, duration, treatment received, success of treatment, and season of year in which attacks occurred. General information should include a family history of congenital defects, a history of sore throats or nasopharyngeal pain, swollen, tender glands, postnasal discharge, nasal obstruction, stopped-up ears, earache, ear discharge, change in hearing, cough or hoarseness, swelling of the salivary glands, dental problems or midline neck swelling, description of nasal obstruction, headaches, previous sinus infections, and description of any previous surgery on the nose, sinuses, or throat.

3. *Physical examination*. The temperature should be taken. To facilitate examination of the mouth, pharynx, and nose, the patient should be sitting in the erect position with head thrust slightly forward and chin slightly depressed. The head should never be thrown back during examination. When the throat is examined, the patient should be instructed to breathe through his mouth. If a tongue depressor is employed, it should be placed on the anterior two-thirds of the tongue and pressed down and forward. A beam of light either reflected from a head mirror or a head light offers the best illumination for examination of the mouth and pharynx. The following steps should be included in the examination.

a. Neck. Examination of the neck should include inspection of the skin over the neck and a search for draining sinuses as well as palpation of the cervical, submental, postauricular, occipital, and suboccipital areas for enlarged glands. The anterior and posterior cervical chains should be palpated, as should the glands along the course of the jugular vein. The parotid gland and submaxillary glands should be palpated to determine enlargement and to identify masses in the glands or along their ducts. The larynx should be checked for free mobility and local masses. Any midline swelling should be carefully examined.

b. Mouth. The lips should be examined for unusual color, prominent blood vessels, ulceration, or induration. The temporomandibular joint should be palpated on opening and closing the mouth to rule out subluxation or crepitus. The teeth should be examined to determine the condition of the gums, and notation should be made of dental caries, missing teeth, and malocclusion. The buccal mucous membrane, gums, tongue, sublingual region, palate, and pharynx should be inspected (Fig. 5-4). The orifices of the parotid and submaxillary ducts should be checked. The hard palate should be inspected for midline cysts, a torus palatinus, clefts, and submucous clefts. The movement of the soft palate should be checked, and abnormalities of the uvula noted. Tongue movement should be tested for deviation at rest, in retraction, and in extension, for elevation, and for lateral movement. Any abnormalities on tongue surface should be noted. Size and color of the tonsils, discharge from the crypts, ulceration, any pseudomembrane or membrane formation on their surfaces, and any displacement of a tonsil anteriorly or medially should be noted. The anterior pillar of the tonsil should be checked for unusual color or bulging that might suggest peritonsillar abscess formation.

c. Oropharynx. Examination of the oropharynx is greatly enhanced by depressing the dorsum of the tongue with a spatula or spoon, followed by gentle elevation of the soft palate with a palate elevator or spatula. Inspection of the oropharynx should

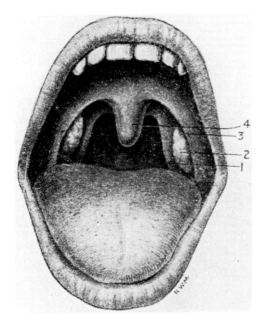

FIG. 5-4. Normal pharynx. (*1*) posterior pillar. (*2*) tonsil. (*3*) anterior pillar. (*4*) uvula. (From Hall, I. S., and Colman, B. H.: *Diseases of the Nose, Throat, and Ear*, p. 128. Livingstone, Edinburgh, 1969. With permission).

include notation of any unusual redness, ulceration, or swelling of the mucous membrane, the presence of lymphoid tissue (lateral bands) on the posterior wall, and any bulging of the posterior wall. Postnasal discharge should also be noted.

d. Nasopharynx. For the inexperienced, satisfactory inspection of the nasopharynx can be difficult. The usual method is to depress the back of the tongue with a spatula and then introduce a small mirror (6–8 mm) into the oropharynx, taking care not to press it against the posterior wall (gag reflex) (Fig. 5-5). A beam of light is directed against the mirror so as to illuminate the nasopharynx. If the patient is a persistent gagger, the use of a light local anesthetic sprayed on the posterior wall of the oropharynx sometimes makes examination easier.

On mirror examination, the adenoids can be seen extending from the vault of the nasopharynx down the posterior wall to a line about 5 to 6 mm above the lower border of the soft palate. They appear as a red lobulated mass. When the adenoids are very hypertrophied, they may extend so far laterally as to obscure the cartilaginous torus tubarius, which surrounds the eustachian tube orifice, and the recess posterior to this, the fossa of Rosenmüller. Very enlarged adenoids can obstruct the entire nasopharyngeal airway (Fig. 5-5). When adenoids are moderate to small in size, the examiner should see the vault of the nasopharynx, which anteriorly is divided by the posterior end of the nasal septum; the rounded posterior tips of the turbinates should also be visible in the anterior nasopharynx. Below the vault and forming part of the lateral walls are the eustachian tube orifices and the fossae of Rosenmüller. Occasionally a depression is seen in the midportion of the adenoids; this is the nasopharyngeal bursa around which, when it is infected, may be a thick, sticky, yellowish discharge with some crusting. This is a remnant of Rathke's pouch,

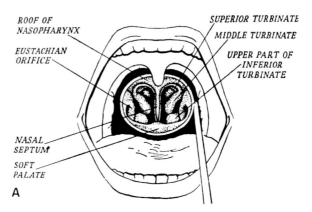

ROOF OF
NASOPHARYNX

SUPERIOR TURBINATE

MIDDLE TURBINATE

EUSTACHIAN
ORIFICE

UPPER PART OF
INFERIOR
TURBINATE

NASAL
SEPTUM

SOFT
PALATE

A

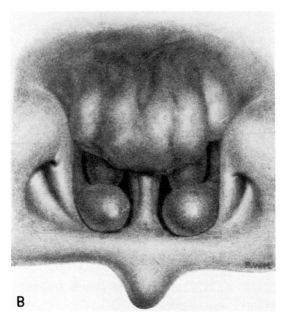

B

FIG. 5-5. Posterior rhinoscopy. **A:** Nasopharynx, without adenoids, showing the posterior ends of the turbinate bones, the arch of the nasal septum, and the eustachian tube orifices surrounded by the cartilagenous torus tubarius. The mirror is in place behind the soft palate. In practice it is quite impossible to obtain a view of the entire area at one examination. One has to manipulate the mirror to bring all these structures successively into view. **B:** Posterior rhinoscopy showing the adenoids and their relationship to the torus tubarius and the eustachian tube orifices. (**A** from Reading, P.: *Common Diseases of the Ear, Nose and Throat,* 3rd ed. Churchill, London, 1961. With permission. **B** from Hall, I. S., and Colman, B. H.: *Diseases of the Nose, Throat and Ear,* p. 132, 9th ed. Livingstone, Edinburgh, 1969. With permission.)

which is a diverticulum of the embryonic buccal cavity from which the anterior lobe of the pituitary gland develops. Polyps descending into the nasopharynx from the posterior nares and tumors forming in the nasopharynx can also be identified by mirror examination.

A second method for examining the nasopharynx consists of passing a nasopharyngoscope along the floor of a nostril into the vault of that cavity. The flexible scope can be passed very easily and gives an excellent view of the eustachian tube orifices, the fossae of Rosenmüller, and the posterior and anterior walls of the nasopharynx.

e. Laryngopharynx (hypopharynx). Examination here is also facilitated by a mirror examination. A large mirror is employed (about 1.5 cm) than for examination of the nasopharynx. The laryngopharynx should first be inspected by depressing the posterior surface of the tongue with a tongue depressor, then placing the mirror high in the oropharynx. This gives a good view of the posterior wall of the laryngopharynx (Fig. 5-6). Next, the tongue should be grasped with a piece of gauze and drawn forward with the mirror in the oropharynx. The patient should be instructed to breathe rapidly through the mouth. This affords a view of the base of the tongue, with the depression of the foramen caecum in the midline of the dorsum of the tongue, the circumvallate papillae, and the lingual tonsils on its lateral margins. The epiglottis and the supraglottic larynx can also be seen below the base

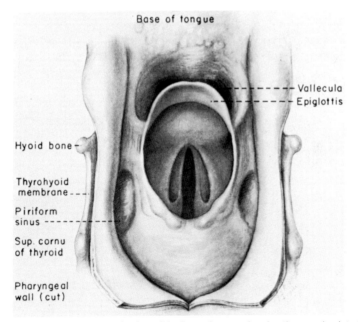

FIG. 5-6. Indirect or mirror examination of the hypopharynx showing the opening into the larynx and the vocal cords, the epiglottis, and the piriform sinuses. (From Deweese and Saunders: *Textbook of Otolaryngology,* p. 50. Mosby, St. Louis, 1968. With permission.)

of the tongue, forming the upper end of the larynx; on each side of it are the pyriform sinuses. The lateral and posterior walls of the laryngopharynx are smooth and covered with nonciliated mucous membrane. Foreign bodies in the hypopharynx can be visualized by mirror examination.

f. Digital examination. In infants and in some children, when mirror examination is unsatisfactory, a great deal can be learned from a digital examination of the nasopharynx and the laryngopharynx. Care should be taken to prevent forceful closure of the jaws on the investigating finger. This can be done by inserting a bite block or by wedging the mouth open with three or four spatulas. The finger is then inserted at the corner of the mouth; to examine the nasopharynx, it is passed alongside the tongue behind the soft palate and directed upward. The eustachian tube orifices and fossae of Rosenmüller can be palpated on the lateral walls, and the vault can be reached with the fingertip; the adenoid mass in the vault and on the posterior wall can easily be estimated by this method, and tumors can be palpated.

Digital examination of the hypopharynx permits palpation of the base of the tongue, the lingual tonsils, the epiglottis, and the pyriform sinuses. It can also detect tumor masses in these regions.

DISORDERS AND DISEASES OF THE MOUTH

Dental Problems

The most common problems related to the teeth of children are (a) developmental anomalies that are usually associated with congenital harelip and cleft palate; (b) apical or alveolar infection; (c) cysts of dental origin; and (d) malocclusion.

Harelip

In cases of harelip there is failure of the frontal and maxillary processes to unite on one or both sides, resulting in a single or a double cleft (single or double harelip). The cleft lies between the upper canine teeth and upper lateral incisors. In these children the lateral incisors are missing on the side involved (see "Congenital Deformities," below).

Infections

Dental infection or alveolar abscess can occur in both milk and permanent teeth. Infection around the tooth penetrates the pulp and from there extends to the apical space surrounding a tooth root. When this space becomes expanded by pus formation, it erodes the neighboring alveolar bone. Pain occurs along the distribution of the fifth cranial nerve, and it may become so general that localization of the infected tooth is difficult. The pain associated with such infections is increased if the patient introduces hot liquids into his mouth and can be reduced slightly by the presence of cold liquids.

Osteomyelitis

Dental infections may spread into the surrounding bone of the upper or lower jaw, resulting in osteomyelitis and bone destruction (Fig. 5-7). In the maxilla, the osteomyelitis usually has an upward course following thrombosis of the infraorbital artery and vein. In the mandible, destruction is more local. Extraction of infected teeth often precipitates this condition. Treatment consists of aggressive antibiotic therapy and surgical removal of infected bone.

Cysts

There are two dental cysts of great interest to the otolaryngologist. (a) The dentigenous cyst is formed by expansion of the tooth follicle with retention of the tooth, which is usually deformed inside it (Fig. 5-8). Such cysts can expand in the roof of the mouth or the cheek as a smooth swelling that on pressure is slightly compressible and produces a crepitus. (b) The radicular cyst forms around a tooth root after the crown has developed. It is epithelium lined and contains dentine and cementum. It can elevate the floor of the nose or extend into the maxillary sinus.

Malocclusion

Occlusal difficulties and mild facial deformities can result from narrowing of the palatal arch. This can be corrected by orthodontic rehabilitation and maintenance of a patent nasal airway.

Lead Poisoning (Plumbism)

Usually found in children living in poor sections of cities where there is deteriorated housing, lead poisoning is caused by ingestion of small amounts of lead paint flaking from the walls or from lead-glazed china. As many as 2% of preschool children in some communities have developed the symptoms of plumbism. Multiple cases are found in the same family, so examination of siblings is advisable. If enough lead is ingested it is life threatening, and the child may develop lead encephalopathy or other brain damage. The condition begins with anorexia and increased intercranial pressure. Incoordination is followed by ataxia, and the child shows signs of anemia. In many children a bluish line develops in the gums (lead line), which is often accompanied by swollen mucous membranes and low-grade infection around the teeth.

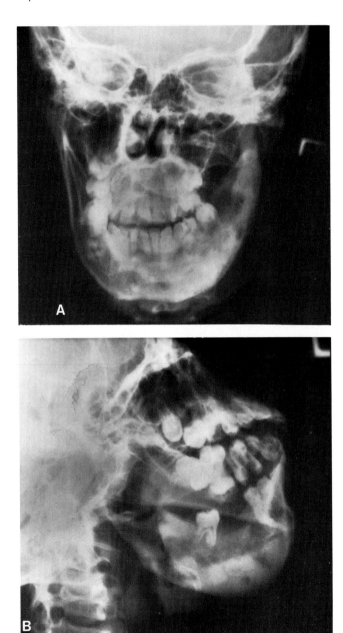

FIG. 5-7. Anteroposterior **(A)** and lateral **(B)** views of osteomyelitis of the left mandible in a 15-year-old boy. There was a history of extraction of the left molar tooth 6 years previously, followed by recurrent draining sinus. Note the thickening and moth-eaten appearance of the mandible with loss of bone around the remaining molar tooth in this region.

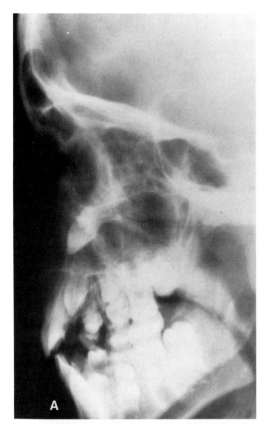

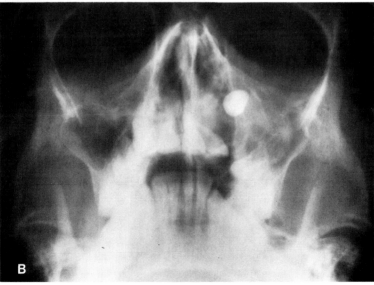

FIG. 5-8. Lateral **(A)** and anteroposterior **(B)** views of an infected dentigenous cyst in the left antrum of a 10-year-old boy with a history of fullness of the left cheek,. Note the unerupted canine tooth in the cyst; the same tooth on the opposite side has descended.

Congenital Deformities

Congenital deformities result from faulty development of the embryo or fetus and may be of such serious nature as to require almost immediate repair or so inconsequential as to require only reassurance for the parent.

Clefts

The most obvious deformities around the mouth are those of the lips and teeth. Such deformities are only the outward signs of considerably more extensive changes in the mouth. They can be classified as clefts.

Cleft or harelip

Cleft or harelip may be unilateral or bilateral and may extend upward to the floor of the nose or into the nose. It is caused by failure of the frontonasal process to fuse fully with the maxillary processes (Fig. 5-9). This can also leave an orbital fissure that extends from the orbit into the mouth passing lateral to the nose, and it can be unclosed or only partially closed. Bilateral clefts leave a floating premaxilla.

It has been theorized that this malformation (cleft) results from an absence or a decrease in the size of the lateral mesodermal masses on the anlage of the upper lip and premaxilla, resulting in unilateral or bilateral clefting of the lip and lateral incisor regions of the alveolus. A decrease in mass of the medial mesodermal mass

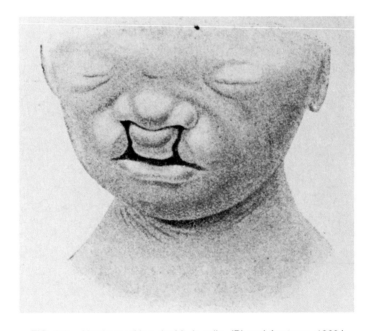

FIG. 5-9. Newborn with a double harelip. (Piersol Anatomy, 1923.)

of the anlage may also result in a rare median cleft lip and clefting of the central alveolar region.

In some cases, a central cleft can result from failure of the two lateral downgrowths of the frontonasal process (globular processes) to fuse. This fusion ordinarily is completed during the second month of intrauterine growth. Such failure has been attributed to the failure of the tongue to recede from its original position or to the possibility of a fetal intrauterine infection. The incidence of cleft lip is about one in every 700 to 1,000 births.

Clefts extending into the nose make it almost impossible for an infant to nurse. Repair of the cleft lip is usually done as soon after birth as possible, not only to make nursing possible but also because the cosmetic deformity may have an adverse effect on parental acceptance.

Repair requires mobilization of tissues of the lip, premaxilla, and maxilla in order to provide the necessary tissue for a careful closure with a well-matched vermilion line of the lip. Present surgical methods of repair offer the opportunity for a very acceptable result.

Cleft palate

Cleft palate is the result of the failure of one or both of the palatal plates to reach the midline as the roof of the mouth is formed (Fig. 5-10). It is one of the oldest

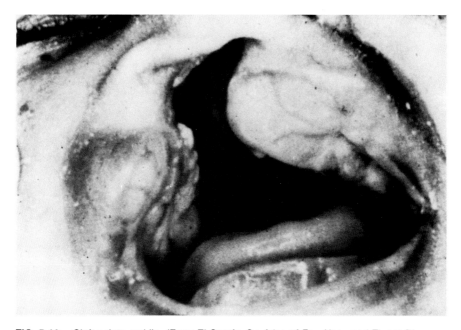

FIG. 5-10. Cleft palate and lip. (From El Sarafy, S.: *Atlas of Ear, Nose and Throat Diseases*, p. 125. Ali Bin Ali, Doho, Qatar, Egypt, 1977. With permission.)

recognized congenital defects, and some surgical success was first obtained by closing the cleft with sutures as early as the 18th century. Cleft palates with or without cleft lips occur in about one in 650 births. Approximately one-third of cleft palates are bilateral. These are associated with cleft lips more commonly in males than females, whereas isolated cleft palates are more common in females. The anomalies around the mouth associated with cleft palates are microglossia, macroglossia, and micrognathia. Such anomalies are frequently associated with other defects such as hypertelorism, congenital heart defects, and extremity abnormalities (Fig. 5-11).

Davis, Richie, and Veau classified clefts as follows: (a) isolated cleft lip; (b) cleft lip and cleft palate unilateral or bilateral, complete or incomplete; and (c) isolated cleft palate. Cleft palates involve the uvula and may consist of a deficiency of the medial portion of one or both palatine bones; however, the vomer and septum remain intact. Occasionally, there is an incomplete cleft palate that results from a midline posterior hard palate deficiency that leaves the vomer hanging free. Isolated clefts usually involve the uvula and soft palate.

Deficiencies of the palatine bone may be very small and may be covered by mucosa. Such a submucosal cleft is often difficult to identify, but it may have an adverse effect on voice quality and may also be associated with recurrent ear infections.

In addition to the cosmetic effect and the feeding difficulties encountered with cleft palates, ear problems are also very common because almost anything taken

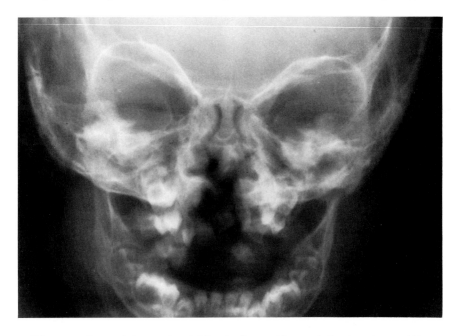

FIG. 5-11. Congenital anomaly: cleft hard palate and hypertelorism in a 4-year-old boy.

in the mouth will be pushed up into the unprotected eustachian tube orifices during attempts to swallow. This results in frequent attacks of acute otitis media and chronic serous otitis media, which may be followed by conductive hearing loss. Speech is also very distorted because of the loss of sphincter action of the soft palate and the free communication between the nose and the mouth through the palatal defect. It is very important that the surgeon reconstruct the soft palate so that there is not too great a space between the soft palate's posterior border and the posterior wall of the nasopharynx. Too much postpalatal space can result in regurgitation of food through the nose, and it always results in a marked increase in voice nasality. Because of the importance in establishing the proper postpalatal space after repair, the adenoids should never be removed before a cleft palate repair. The bulk of the adenoids may act to help close this space and in many cases make it possible to avoid a secondary "push-up" operation of tissues on the postpharyngeal wall for additional closure of the postpalatal space after primary correction of a cleft palate. When necessary, partial or complete adenoidectomy can be performed after palate closure. Speech lessons are very important after correction of the cleft in order to get the child started in the production of good speech.

Pierre Robin Syndrome

Pierre Robin syndrome consists of a cleft palate, an underdeveloped mandible (micrognathia) (Fig. 5-12), and a tongue displaced backward in the "retroposition." This results in airway obstruction, especially when the infant is recumbent and/or sleeping. The severity of this condition varies with the size of the tongue and the

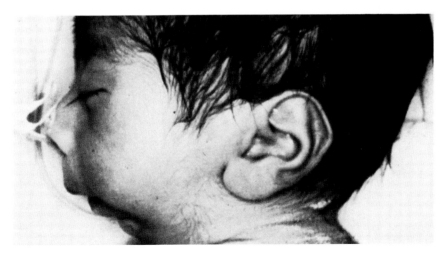

FIG. 5-12. Pierre Robin syndrome. (From El Sarafy, S.: *Atlas of Ear, Nose and Throat Diseases,* p. 280. Ali Bin Ali, Doho, Qatar, Egypt, 1977. With permission.)

degree of micrognathia. Mild conditions can be handled by placing the child face down in the prone position. In severe cases the tongue should be brought forward and sutured to the inside of the lower lip until the lower jaw grows forward enough to relieve crowding. In most instances this condition gradually improves as the general body growth pushes the mandible forward, reducing the relative mass of the tongue.

Mandibulofacial Dysostosis (Treacher Collins Syndrome)

Mandibulofacial dysostosis is a hereditary malformation of the face characterized by altered growth of the maxillary and mandibular complexes. There is failure of development of the outer inferior quadrant of the bony orbit resulting from failure of growth of the malar complex. The zygoma is much attenuated or lacking. Frequently associated with this are clefting of the palate, micrognathia, and separation of the teeth because of lack of room for the tongue. The frontonasal elements develop normally, giving the midface marked prominence; the neuromusculature is not affected by this condition. It has been theorized that the alteration in bony growth may be secondary to the defective development of the maxillary arteries

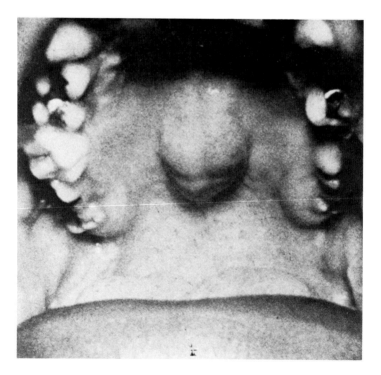

FIG. 5-13. Torus palatinus. Note the midline location. (From Paparella, M. M., and Shumrick, D. A.: *Otolaryngology*, p. 370. Saunders, Philadelphia, 1973. With permission.)

beyond the pterygomaxillary fissure as a result of a disturbance of the embryonic blood supply. The appearance of these children can be improved by orthodontic procedures, bone grafts to replace lacking malar bone, and plastic surgery.

Forms of micrognathia such as mandibulofacial dysotosis are not self-correcting and require surgical corretion. Injury to the growth sites in the condyles may lead to serious deformities of the jaw and interfere with function.

Additional bony deformities seen in the mouth are the torus palatinus (Fig. 5-13) and the torus mandibularis, which are exostoses that appear as bony tumors in the midline of the hard palate and along the lingual border of the mandible. The torus mandibularis is usually bilateral, and the swellings are smaller than those of the torus palatinus. They appear as one or a number of mucous-membrane-covered, smooth, firm nodules along the inner aspect of the lower jaw. Neither of these growths progresses much after birth. They are benign, and the common treatment is parental reassurance.

Tumors of the Jaw

The cystic tumors of dental origin have been described in the section on dental problems. The nasopalatine cyst (midline anterior maxillary cyst) is a nonodontogenic cyst appearing in the anterior midline of the hard palate. It can be congenital in origin and is usually very slow in growth (Fig. 5-14). X-ray studies are helpful but of questionable value for diagnosis of tumors of the jaw.

Ossifying Fibroma/Fibrous Dysplasia

Ossifying fibroma and fibrous dysplasia are frequently considered to be of the same origin. They are nonencapsulated tumors composed of fibro-osseous tissue and occur in the facial bones (Fig. 5-15). The tumor is considered more aggressive when originating in the maxilla than in the mandible (see Chapter 4, Nasal Disorders section). Histologic sections show a mixture of cancellous bone spicules in masses of connective tissue. A slow-growing tumor that occurs in childhood but usually is not discovered until late adolescence, it appears as a nontender swelling in the mandible that causes local pain. It has been theorized that these lesions may be caused by trauma.

Fibrosarcoma

Fibrosarcoma occurs in the jaws of young children. It arises from the endosteum, and X-ray studies show marked bone destruction. The first symptom is nontender swelling of the jaw; as the tumor grows, the teeth are displaced and later lost. Wide surgical excision is the method of treatment.

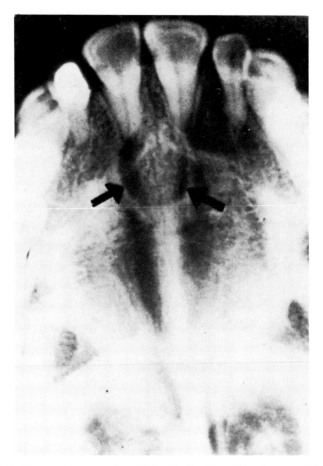

FIG. 5-14. Median maxillary cyst. (From El Sarafy, S.: *Atlas of Ear, Nose and Throat Diseases,* p. 129. Ali Bin Ali, Doho, Qatar, Egypt, 1977. With permission.)

Sarcoma

Sarcomas are reported to invade the upper and lower jaws of very young children (Fig. 5-16). They cause rapid and marked swelling of the jaw, and X-ray studies show much bone destruction and displacement of teeth. Pain is often a serious complaint. Surgical removal is the treatment of choice. These tumors have been reported to metastasize rather early.

Actinomycosis

See description in Chapter 6.

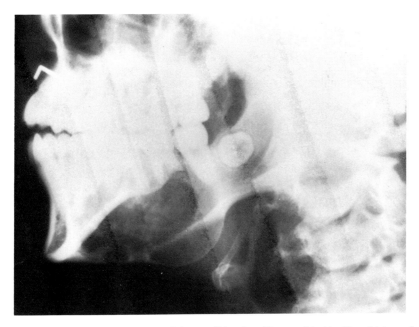

FIG. 5-15. Ossifying fibroma in the left mandible of a 13-year-old girl with a history of an enlarging, painless lump in the left jaw for 6 months. Note the cyst-like loss of bone in the mandible.

Abnormalities of the Tongue

Congenital Macroglossia

Congenital macroglossia is a disorder in which the lymph channels and spaces of the tongue become dilated. There is also an increase in the lymphoid tissue, especially at the base of the tongue. The deformity occurs in Down's syndrome (mongolism) and may occur in other conditions or as a separate entity. In this disorder, the tongue may become so large so as to interfere with normal respiration and can cause deformities of the alveolar arch and teeth by the pressure of its bulk. In such patients, oral hygiene is necessary but difficult to maintain; infections of the tongue are common (Fig. 5-17). Surgery is seldom advisable, but a number of procedures have been devised to reduce the size of the tongue when respiration is dangerously interfered with.

The tongue, because it is suspended primarily from the hyoid bone by the attachment there of its principal muscles, has a natural tendency to fall backward into the hypopharynx when a child is placed on his back. When a tongue is enlarged, this can happen during sleep and can seriously endanger the airway. The same danger exists in the presence of a normal-sized tongue during general anesthesia. In both instances it is advisable to devise a method to hold the tongue forward.

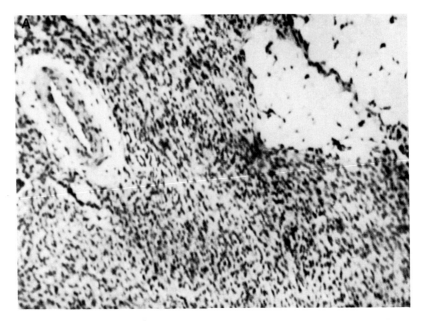

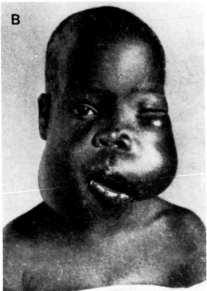

FIG. 5-16.   A: Sarcoma of the right jaw in a 3-year-old boy that metastasized to the lungs. **B:** Section of tumor showing its invasion of adjacent fat. (From Benson, C. D. et al.: *Pediatric Surgery,* Vol. 1, p. 151. Year Book, Chicago, 1962. With permission.)

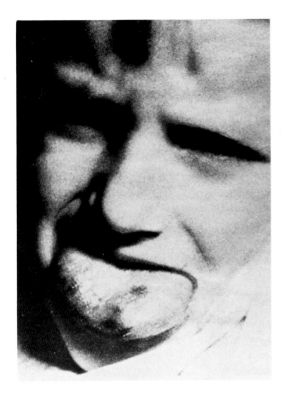

FIG. 5-17. Macroglossia from lymphangioma. This 2-year-old has his tongue at rest and not protruded. (From Paparella, M. M. and Shumrick, D. A.: *Otolaryngology,* p. 179. Saunders, Philadelphia, 1973. With permission.)

Hairy Tongue

Hairy tongue is not congenital but seems to be associated with some types of medication, especially antibiotics. Some cases cannot be explained. It may be localized or cover the surface of the whole tongue. The dark, hairy appearance is caused by increased keratinization and pigmentation of the papillae; cultures frequently identify *Monilia*. To treat this condition, the cause must be identified if possible and eliminated. Vitamin B is helpful if associated with antibiotics, and oral hygiene must be maintained.

Burns of the Mouth and Oropharynx

Caustic Burns

Burns of the lips and mouth by caustic agents are encountered regularly despite the safety measures that have been developed. An important rule that should always be followed when presented with a patient suffering from lip or mouth burns from contact with a caustic substance is to arrange to have hypopharyngeal, laryngeal, and esophageal examinations by a competent endoscopist to ascertain that there are not also burns in these areas. Usually by the time the child is seen by the pediatrician or a general practitioner, it is too late to attempt to neutralize the action (acid or alkaline) of the caustic. The local oral burns can be treated with sterile mineral oil, and if there is a severe local reaction, the child can be put on antibiotics and a cortisone preparation. Such lesions involving only a small portion of the mouth heal very well; however, lesions of the hypopharynx, larynx, and esophagus require prolonged care by an endoscopist. If neglected, a burn around the larynx can cause permanent respiratory problems, and those of the esophagus can result in perforation or later in serious esophageal stenosis (see Chapter 7).

Electrical Burns

Electrical burns of the mouth occur more commonly in children before the age of 4 years. They are frequently associated with crawling, and the burns are the result of contact with electrical connections in or near a baseboard. Unless the child is connected to an efficient ground, he is not electrocuted, but there is usually wide destruction of tissue, much greater than first examination suggests. Immediate hospitalization is usually required, and the child should remain there until all slough has separated because severe hemorrhage is common following electrical burns of the tongue. Any efforts at plastic surgical correction of the damage following electrical burns should be deferred for at least 12 months after recovery.

Infections of the Oral Cavity

Noma

Noma is a severe necrotizing lesion that appears during the first decade of life. It is caused by a mixed infection in which Vincent's organisms usually occur. It can appear in the nose, eyes, or vulva but is most often seen in the mouth. It develops in children with greatly lowered resistance as a result of malnutrition, blood, dyscrasias, etc. It starts in the mouth with ulceration of the buccal mucous membranes, progresses to necrosis, and perforates the cheek; if not controlled, it can destroy much of the face (Fig. 5-18). The destruction of tissues is accompanied by a very foul odor. Treatment is by heavy broad-spectrum antibiotic therapy and surgical debridement. Supportive treatment of the general condition of the child should be carried out as rapidly as possible.

The following conditions, although causing changes elsewhere in the mouth, are also associated with ulcerative tonsillitis.

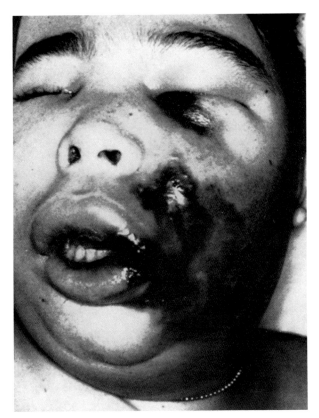

FIG. 5-18. Gangrenous stomatitis, noma, destroying the left check in a 10-year-old suffering from leukemia. (From Benson, C. D., et al.: *Pediatric Surgery,* Vol. 1, p. 153. Year Book, Chicago, 1962. With permission.)

Plaut Vincent's Infection (Trench Mouth)

Trench mouth is an infection that invades the gingiva and oral mucous membrane and may involve the tonsils. The organisms identified with it are fusiform bacilli and spirochetes, which can be identified on smears taken from the lesion. Symptoms are sore gums and, if the tonsils are involved, a sore throat. Fever can accompany the infection. The patient complains of a very bad taste and occasional blood-streaked sputum; cervical adenopathy is seen on the side of the infection. The lesion is a punched-out ulcer with raised edges 2 to 10 mm in diameter, the base of which is covered by a dirty gray pseudomembrane; when this is removed, a very rough, red, easily bleeding raw surface is revealed. This infection may occur in epidemic form in institutions for children. Penicillin is the specific treatment. Vincent's infection therapy should be followed up by a dental referral for oral hygiene and removal of all tartar deposits from the teeth (see Fig. 5-21, below).

Oral Candidiasis (Thrush)

Oral candidiasis occurs in about 5% of infants. The etiologic agent is *Candida albicans,* and the lesions consist of grayish-white plaques that occur on the buccal mucous membranes, tongue, soft palate, and tonsil. Removal of the membrane reveals a rough, eroded base that bleeds easily. The infection occurs most often in the infant population but can be seen in older children who are under steroid therapy or who suffer from debilitating disorders and blood dyscrasias. Gram-positive budding spores and myceles can be identified in smears taken from the lesion. Local treatment with gentian violet is sometimes helpful, but the specific therapy is by oral administration of nystatin or amphotericin.

Coxsackie Virus

Coxsackie visus is associated with pharyngotonsillitis in which small vesicles develop on the mucous membrane surface. These break down into small, punched-out, painful ulcers. One form appears during late summer as a febrile disease in children.

Herpes Hominis Virus

The herpes hominis virus usually attacks the anterior oral cavity and spreads to the oropharynx, involving the soft palate and tonsil. The lesions, which are very painful, start as a series of vesicles on the membrane surface that break down into ulcers. This disease may be accompanied by fever, and the virus, despite the fact that neutralizing antibodies appear between the fourth and seventh days after onset, usually remains in the patient's tissues and may subject him to recurrent attacks. Multinucleated giant cells with inclusion bodies can be identified in smears. Treatment is nonspecific. Rest, mouthwashes, and an analgesic may make the patient more comfortable.

Behcet's Disease

Behcet's disease is an inflammatory condition of undetermined origin that affects the mouth, eyes, and genitalia; it occurs in both children and adults. First described by Behçet in 1937, its symptoms are oral ulceration, ocular inflammation, and ulceration of the genitalia. The lesions consist of perivascular infiltrates with mononuclear lymphocytes and endothelial swelling that obstructs the lumen of small vessels. Perivasculitis is seen in all lesions, but it becomes necrotizing in the retinal arteries. The cause of this condition is undetermined, but a slow virus has been suggested by some investigators as the causal agent, although others believe that immunologic abnormalities may be the cause. These include elevated serum α_2- and γ-globulins with increased circulating antibodies. The condition has frequently been described as herpes simplex, pemphigus, lupus, or Crohn's disease. It usually presents as multiple aphthous ulceration of the buccal surfaces and the tongue, associated in most cases with genital ulceration and eye inflammation—all with negative bacterial, fungal, and viral cultures (Fig. 5-19). The eye inflammation may be anterior or posterior uveitis with retinal vessel occlusion. In some cases, blindness has been reported. Aseptic meningitis and cerebellar ataxia can occur. Treat-

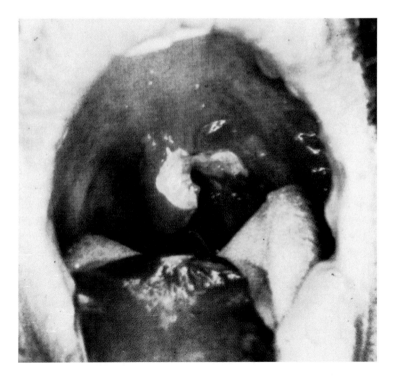

FIG. 5-19. Behcet's syndrome. Painful ulcerative lesions on the uvula and soft palate in a boy who also suffered from skin and genital lesions. The oral lesions are suggestive of Vincent's infection. (From El Sarafy, S.: *Atlas of Ear, Nose and Throat Diseases,* p. 142. Ali Bin Ali, Doho, Qatar, Egypt, 1977. With permission.)

ment with steroids has been tried for relief of pain, but to date there is no specific therapy.

Tuberculous Lesions

Primary tuberculous lesions of the mouth are rare in children today, although they can occur in the form of small transient ulcers on the tonsils or small nodules in the tonsils with ipsilateral glandular enlargement. These lesions are said to occur in communities where bovine tuberculosis is present. There is very little inflammatory reaction around the lesions. There have been numerous reports of isolation of tuberculosis organisms from children's tonsils and the hypopharynx. Ulcerations do occur in the mouth and around the tonsils in individuals suffering active pulmonary tuberculosis. Both conditions are accompanied by cervical adenitis. Diagnosis can be made by sputum studies and smears from the ulcers. In those patients suffering from a pulmonary infection, the diagnosis can be confirmed by chest X-ray studies. Treatment is specific drug therapy.

Blood Dyscrasias

A number of blood dyscrasias cause ulcerative conditions of the mouth and pharynx that also involve the tonsil.

Agranulocytosis is a leukopenia in which neutrophil polymorphonuclear cells are seriously reduced in number or dissapear from circulation. This results in multiple necrotic ulcerative lesions around the gums and on the buccal surfaces, soft palate, and tonsils. This disease can occur spontaneously from no known cause as well as after long serious bacterial infections, but most commonly it is caused by the action of certain drugs, e.g., arsphenamine, aminopyrine, some sulfonamides, and certain antibiotics, and by a number of chemical combinations used for treating malignancy. Agranulocytosis frequently begins with marked anorexia, relatively high fever, and a sore throat. The blood picture shows a marked diminution of polymorphonuclear forms and a marked increase of mononuclear cells. The pharynx and tonsils are partially covered with a grayish membrane and exhibit superficial ulcerations. The uvula and soft palate are edematous and are covered with a number of small, ragged ulcers. Treatment consists of withdrawal of all possible cytotoxic drugs and the institution of supportive measures such as transfusions and a course of penicillin therapy.

Leukemia also can cause sore throats and ulcerative lesions in the mouth and on the tonsils. As in agranulocytosis, the patient appears very ill, local measures for treating a sore throat are ineffective, and the condition usually progresses. The diagnosis is made by careful blood studies. Treatment is medical.

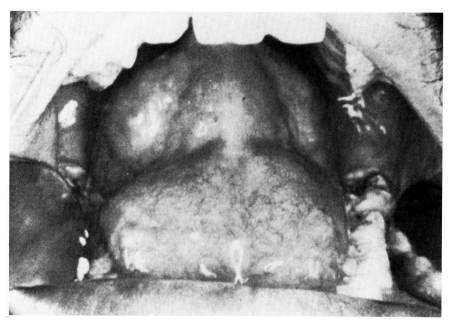

FIG. 5-20. The ranula is a thin-walled cyst filled with mucus that forms under the tongue, elevating its anterior half. (From El Sarafy, S.: *Atlas of Ear, Nose and Throat Diseases*, p. 158. Ali Bin Ali, Doho, Qatar, Egypt, 1977. With permission.)

Tumors in the Mouth

Ranula

Ranula is a cystic mass presenting under the tongue, usually unilaterally. It is soft and fluctuant, elevating the anterior tongue. It has a thin wall, contains mucus, and is painless (Fig. 5-20). There are two types reported. The first results from obstruction of a salivary duct and is limited to the sublingual space. A second type is thought to arise from a bronchogenic structure; this extends into the neck. These are benign lesions and are best treated by surgical removal or by marsupialization. Incision and drainage is inadvisable.

Hygroma

The hygroma can extend under the tongue from the parotid or form a classic collar-like growth. It is cystic, soft, and painless, and it elevates the tongue. It has some of the appearance of a ranula. Total surgical extirpation of the tumor is the best treatment, but the tumor is usually so involved in surrounding structures that subtotal removal is frequently the only practical method.

Papilloma

Papilloma, a benign tumor, appears on the tongue, the soft palate, and the tonsil. It is sessile, covered by normal-appearing mucous membrane, and painless. Simple surgical excision is advised (see Chapter 4).

Mixed Tumors of Salivary Origin

Mixed tumors of salivary origin are rare in children but are considered to have more malignant potential in this age group than in adults. They most frequently appear in the palate as a smooth, round, painless mass. They seldom ulcerate. Such tumors in the palate have a less-well-defined capsule than mixed tumors elsewhere in the mouth and are more likely to recur after surgical removal unless a wide excision is performed. Although they appear benign, there are reports of metastasis to the cervical glands. The tumor contains both epithelial and mesenchymal elements. The epithelial elements range from well-differentiated glandular types to undifferentiated basal types. The mesenchymal elements range from developed bone to simple mucin.

TONSILS AND ADENOIDS

Role in Immunity

For years there has been an ongoing discussion concerning the possible role of the tonsils and adenoids in the developing child. It has been known that the lymphoid tissue of Waldeyer's ring, of which the tonsils and adenoids compose the largest part, is relatively small at birth. After the age of 6 to 8 weeks to 1 year, there is an accelerated growth that continues until 8 to 9 years of age. Atrophy of the tonsils and adenoids begins at about the time of puberty unless the child is exposed to an unusual number of infections, and it continues for the next 10 to 15 years. In regions where upper respiratory infections and streptococcal infections are rare in children, many adults have very small tonsils and adenoids.

The location of these lymphoid masses in the pharynx at the juncture of the nasal and oral airways naturally exposes them constantly to airborne infections. Much effort has been expended to prove that the tonsils and adenoids play an important role in the developing immunity of a growing child. Studies have suggested that three cell types play a critical role in the immunologic processes: B cells, T cells, and monocytes or macrophages. The B cells are small lymphocytes that under certain stimuli can become immunoglobulin-secreting cells. The T cell is also a small lymphocyte and is believed to be a product of the neonatal thymus gland. It interacts with the B cell, and many of the immune responses depend on this inter-action. The B cells have surface receptors for the Fc portion of the immunoglobulin and receptors for IgG, IgE, and IgM; the monocytes carry a large complement of lysosomal enzymes.

It has been noted that each tonsil crypt is surrounded by a layer of small lym-phocytes, and the connective tissue of the tonsillar capsule is often infiltrated with monocytes, lymphocytes, and polymorphonuclear leukocytes. The tonsil contains a large number of B cells but relatively few T cells and monocytes. Although removal of a child's tonsils has no apparent effect on his immunity, Muchmore, in an excellent article on the immune role of the tonsils and adenoids, stated that in Bruton's type agammaglobulinemia, which occurs in young males, there is an absence of circulating B cells and extremely low levels of serum immunoglobulin and that these young males lack tonsils. They are highly subject to sinusitis and pulmonary infections and show little resistance to the encapsulated bacteria. These individuals are greatly helped by the administration of γ-globulin. Muchmore con-cluded by stating, "By its anatomic position in the oral cavity and from its cellular composition, it is believed that the tonsil acts as an antigen trap and may be an important site for antibody production, especially those antibodies against mouth and respiratory pathogens." Other lymphoid sites must also produce such antibodies because the antibody level in a child is not decreased measurably following ton-sillectomy. Studies by Reichmeyer (*personal communication*) indicated that the tonsil is capable of producing interferon.

Hypertrophy of the Tonsils

Normally tonsils are small at birth and begin to hypertrophy at a few weeks of age. This hypertrophy is accelerated at 6 months and continues until puberty, when hypertrophy stops; in most cases, the tonsils then begin to atrophy slowly. The cause of this hypertrophy is not completely understood. Since it begins at the time an infant starts its exposure to airborne infection and stops at about the time these exposures are reduced and antibodies have reached a relatively high level, one explanation for hypertrophy is that the tonsils play a role in the early production of antibodies or fill some other protective role during the early years. Another possible factor is that growth hormones may monitor tonsil hypertrophy. It has also been noted that repeated acute infections result in additional hypertrophy and that certain generalized bacterial or viral infections such as scarlet fever and chickenpox are followed by a moderate increase in tonsil size. There appears to be an increase in the connective tissue and lymphoid elements, which show an increase in the size and number of germinal centers accompanying hypertrophy. In some cases after repeated infection, the crypts become distended by epithelial debris and calculi.

Tonsil hypertrophy varies greatly in growing children, and in some cases one tonsil becomes larger than the other. Often the children with the largest tonsils have very little history of tonsillitis, generalized infections, or glandular enlargement. Hypertrophy can become life threatening in those infants or very young children in whom the tonsils become so large as to interfere with respiration. Often such children have little evidence of infection, but the obstruction from the enlarged tonsils becomes so severe that the child can sleep only in a sitting position and even then has marked stridor. On inspection, the tonsils may not appear infected but are so enlarged that they meet in the midline. Such a condition can result in the child's developing a "cor pulmonale"; to prevent this, the tonsils should be removed. As a general rule, hypertrophy of the tonsils alone is not an indication for tonsillectomy (see obstructive sleep apnea in the section "Nasopharynx," below).

Infections of the Tonsils and Adenoids

Acute and chronic infections of the tonsils and adenoids are considered in this section. The infecting agents and the medical measures to be employed to control these infections are discussed. Because the adenoids are subject to the same types of acute and chronic infections as the tonsils, they are included in this section as well as in the section of the nasopharynx.

Acute tonsillitis is characterized by malaise, fever, cervical adenitis, dysphagia, and a severe sore throat. It may accompany an acute respiratory infection or develop without associated infection. On examination, the patient appears flushed and hot to the touch. The cervical glands are usually enlarged and tender. There are marked injection and swelling of the tonsils, the anterior tonsillar pillars, and the posterior wall of the pharynx. Acute tonsillitis may be broken down into four categories. (a) Inflammatory tonsillitis is characterized by marked erythema, injection, and swelling of the tonsils. The anterior pillars and postpharyngeal walls are red and somewhat swollen. There is no discharge around the crypts, and no membranes develop on the surface of the tonsil. (b) Exudative or follicular tonsillitis presents an inflamed tonsil with a film or thin, nonadherent, grayish membrane in small plaques over its surface. The crypts contain a yellowish exudate, and the edges of their orifices are very swollen (Fig. 5-21). This exudate should be differentiated from the epithelial debris often seen in crypts. The membranes can be wiped away easily, and their removal does not cause bleeding. (c) Membranous (pseudomembranous) tonsillitis is typified by a grayish, rather thick pseudomembrane that is adherent to the mucous membrane surface of the tonsil. It is difficult to remove, and the surface under it bleeds after removal. The membrane is not limited to the tonsil surface but is confluent and may "spill over" onto neighboring mucous membrane surfaces. (d) Ulcerative tonsillitis may present as a rather localized erythema within which is a punched-out ulcer covered by a thick, gray, necrotic pseudomembrane, or it may be more generalized with numerous small ulcers on the tonsillar surface (Fig. 5-21) (see "Plaut Vincent's Infection," above). Each of the types described above may be accompanied by cervical adenitis.

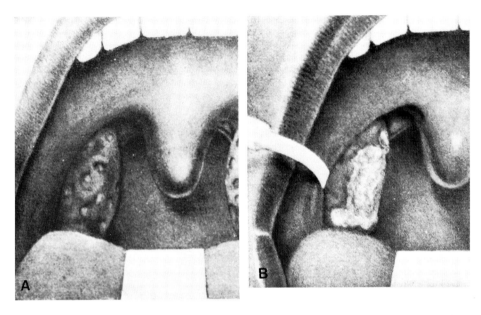

FIG. 5-21. A: Acute follicular tonsillitis. **B:** Vincent's infection of the tonsil. (From Hall, I. S., and Colman, B. H.: *Diseases of the Nose, Throat, and Ear,* p. 139. E. & S. Livingstone, Edinburgh, 1969. With permission.)

Chronic tonsillitis is found in adults more frequently than in children. It results from recurrent attacks of acute tonsillitis or repeated subclinical infections. The condition is manifested by low-grade sore throats when the weather changes or when the patient is overtired or debilitated by other illnesses; it may cause low-grade fevers at time and be accompanied in some individuals by enlarged glands in the anterior cervical chain. As a result of repeated infection, the tonsil may become enlarged, but longstanding chronic tonsillitis often causes a decrease in tonsil size as the tonsil becomes more fibrotic. On examination, the tonsil is moderately inflamed, and there is a corona of redness outlining the tonsil on the anterior wall of the anterior pillar. The anterior pillar itself is tightly adherent to the tonsil. The surface of the tonsil is smooth and glistening, and crypt openings are very small and seem reduced in number. Occasionally, a chronic infected tonsil exhibits an enlarged crypt or two with some purulent discharge at the orifice, or it may exude whitish paste-like epithelial debris. The latter type of tonsil is larger than the average chronically infected tonsil.

The adenoids are subject to acute and chronic infections just as the tonsils are, but they also present other problems that must be considered when their removal is contemplated.

Acute adenoiditis is accompanied by fever, pain in the nasopharynx, restricted nasal breathing, postnasal discharge, stuffy ears or earache, occasional mild conductive hearing loss, and increased nasality in speech. It may also cause swollen tender cervical glands. On examination, the posterior wall of the oropharynx is red and may be covered by mucopurulent discharge seen coming down the posterior pharyngeal wall from behind the soft palate. With a postnasal mirror, a red mass can be seen almost to fill the superior nasopharynx. This mass may be blanketed by mucopurulent discharge, or it may be covered by an exudate or a membrane. The eustachian tube orifices may be completely enveloped by this mass of adenoids. Bilateral swollen glands are usually present in the posterior cervical chain.

Chronic adenoiditis often is the cause of chronic postnasal discharge, mild sore throats, and enlarged cervical glands. This condition is a frequent cause of a night cough in children. Such infections can be instituted or prolonged by the presence of an infected bursa (Thornwaldt's disease), which lies in the posterior wall of the nasopharynx in the center of the adenoid mass. Thornwaldt's disease is characterized by postnasal crusting, a fetid odor, and a bad taste.

Acute tonsillitis and adenoitis occur as a result of invasion by pathogenic bacteria and/or viruses. The virus infections, which cause about 15% of all childhood acute throat infections, usually become established at the time of an acute upper respiratory infection. Bacterial infections may or may not accompany respiratory infections. Streptococcal infections account for about one-third of all acute tonsillitis and adenoiditis in children. In most children the group A *Streptococcus* is the predominant organism, but in children under 3 years of age *Hemophilus influenzae* is probably a more common cause of tonsillitis and adenoiditis than the *Streptococcus*. The pneumococcal organism occurs rather infrequently in cultures from acute infections, but it contributes to the number of cases seen each year. The incidence of pneumococcal tonsillitis varies greatly from year to year.

Acute viral tonsillitis and adenoiditis fall in the classification of inflammatory tonsillitis. It is usually caused by an adenovirus and precedes the appearance of coryza by 24 to 48 hr. Its first symptom may be the sudden onset of fever followed by a severe sore throat. The tonsils and pharynx look beefy red and swollen, and the patient may complain of fullness in the nasopharynx and have some voice change. There may be cervical gland enlargement. No exudate is seen around the tonsil crypts, any membrane formation is rare, and there is no postnasal discharge. The sore throat and fever usually subside within 2 to 3 days, but the coryza persists with a cough for 4 to 5 days longer. A secondary bacterial infection may develop following the acute phase, signaled by marked mucopurulent nasal and postnasal discharge. The treatment advised for a viral acute tonsillopharyngitis is rest in bed for 3 days with humidified air, forced fluids, and a warm saline gargle. In the cold winter season of the year, the windows should be kept closed day and night. Analgesics should be given during the febrile period. Antibiotics should be withheld unless the secondary bacterial infection becomes serious. Local complications of a viral sore throat are minimal.

Streptococcal infections begin with a moderate to severe sore throat, which at first may be unilateral. The temperature rises rapidly to 103° to 104°F, and younger children may develop convulsions during this temperature rise. Younger children may also suffer a severe loss of fluids from vomiting. There is marked dysphagia. The pulse rate rises along with the temperature, and the pulse is strong and bounding. On examination one finds the picture of acute follicular or exudative tonsillitis and adenoiditis. The tonsils are red and swollen, and there is exudate at the crypt orifices. A thin, grayish, nonadherent exudate may cover portions of the tonsils and adenoids. The pharynx is very red and somewhat swollen, and there is very little postnasal discharge. Postnasal examination of the adenoids shows much of the same picture as that seen in the tonsils. The cervical glands in both adenoiditis and tonsillitis are movable, swollen, and tender.

In a healthy child treatment of such acute infections by simple bed rest, forced fluids, humidity, closed windows (in winter), and administration of analgesics is usually successful in alleviating the acute symptoms, and the infection clears in a week to 10 days. A culture should be obtained at the onset of the illness as a guide for specific antibiotic therapy if needed. Children debilitated because of some other causes will probably require antibiotic therapy at the onset of a streptococcal tonsillitis or adenoiditis in order to prevent any complications.

Complications associated with acute streptococcal tonsillitis or adenoiditis can be dangerous. Locally, such infections can result in abscessed ears, a retropharyngeal abscess, peritonsillar abscess, or a parapharyngeal abscess. The systemic complications of septicemia, vascular thrombosis, and scarlatina rash can also result from such infections.

Hemophilus influenzae (influenza bacillus) infection can be identified very early in infancy. Antibodies can be recovered from infants at 6 to 9 weeks of age, and it is recognized as occurring frequently in acute upper respiratory infections where influenzal tonsillitis and fever complicate the illness. Some antigens have been shown to be common to both the *Hemophilus influenzae* and the pneumococcal organisms, and crossing reactions confuse the diagnosis. It is therefore important to identify the organism by microscopic examination and gram stain.

The clinical picture of acute tonsillitis caused by *Hemophilus influenzae* is much the same as that caused by *Streptococcus* or pneumococcus. It is an exudative or follicular tonsillitis. There are fever, dysphagia, sore throat, occasional change of voice, and cervical glandular enlargement with tenderness. The tonsils and pharynx are very red and somewhat swollen; exudate appears within about 24 hr. At first the exudate is thin and liquid, but it rapidly thickens and becomes moderately adherent to the tonsil. Yellow plugs of exudate form in the orifices of the crypts. Treatment is the same as that for acute streptococcal tonsillitis.

Pneumococcal infection of the tonsils and adenoids clinically resembles that of *Streptococcus* group A. However, it is usually milder and accompanied by greater postnasal obstruction and postnasal discharge. Complications are much less frequent unless the pneumococcus is a heavily encapsulated strain. This frequently causes ear and mastoid infections and progresses rapidly to meningitis. Identification of the heavily encapsulated pneumococcus calls for administration of antibiotics; otherwise treatment is the same as that for streptococcal tonsillitis.

One form of pseudomembranous-type tonsillitis is that resulting from diphtheria (*Corynebacterium diphtheria,* Klebs-Löffler bacillus) infection. Onset is marked by a moderate to severe sore throat, initially unilateral, or by pain in the nasopharynx accompanied by a low-grade fever. There are marked anorexia and circumoral pallor, and the pulse is rapid and weak. Examination shows (a) a thick, adherent, gray pseudomembrane on one or both tonsils spilling over onto the adjacent mucous membrane; (b) a similar membrane in the nasopharynx partially obstructing the choana; or (c) a membrane extending from the lower pole of the tonsil or lingual tonsil down into the hypopharynx and larynx. The throat is mildly red and rather edematous. The pseudomembrane is confluent and adherent, and removal causes bleeding. As the disease progresses, the patient appears very ill considering the rather mild involvement seen in the throat and pharynx. Diagnosis is confirmed by throat culture, but the physician should be warned that a negative culture in the presence of suggestive clinical symptoms should not be accepted as ruling out diphtheria. This is especially true if the patient has received an antibiotic, because the drugs appear to suppress growth of the bacillus in a culture. In such a case, miroscopic study of a smear may be helpful. Reculture should always be done when cultures are negative if the patient's condition clinically suggests diphtheria. Treatment consists of diphtheria antitoxin and supportive measures. This is a dangerous disease that appears sporadically and can easily be missed on a routine examination. One of the authors has seen more than 30 laboratory-identified cases of diphtheria since 1942. Three of these patients were on antibiotic therapy, and repeated cultures were negative; by the time a positive culture was obtained, the patients were very ill (also see "Plaut Vincent's Infection," above).

Lingual tonsillitis in its acute form is of primary interest in children. The infecting agents are nearly always *Streptococcus, Staphylococcus,* or pneumococcus except in very young children, where *Hemophilus influenzae* predominates. In acute lingual tonsillitis, examination reveals swollen, red lymphoid masses lying on each side of the tongue base. In some instances, small yellow or gray plugs can be seen in the crypt orifices, or a small amount of exudate is visible on the tonsil surface. The acute infection usually is accompanied by a moderate fever, unilateral or bilateral sore throat, some voice change, and malaise. Treatment is bed rest, forced fluids, and analgesics for fever and malaise. A specimen for culture should be taken. The infection lasts about 5 days. If it is severe or the child is debilitated, antibiotic therapy can be employed.

Tonsilloliths are formed by deposits of lime salts in the crypts of the tonsil, particularly in those crypts that harbor fungi. These deposits may accumulate to the degree that they form stones up to a centimeter in diameter. Such stones harbor chronic infection, which results in chronic inflammation of the tonsil and discharge from the crypts. The tonsil is frequently enlarged. Stones occasionally produce acute flare-ups of infection, resulting in acute sore throat, fever, and glandular enlargement. Sections of tonsils obtained from routine tonsillectomies have shown calcareous deposits in 8% of those examined. The majority of these were microscopic in size. When stones are identified, they can be removed by local incision or by removal of the tonsil.

Pseudotonsillitis

Tangier disease was first observed on Tangier Island in Chesapeake Bay. It appears with α-lipoprotein deficiency and hypocholesterolemia. The patients exhibit low lipoprotein levels. The tonsils present with orange and red striations; the peripheral lymph glands, spleen, and liver are enlarged. The prognosis of this condition is not fully known.

Infectious mononucleosis (glandular fever) is associated with generalized lymphadenopathy, sore throat, general malaise, and fever. It occurs most frequently in older children but has been identified in children as young as 2 to 3 years of age. It is frequently confused with acute tonsillitis of bacterial origin or diphtheria. The changes seen in the throat vary a great deal, leading some observers to classify the symptoms as glandular in children under 5 or anginal in older children. The tonsils are dull red and greatly swollen. The lingual tonsils appear very large. Lymphoid plaques on the posterior pharyngeal wall are greatly enlarged and beefy red. A white membrane may occur on the tonsil and in the nasopharynx, which is somewhat adherent to the underlying mucous membrane. There is marked bilateral cervical glandular enlargement and palpable epitrochlear and axillary glands. In severe cases ulcerations may occur on the tonsils and/or the postpharyngeal wall. The spleen is enlarged. Blood studies show an increased number of lymphocytes with many atypical forms, and during the early course of the disease, heterophil antibodies appear. There is no known specific therapy available, so the patient must be given as much rest as possible; the use of hot gargles and aspirin may alleviate the more acute symptoms.

In all instances when sore throats fail to improve under therapy or the patient appears more ill than he should be from the appearance of his throat, it is advisable to perform a careful blood study to identify mononucleosis or blood dyscrasias. It is also well to obtain throat cultures to eliminate the possibility of diphtheria.

INFECTIONS INVOLVING THE PHARYNGEAL SPACES

Infections involving potential spaces in the head and neck are secondary to primary infections elsewhere, and they range from infections beginning in the mouth to deep neck infections. In this section infections of the submental space, the peritonsillar space, the retropharyngeal space, the pharyngomaxillary space (parapharyngeal space), and infection in the floor of the mouth are discussed, as they form the group that occur most commonly in children. Moreover, when they occur, their symptoms are sufficiently clear to permit early recognition by the pediatrician and general practitioner.

Submental Space Infection

Infections of the chin and the midportion of the lower lip drain into the submental glands lying on the mylohyoid muscle between the anterior bellies of the digastric muscles. Infection entering these glands causes marked swelling of the chin and the submental region. Abscesses can form in the submental region when a gland breaks down. Such an abscess can be distinguished from thyrohyoid tissue disease because it lies anterior to and above the hyoid bone. Treatment consists of incision, drainage, and administration of antibiotics.

Peritonsillar Space Infection

Peritonsillar abscesses form in the loose connective tissue that lies in the potential space between the capsule of the tonsil and the fascia of the superior constrictor muscle. They are secondary to tonsillar infection, which involves a crypt lying against the tonsillar capsule. Penetration of the capsule allows the infection to expand into the peritonsillar space, dissecting the tonsil away from the constrictor muscles. The symptoms are fever, great pain, especially on swallowing, that is frequently referred to the ear, dysphagia, trismus, change of voice, drooling, and often a very stiff neck. On examination there is difficulty in opening the mouth sufficiently for a satisfactory view of the tonsils. There are marked redness and swelling of the tonsillar mucous membrane, often with exudate on the tonsil. The anterior pillar of the tonsil is bulging; the tonsil is pushed toward the midline; and the soft palate and uvula are swollen (Fig. 5-22). The cervical glands on that side are swollen and tender. The infecting organisms are usually *Streptococcus* or *Staphylococcus*.

Treatment consists of hot gargles, analgesics, and an antibiotic. As the abscess forms, the anterior pillar develops some pallor, and there is some fluctuance. When

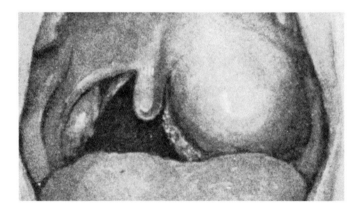

FIG. 5-22. Peritonsillar abscess, left. Note forward displacement of the anterior pillar and medial displacement of the tonsil. (From Ballenger, H. C., and Ballenger, J. J.: *Manual of Otology, Rhinology, and Laryngology*, p. 131. Lea & Febiger, Philadelphia, 1959. With permission.)

the abscess is established, the child should be seen by an otolaryngologist, who should drain it. Care must be exercised to have the child's head in a dependent position to prevent inhalation of the purulent discharge released when the abscess is incised. Antibiotics should be continued for 4 to 5 days after the fever and symptoms have subsided. Serious complications can develop if this condition is not treated properly, especially spread of infection into the pharyngomaxillary space and from there into the mediastinum.

Retropharyngeal Space Infection

The retropharyngeal abscess, which is frequently associated with acute adeno-iditis, has occurred only rarely since the advent of antibiotics. It is seldom seen in adults because the retropharyngeal glands, which lie in the loose alveolar tissue that separates the posterior wall of the pharynx from the prevertebral fascia covering the first five cervical vertebrae, usually disappear during adolescence. These glands may become involved by infection through the posterior wall of the pharynx or through the lymphatics that drain the vault of the nasopharynx and the prevertebral area. Infection in the retropharyngeal space may result from acute infections in the nasopharynx caused by *Streptococcus, Staphylcoccus,* and pneumococcus organisms, or it may be caused by a tuberculous infection originating in a cervical vertebra that breaks through the prevertebral fascia. As the retropharyngeal glands break down, an abscess forms, which pushes the posterior wall of the pharynx foward.

As the infection spreads, the abscess extends further inferiorly and can cause respiratory obstruction. Abscesses in the retropharyngeal space can also dissect downward into the mediastinum or can spread into the parapharyngeal spaces. As the abscess forms, the child develops nasal obstruction, a muffled cry, increasing dyspnea, and stridor, and lies with the head extended. Examination reveals a smooth, rounded, red swelling of the posterior wall of the oropharynx extending upward into the nasopharynx (Fig. 5-23). If the gland has broken down, this mass is fluctuant. Lateral X-ray films show bulging of the posterior wall, and if the abscess is large there will be some forward displacement of the larynx (Fig. 5-24). Treatment requires an incision through the posterior pharyngeal wall and drainage of the abscess. This should be carried out with the child's head dependent and with active suctioning of the pharynx in order to avoid aspiration. The child should be placed on antibiotics. These abscesses should not be allowed to rupture spontaneously because of the danger of aspiration and/or suffocation.

Parapharyngeal Space Infection

Parapharyngeal (pharyngomaxillary) infections may be caused by peritonsillar infections, retropharyngeal infections, or infections around the parotid gland. The most common sources of such infections are the tonsils and adenoids. This potential space forms in the loose connective tissue that lies internal to the fascia of the

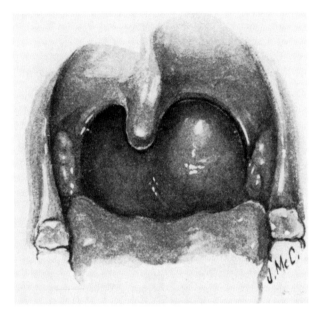

FIG. 5-23. Retropharyngeal abscess, left. Note swelling of the left posterior pharyngeal wall behind the posterior tonsillar pillar. (From Ballenger, H. C., and Ballenger, J. J.: *Manual of Otology, Rhinology, and Laryngology,* p. 150. Lea & Febiger, Philadelphia, 1954. With permission.)

parotid gland and internal pterygoid muscle and external to the fascia of the superior constrictor muscle. It constitutes a gutter in which lie the internal carotid artery, the 12th cranial nerve, the ninth cranial nerve, and the styloid muscles; this gutter continues inferiorly along the course of the vessels into the mediastinum (see description in the section on the anatomy of the pharynx).

The styloid muscles and the styloid bone divide this space into anterior and posterior compartments. The anterior compartment lies adjacent to the tonsillar fossae medially and the internal pterygoid muscle laterally. The posterior compartment contains the carotid sheath and the ninth and 12th cranial nerves. Posteriorly this potential space can communicate with the retropharyngeal space, and laterally it may become infected from the parotid space. The symptoms of infections of the pterygomaxillary space vary according to the compartment involved. Anterior compartment infection causes swelling at the angle of the jaw and trismus. There is some induration of the upper neck, and the tonsil and lateral wall of the pharynx are pushed medially, somewhat resembling a peritonsillar abscess (Fig. 5-25) but without the inflammatory reaction of the tonsil or the bulging of the anterior pillar seen in peritonsillitis. Posterior compartment infection displaces the posterior portion of the tonsil and the lateral and posterior wall of the pharynx toward the midline. The concave portion of the neck behind the jaw is obliterated by indurated swelling. There is no trismus involved in posterior compartment infection. Infections in both

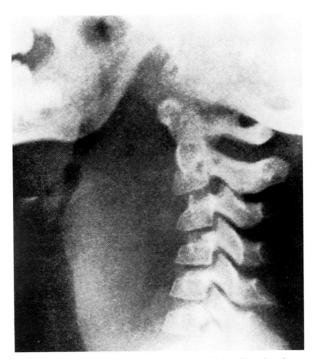

FIG. 5-24. Retropharyngeal abscess. Lateral soft tissue X-ray film showing massive prevertebral swelling, displacing the trachea and larynx and narrowing the hypopharynx. (From Seid, A. B., et al.: Retropharyngeal abscesses in children revisited. *Laryngoscope,* 89:1722, 1979. With permission.)

compartments manifested as fever, sore throat, dysphagia, inability to flex the neck, and pain in the ear.

Treatment consists of antibiotic coverage and surgical drainage of the abscess by incision and blunt dissection in the lateral neck below the angle of the jaw and, if the abscess is extensive, an additional incision lower down along the carotid sheath. A complication seen in such an infection is sudden drainage of pus and/or fresh blood from the external auditory canal. The blood might indicate a rupture of the carotid artery. Parapharyngeal abscesses can also rupture and drain spontaneously through the tonsillar fossae. If drainage is not carried out, the infection can spread into the mediastinum or may set up a thrombosis in the jugular vein or erode the carotid artery.

Submaxillary Space—Ludwig's Angina

Infection of the submaxillary space, or Ludwig's angina, is usually secondary to a dental infection or to infection of the floor of the mouth or the base of the tongue. It is occasionally the result of infiltration of the posterior portion of the inner aspect of the mandible with infected solution injected during local anesthesia for tooth extraction, which penetrates below the mylohyoid muscle. Ludwig's angina

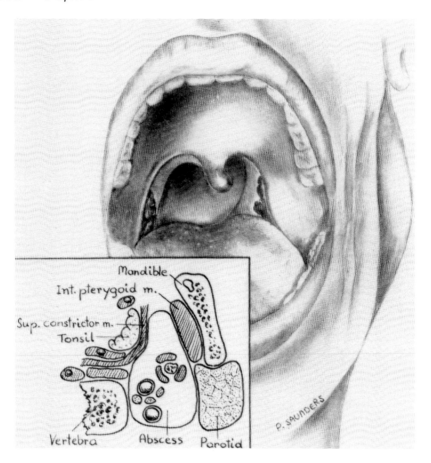

FIG. 5-25. Pharyngomaxillary abscess causing swelling behind the ramus of the mandible and the lateral pharyngeal wall without the marked bulging of the anterior tonsillar pillar that is seen with a peritonsillar abscess. **Inset:** Anatomic location of the abscess medial to the internal pterygoid muscle. (From Deweese and Saunders: *Textbook of Otolaryngology,* p. 62. Mosby, St. Louis, 1968. With permission.)

usually presents as a phlegmon rather than an abscess. The infection begins above the mylohyoid muscle, with increasing swelling of the floor of the mouth and gradual upward displacement of the tongue. At first there is no swelling of the neck. Surgical interference by drainage at this time through the floor of the mouth may avoid the second phase, which is when the infection penetrates through the mylohyoid muscle into the submaxillary space (Fig. 5-26). Such an extension involves the tissues of the neck and was described by Ludwig in 1836. Infection in the submaxillary space proceeds rapidly and is life threatening. The posterior tongue is pushed upward and forward and cannot be depressed. There is marked swelling under the chin extending over the upper anterior and lateral neck (Fig. 5-27). On palpation there is a board-like feeling of the areas under the mandible and

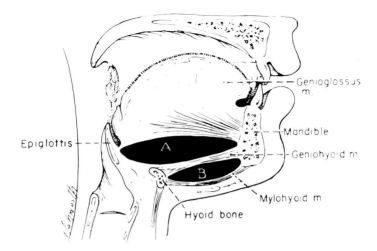

FIG. 5-26. Subglottic spaces in which Ludwig's angina may begin, either above or below the geniohyoid muscle. As the infection spreads, it penetrates the mylohyoid muscle, involves the submaxillary spaces, and spreads into the neck. (From Deweese and Saunders: *Textbook of Otolaryngology,* p. 63. Mosby, St. Louis, 1968. With permission.)

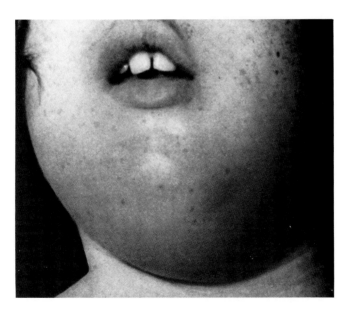

FIG. 5-27. Ludwig's angina in an 11-year-old, showing the brawny edema in the submental and submandibular regions. Elevation and retroposition of the tongue also caused respiratory distress. (From Benson, C. D. et al.: *Pediatric Surgery,* Vol. 1, p. 152. Year Book, Chicago, 1962. With permission.)

in the anterior neck. As the infection spreads, edema of the larynx can occur. The patient experiences a rapid increase in temperature, and he holds his mouth open and drools. Palpation over the hyoid is extremely painful, and modeling around the angles of the jaws is obliterated by swelling. The patient is very ill.

Treatment consists of very aggressive antibiotic therapy and supportive measures. If the patient begins to have a noticeable voice change or signs of respiratory distress, surgical intervention is indicated. A tracheotomy may be necessary before the neck is incised for drainage. Usually incision and drainage produce only some foul, serous material with little or no pus, but it does help to relieve the tension in the infected tissues. The complications of Ludwig's angina can be a mediastinal extension of infection or invasion of the pharyngomaxillary space.

TUMORS OF THE TONSILS

Benign Tumors

Papillomas occur on the tonsil, the anterior tonsillar pillar, or the soft palate as pedunculated mucous-membrane-covered masses. They may appear slightly bluish in color. They are painless and can be easily removed surgically (Fig. 5-28).

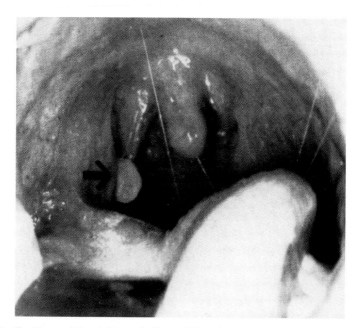

FIG. 5-28. Papilloma of the right tonsil. (From El Sarafy, S.: *Atlas of Ear, Nose and Throat Diseases*, p. 172. Ali Bin Ali, Doho, Qatar, Egypt, 1977. With permission.)

Inclusion cysts on the tonsil surface occur rather frequently. They expand slowly but are not considered a serious condition.

Hemangiomas may occur in the subcapsular region of the tonsil, pushing the tonsil toward the midline. Diagnosis is usually made during tonsillectomy.

Malignant Tumors

Lymphosarcomas can occur as primary tumors in the tonsil and are the most common tonsillar malignancy in children. They appear in the tonsil as a dull, red, round or nodular mass, firm to the touch and painless. As they grow they may ulcerate, but this is usually late. Firm, fixed cervical glands may be an early finding. On biopsy the cells may show various shapes and forms with no orderly arrangement. Mononuclear cells predominate. There is very little fibrous stroma. Blood vessels appear very fragile, and bleeding is common.

Lymphoepitheliomas are frequently clinically classified as lymphocarcinomas. They are very firm and painless on palpation, frequently with a whitish-gray, glazed appearance. The ipsilateral cervical gland is enlarged. They differ from lympho-sarcomas in that they ulcerate early, but bleeding is a late symptom. Infiltration of surrounding tissues occurs early. This tumor in its early stages has much the appearance of Vincent's infection of the tonsil. Oncologic consultation should be sought concerning any decision for therapy for either of these lesions.

Carcinoma of the tonsil is very rare in children but can occur. Infiltrative lesions of the tonsils should be biopsied for early identification. When enlarged cervical glands contain carcinoma cells, a careful tonsil examination should be included in the subsequent survey.

NASOPHARYNX

The nasopharynx functions as a passage for nasal respiration. It is into the nasopharynx that the nasal secretions are emptied; in it the eustachian tube opens to empty the mucous discharges of the middle ear, and through this tube air also passes to equalize the middle ear pressure with that of the local environment. On its posterior wall, a portion of Waldeyer's ring grows in the form of the adenoids. The nasopharynx is therefore involved in nasal respiration, postnasal drainage, and middle ear function as well as its own local disorders.

Disorders of the Nasopharynx

Disorders related to the adenoids are the most frequently occurring problems in the nasopharynx of children. Infections of the adenoids can be acute or chronic. They have been discussed in the section on tonsillar infections.

Hypertrophy of the Adenoids

This is influenced by age and infection and possibly by some growth factor. Certainly a potent factor in hypertrophy is the adenoids' exposure to infection. Hypertrophy usually begins at 6 to 8 weeks after birth and reaches a peak about the second or third year of school; atrophy begins at about 13 or 14 years of age, when the adolescent has accumulated a vast store of antibodies and when he is less exposed to infection in school. This is also the period that body growth rates are significantly altered. Hypertrophy of the adenoids does not necessarily mean that they are in an active state of infection, and they do not often act as a focus that results in debilitation of the child, but their hypertrophy may lead to surgical removal more often than hypertrophy of the tonsils requires their removal. Hypertrophied adenoids can affect a child adversely in many ways. If the adenoids are large enough to fill the airway of the nasopharynx completely, all nasal respiration stops. If mouth breathing persists over a prolonged period, there is a tendency to alter facial development (see paragraph on sleep apnea, below).

1. *Effect of adenoid hypertrophy on facial development.* Long-term studies have established that obstructive adenoid hypertrophy can produce elongation of the growing face, relative shortening of the upper lip, a grooved tongue, narrow nostrils, prominent upper incisor teeth, a high-arched narrow palate, a shortened mandible (receding chin), and mouth breathing. Because of the shortened mandible, there is decreased space for the tongue, which results in a forward tongue thrust, causing malocclusion. Such children have an increased tendency to ear infections and hearing impairment. Measurements of the anteroposterior (AP) nasopharyngeal space have shown significant reduction from normal. Children suffering from adenoid hypertrophy who exhibited the above changes showed marked improvement after adenoidectomy. There were widening of the face, lengthening of the upper lips, and improvement in the nasal airway. The nasopharyngeal AP space increased significantly, and occlusion improved. Adenoidectomy is indicated in such children.

2. *Hypertrophied adenoids and obstructive sleep apnea.* This syndrome appears in young children at night because of partial or intermittent obstruction of the upper airway above the hypopharynx. It is thought to be a contributing factor in crib deaths. It can be caused by defective CNS control of the pharyngeal muscles or by severe tonsil and/or adenoid hypertrophy. The latter condition is by far the most common cause of this apnea.

The symptoms during sleep are labored breathing and/or snoring followed by periods of silence of up to 10 to 15 sec when there is no respiratory exchange. Sleep is much disturbed, and frequently there is enuresis. Cyanosis occurs during sleep, and there is a rise in the P_{CO_2}. There is slow arousal from sleep when the child is awakened, which may be followed by periods of disorientation. The child frequently complains of headache; he falls asleep while performing simple tasks; and he appears to be slowed mentally. This type of apnea occurs more frequently in males.

Diagnosis is difficult because it occurs at home at night when no professional observer is available. Such children can be studied in a sleep laboratory where multiple records can be obtained to establish the diagnosis, but this is hard on the child and expensive. A simpler method is for the parents to use a tape recorder and pick several periods during the night to record the respiratory pattern; the tape is then given to the pediatrician for analysis. The treatment for obstructive sleep apnea in the presence of adenoidal and/or tonsillar hypertrophy is adenoidectomy and/or tonsillectomy.

3. *Hypertrophied adenoids and sinus disease.* Obstructive adenoids can cause a pooling of nasal secretions above them, and this may result in recurrent or chronic sinus infection. Two theories explain how this may occur: the first is that pooled infected secretions may reflux into the posterior ethmoid sinuses and cause repeated flare-ups of sinus infection; the second is that infected material sets up a chronic infection in the adenoids that, under proper conditions, spreads into the posterior ethmoid sinuses.

4. *Hypertrophied adenoids and ear disease.* Another problem associated with adenoid hypertrophy is obstruction of proper drainage of the eustachian tube and interference with its function of equalizing middle ear pressure. Enlarged adenoids can overgrow and obstruct the eustachian tube orifice, causing a reflux of middle ear mucous secretions, and may result in serous otitis media, which in turn causes a fluctuating conductive (middle ear) hearing loss. When there is active infection in the nasopharynx, it can travel up the tube in the pooled secretions and cause acute otitis media with all of its attendant problems. Many otologists believe that the adenoids need not completely obstruct the eustachian tube orifice to cause serous otitis media and hearing loss, but infected adenoids in the fossae of Rosenmüller can cause edema of the mucous membrane around the orifice, interfering in lymphatic drainage and causing partial obstruction of the tube and a stasis in the tube resulting in conductive hearing loss.

Foreign Bodies in the Nasopharynx

Various foreign objects have been found in the nasopharynx. In many instances such objects are pushed into a nostril, and attempts to remove them force them posteriorly; hence they may become lodged in the vault of the nasopharynx above the adenoids, especially if a large adenoidal mass is present (Fig. 5-29). The presenting symptoms are increased voice nasality and nasal and postnasal muco-purulent discharge with a fetid odor. Occasionally the discharge is blood streaked. Metal or radiopaque objects can be identified by X-ray studies. Removal is best performed by a trained otolaryngologist.

Tumors of the Nasopharynx

Nasopharyngeal tumors are rare in children. They represent less than 2% of those occurring in adults.

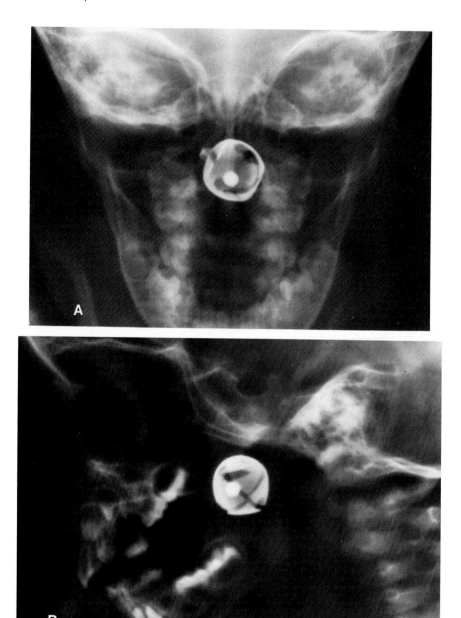

FIG. 5-29. Anteroposterior **(A)** and lateral **(B)** views of a foreign body in the nasopharynx of a 2-year-old girl.

Benign Tumors

Choanal polyps are those that form in the nose or sinuses, extend into the back of the nose as they grow, and slowly descend into the nasopharynx. The early symptoms of these polyps are usually postnasal obstruction and discharge with a history of unilateral nasal obstruction and/or discharge. As they grow, they may cause the sensation of a mass in the upper oropharynx and indice a gagging sensation or a feeling of fullness in an ear; a change in voice may also take place. A polyp may become so large as to present as a smooth, yellowish-gray, avascular, rounded mass in the upper oropharynx (Fig. 5-30). Otherwise, it can be identified by the use of a postnasal mirror. Such a polyp should be removed surgically by severing the stalk at the orifice of the sinus if it originates in an ethmoid cell or by surgical removal from the maxillary sinus if it originates there and then insuring adequate drainage of the infected sinus.

Fibromas may also descend into the nasopharynx from the nose. These may be quite vascular. Such tumors are sessile with relatively long stalks, but they rarely appear in the lower nasopharynx. On mirror examination they are smooth, pinkish masses on the surface of which small vessels can be seen. Removal here is also done through the nose. Because of its vascularity, there is a distinct risk of bleeding.

Juvenile angiofibromas, although considered benign, have been reported as showing some malignant changes on rare occasions. As it grows, this tumor is very

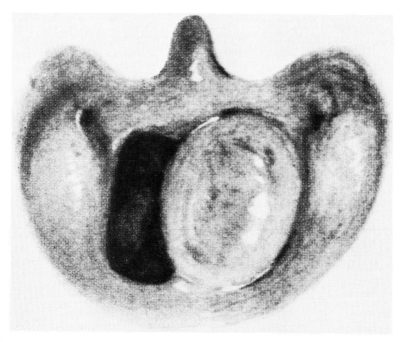

FIG. 5-30. Postpalatal view of a left choanal polyp. (From Hall, I. S., and Colman, B. H.: *Diseases of the Nose, Throat, and Ear,* p. 56. Livingstone, Edinburgh, 1969. With permission.)

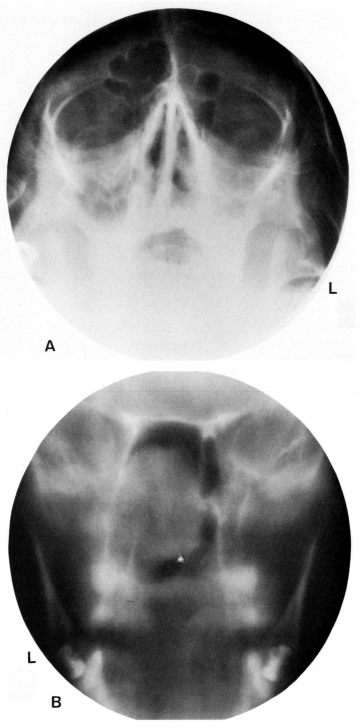

FIG. 5-31. Anteroposterior **(A)** and lateral **(B)** tomographic views of juvenile angiofibroma arising in the nasopharynx of a 10-year-old boy with a history of severe repeated epistaxis. The tumor has extended into the nose and left maxillary sinus.

destructive of the surrounding structures. Clinically it is identified in the nasopharynx of males as early as 8 to 9 years of age, but its origin may be during early infancy. It originates in the sphenoethmoid recess or the basiocciput from the periosteum or perichondrium of that region. Its rate of growth varies, and it is reported to atrophy somewhat as the patient passes the second decade; however, the administration of testosterone has little effect on its size. It is composed of masses of large vessels deficient in contractile elastic tissue that grow in masses of fibroblasts and connective tissue. Some pathologists feel that this is basically an angioma (Fig. 5-31).

As an angiofibroma grows, it spreads into the choanae of the nose, expanding into the sinuses and in some instances growing into the pterygomaxillary space (Fig. 5-32). Early symptoms are fullness in the ears, obstruction to nasal respiration, voice nasality, postnasal discharge, and epistaxis. On examination there may be some retraction of the eardrums and slight conductive hearing loss; on postnasal mirror examination a grayish-red mass can be seen growing from the vault area of the nasopharynx. If the tumor has become extensive, it is sometimes seen on examination through the anterior nares. Treatment is surgical removal. This can present a very difficult surgical problem, especially if the pterygomaxillary space has been invaded. Attempts to biopsy this tumor, even if it presents in the anterior nose, should be done by a surgeon prepared to control serious bleeding; it is definitely not an office procedure.

Encephaloceles occasionally present in the vault of the nasopharynx, having

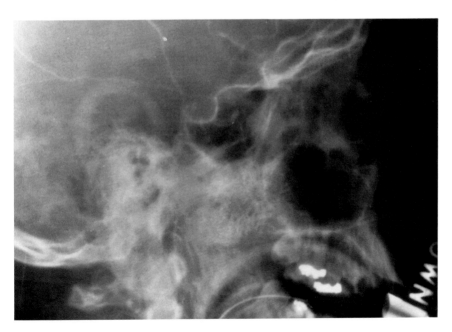

FIG. 5-32. Angiogram of the tumor shown in Fig. 5-31 outlining its position in the nasopharynx and demonstrating the extreme vascularity of the tumor.

penetrated through a defect between the posterior ethmoid complex and the sphenoid sinus. They appear as smooth, dull, red masses that are rather firm and slow-growing. Usually X-ray studies reveal the skull defect through which the herniated brain has descended. These tumors extend under the mucous membrane of the vault of the nasopharynx and appear as broad-based polypoid masses (see Chapter 4).

Chordomas are rarely diagnosed in children. They arise from the site of the embryonic notochord and are destructive to surrounding structures because of their expanding growth; in some cases a chordoma has been reported as spreading to neighboring glands. It presents as a growth from the posterior wall, filling much of the nasopharynx. X-ray studies show marked destruction of bone, especially anterior to the anterior wall of the nasopharynx. Symptoms are headache, postnasal obstruction, ocular changes, and cranial nerve involvement. Posterior mirror examination reveals this tumor, and its extent can be approximated by X-ray examination. This tumor is very resistant to irradiation or chemotherapy, so surgical removal is advised. However, if the tumor has reached large proportions, complete removal may be next to impossible.

Teratomas and dermoid cysts large enough to embarrass respiration have been seen in the nasopharynx at birth. They arise in the midline and often present as a submucosal or polypoid mass. Surgical removal is usually successful (see Chapter 6).

Craniopharyngioma is more common in children than the pituitary adenomas that occur during the teenage years. It is associated with the early development of the hypophysis and lies behind the nasopharynx and below the sphenoid sinus. The symptoms are usually unilateral or bilateral impairment of vision, which develops during late childhood. Vision loss is progressive and may start with a peripheral field cut in one eye. Extraocular palsies may also occur along with optic atrophy from pressure of the tumor in the middle cranial fossa. If the pituitary gland is invaded or compressed, endocrine disturbances take place. The most common are obesity, low metabolism, and lack of sexual development. These tumors appear as small cystic masses in the nasopharynx. They arise from epithelial remnants of the hypophyseal duct. They are usually cystic and lined with epithelium; some, however, are solid. X-ray studies show suprasellar calcification and/or erosion of the sella turcica. The treatment is surgical removal or debulking by a neurosurgeon.

Chromophobe adenoma, which arises in the pituitary gland, may extend through the floor of the sella turcica, occupying the sphenoid sinus, and then erode through the floor of the sphenoid sinus and present as a tumor in the vault of the nasopharynx and partially obstruct the postnasal airway. It may also invade the orbit and the frontal and/or ethmoid sinuses and extend above the sella. First symptoms are frequently ophthalmologic because of involvement of the third, fourth, and sixth cranial nerves with subsequent limitation of eye movement. Pressure exerted on the pituitary gland by the tumor causes hypopituitarism. This is the most common of the intrasellar tumors, accounting for about 70%. The cells of the tumor are the pleomorphic pituitary type, which stain very poorly. X-ray studies show destruction of the sella turcica. Treatment consists of surgical removal by the transsphenoid or the frontal approach. Irradiation is also effective in some of these tumors.

Malignant Tumors

Malignant tumors of the pharynx are said to occur almost four times as frequently in the nasopharynx as in the oropharynx. They occur much less frequently in children than in adults. Malignant tumors in the nasopharynx have a tendency to spread to the cervical glands on both sides of the neck even when the primary site is unilateral. This is because the nasopharynx, containing so much lymphoid tissue, has developed a very rich network of lymphatic channels.

Lymphoepithelioma is the most common nasopharyngeal malignancy in children and is sometimes called a transitional cell carcinoma. These tumors contain varying amounts of lymphoid tissue, which as some have observed is not the malignant component in these tumors. The epithelial elements are poorly differentiated; nuclei are large and vary in size. These tumors spread very early to the glands of the neck, and the first sign of the growth may be enlarged glands in the posterior cervical chain; frequently, glands become enlarged on both sides at about the same time. The most frequent location of the primary tumor is on the lateral wall in the region of the eustachian tube orifice and the fossae of Rosenmüller, and it may spread first to the retropharyngeal nodes and invade the base of the skull, involving the third, fourth, fifth, and sixth cranial nerves. When the primary tumor is on the vault, it has a tendency to spread to the internal jugular nodes. When the latter are involved, distant metastasis may follow rapidly. Fullness in an ear or slight conductive hearing loss may occur about the time glandular enlargement appears. Pain is not one of the early symptoms. Diagnosis is by biopsy, and the present treatment of the tumor is by irradiation and chemotherapy. Although this tumor usually shrinks rapidly after irradiation therapy, it is rarely destroyed completely and recurs as a more resistant growth. Prognosis in these cases is not good.

Rhabdomyosarcoma occurs rarely in children and adolescents. It may be confused with a benign rhabdomyoma or lymphoma in its early stages. It is an embryonal-type tumor with small dark-staining cells lacking in cytoplasm; a number of eosinophils are also present, and there is an embryonal connective tissue stroma. Its primary site is the lateral or posterior wall of the nasopharynx, and it presents as a slightly polypoid, translucent, grape-like tumor that is sometimes pedunculated. It may cause some obstruction to nasal respiration, fullness of the ears, and increased postnasal discharge. Spread to the cervical glands may be very early and may be bilateral. Diagnosis is by biopsy. Treatment is by a combination of irradiation and chemotherapy. As new techniques have evolved, the prognosis has been much improved.

Plasmacytoma (extramedullary) is a nonepithelial malignant tumor that occurs most often in males, rarely in adolescents. It arises in the soft tissues of the nasopharynx, pharynx, palate, or nose and has the appearance of an inflammatory mass. This tumor is composed of plasma cells with multiple nuclei and large amounts of cytoplasm. It presents as a diffuse swelling but can become pedunculated. There are very few symptoms except some postnasal obstruction. The tumor is characterized by early bone invasion, and removal of the primary tumor may be followed years after extirpation by bone involvement. It is not very sensitive to irradiation, and surgical removal appears to offer the best results.

LARYNGOPHARYNX (HYPOPHARYNX)

The laryngopharynx is the most inferior of the three divisions of the pharynx. The anatomic division between the oro- and laryngopharynx is the fold of mucous membrane known as the pharyngoepiglottic fold, which extends from the epiglottis to the lateral wall of the pharynx. For the convenience of examination and discussion, it is easier to include all those structures in the lower pharynx that cannot be seen in most individuals by direct examination of the throat. Such a definition includes the base of the tongue, the foramen caecum, the lingual tonsils, the epiglottis, the supraglottic larynx, the pyriform sinuses, and the opening of the esophagus. Examination of these structures is best accomplished by gently pulling the tongue forward and using a mirror angled to direct the light beam into the laryngopharynx (Fig. 5-6) or by the fiberoptic laryngoscope. Examination shows the following structures: (a) the lingual tonsils extending from the lower pole of the tonsillar fossa across the lateral third of the base of the tongue; (b) the foramen caecum lying just behind the circumvallate papillae in the midline of the tongue; (c) the epiglottis opening against the base of the tongue; and, when elevated, (d) the opening of the larynx behind and below the epiglottis. The pyriform sinuses lie on each side of the larynx, constituting a portion of the floor of the laryngopharynx.

Benign Lesions

A lingual thyroid may grow at the base of the tongue and presents as a dull, red tumor. When a mass that suggests a mass of lymphoid tissue is seen in the midline on the base of the tongue, it should be biopsied before removal. If the mass is thyroid tissue, great caution should be exercised before it is removed. Scans should be obtained to determine the presence (and amount) of thyroid tissue elsewhere. A lingual thyroid may represent the only thyroid gland tissue in the child. If removal of a lingual thyroid is absolutely necessary and no other thyroid tissue has been identified, plans should be made for replacement therapy.

Location of the foramen caecum is important to the pediatric surgeon removing a thyroglossal duct cyst because he must make sure that he is removing all of the thyroglossal duct along with the cyst.

Infections

Infections in the laryngopharynx most often involve the lingual tonsils and the epiglottis (see discussion of lingual tonsillitis earlier in this chapter).

Epiglottitis is an extremely dangerous condition in children and is always life threatening. It may occur at any age but is most common between the second and fifth years. Its symptoms should be well known to the pediatrician and general practitioner because early diagnosis is of utmost importance. Nearly all cases of epiglottitis are secondary to infection by *Hemophilus influenzae* bacillus of the type B strain. Epiglottitis is reported by a number of investigators frequently to be associated with septicemia, and blood cultures from these cases grow out this strain of *H. influenzae*. The disease usually begins when a seemingly healthy child develops a sore throat and suddenly becomes very ill and appears to go into a condition of shock. There may be a muffled voice, and signs of respiratory distress may develop, but these symptoms are frequently not as dramatic as the child's deteriorating general condition, which is accompanied by a sharp rise in polymorphonuclear cell count. Identification of the condition can be made if the back of the tongue is well depressed or the tongue is pulled sharply forward; the epiglottis then comes into view as a cherry-red mass. Direct examination with a laryngoscope shows a greatly swollen cherry-red epiglottis which has encroached on the airway to a point of nearly total obstruction. Treatment, if the condition is diagnosed before severe edema has developed, is intravenous antibiotics (ampicillin or chloramphenicol), forcing of fluids, and increased humidity; constant observation should be maintained for airway obstruction. If the disease has progressed to shock or if there is clinical evidence of airway obstruction, tracheotomy or intubation should be done. At times intubation can be very difficult and dangerous because manipulation around a very edematous epiglottis can cause sudden, complete obstruction of the airway.

Cysts

Cysts in the base of the tongue can develop from the obstruction of mucous glands. They can reach sufficient size to cause respiratory embarrassment and require surgical measures for their removal or marsupialization.

Retention cysts can occur where there is an abundance of mucous glands in the laryngopharynx. They have been found in the vallecular region and on the epiglottis. They may be small and asymptomatic, or they may become obstructive to the airway and may cause voice difficulties. In the newborn, cysts in this region can be so obstructive as to be life threatening. Any such cysts causing obstructive symptoms should be removed or marsupialized as early as possible. It may be necessary to drain a cyst as an emergency measure before attempting any definitive surgery.

Congenital cysts may be present at birth. They may be related to the remanants of the third branchial arch, and the most common site for these cysts is the lateral wall of the laryngopharynx or in the arytenoepiglottic fold. They may become so large before birth that they obstruct the airway of the newborn. Emergency treatment in the delivery room or nursery consists of opening and draining them. This should be followed within a few days or weeks by their removal or marsupialization.

TONSILLECTOMY AND/OR ADENOIDECTOMY: REASONS FOR AND AGAINST

Tonsillectomy and adenoidectomy, although performed less frequently than a few years ago, are still the most frequently performed operations in children. Nearly a million of these procedures were performed in the United States in acute-care hospitals in 1972, and the great majority were performed on children.

The two operations are frequently performed together. Generally, when it is decided that a child needs a tonsillectomy, an adenoidectomy is routinely included; however, when a child needs only an adenoidectomy, the surgeon often performs a tonsillectomy as well. These two operations should be considered separately, and each should be performed only if it is specifically indicated. Both primary physician and surgeon should remember that any operation has its hazards, and these are increased when general anesthesia is required.

Table 5-2 lists conditions that in the past have been considered causes for removal of tonsils but today cannot be accepted as valid reasons for surgery. Tonsillectomy and adenoidectomy should always be avoided when the conditions listed in Table 5-3 are present.

TABLE 5-2. *Conditions not requiring tonsillectomy*

Frequent colds. Many studies have been done to prove that tonsillectomy reduces colds, but it has never been proved; in fact, tonsillectomy may impair a child's resistance to colds.

Poor appetite. This is likewise unproved and so is no indication for tonsillectomy.

Recurrent ear infections. Tonsil removal for this is rarely justified. Adenoid hypertrophy and infection can cause otitis media, serous otitis, and conductive deafness, but moderate-sized tonsils, even with a history of a few acute infections, should not be removed for such a condition. Instead, a careful adenoidectomy should be performed, and a 12-month postoperative period allowed to determine if it has been effective in reducing the incidence of ear infections.

"Big" tonsils. Hypertrophied tonsils without a history of repeated severe infections, unless they are obstructive, should not be removed. Such tonsils begin to atrophy about the time of puberty, and at 25 to 30 years of age they are about the size of the average tonsil.

Allergy. Tonsillectomy is not advised as a relief from allergies.

Simple cough. This is not an indication for tonsillectomy.

TABLE 5-3. *Conditions contraindicating tonsillectomy and adenoidectomy*

Generalized diseases
  Mononucleosis
  Leukemia
  Hodgkin's disease
  Active pulmonary tuberculosis
  Anemias
Conditions affecting bleeding and clotting
  Hemophilia
  Purpura
Acute respiratory infection (postpone surgery)

Indications for Tonsillectomy

Tonsillectomy is indicated for those conditions enumerated in Table 5-4. In addition, in a few cases where children suffer from marked adenopathy that is increased in the presence of a sore throat, and when infections elsewhere have been ruled out, tonsillectomy may be considered. However, operation should be performed only after the parents have been informed that such surgery may well be ineffective.

Indications for Adenoidectomy

Table 5-5 lists major indications for adenoidectomy. Conditions that do not require adenoidectomy include frequent respiratory infections, poor appetite, and allergies. In addition, adenoidectomy should not be performed in children suffering from cleft palate before closure and should be done after such operations only with the greatest reluctance because it may increase the problem of too great postpalatal space.

TABLE 5-4. *Indications for tonsillectomy*

Repeated attacks of acute tonsillitis that recur after proper antibiotic coverage. Three to four such attacks per year should be cause to seriously consider tonsillectomy. If such repeated attacks recur within periods of only a few weeks after the primary attack of tonsillitis and adequate antibiotic therapy, tonsillectomy is indicated.
Peritonsillar abscess or parapharyngeal abscess associated with tonsillitis.
Hypertrophy sufficient to cause respiratory distress (obstructive sleep apnea, cor pulmonale).
Recurrent positive cultures for diphtheria in an individual free from acute symptoms of diphtheria.
Rheumatic fever when repeated cultures of the tonsils show streptococcal infection.

TABLE 5-5. *Indications for adenoidectomy*

Repeated attacks of acute adenoiditis and fever despite correct antibiotic coverage.

Following a retropharyngeal abscess or a parapharyngeal abscess when it is associated with an attack of adenoiditis.

Marked chronic obstruction to nasal respiration with mouth breathing and altered facial development after all other obstructive nasal conditions have been ruled out.

When adenoid hypertrophy is associated with obstructive sleep apnea.

Repeated attacks of acute otitis media, serous otitis media, and/or hearing loss of a conductive type, either chronic or fluctuating, associated with acute respiratory infections.

Recurrent ethmoid sinus infections in the presence of marked adenoid hypertrophy that occur in the absence of acute respiratory infections when all other intranasal contributing causes have been ruled out.

To control a chronic infection of the adenoid bursa (Thornwaldt's disease). When the tonsils are being removed because of evidence of chronic diphtheria infections (repeated positive cultures).

Complications of Tonsillectomy and Adenoidectomy

Tonsillectomy

Immediate complications

Postoperative hemorrhage is the most common early complication. This can result from failure to remove the whole tonsil, failure to locate and control all of the major bleeders, or because a suture breaks or becomes loose. This condition may require a return to the operating room to remove tonsillar remnants or to resuture or recoagulate a bleeder.

Delayed complications

The most common late complication is hemorrhage about the seventh postoperative day from premature separation of the wet scab (slough). If it continues after the child has been put in a head-elevated position and the clot has been removed from the tonsillar fossa, the surgeon should be notified and the child taken to the emergency area.

The most frequent causes contributing to the premature separation of a slough are dehydration because of the child's failure to take fluids or a local infection in the nasopharynx or the tonsillar fossae that extends under the slough. It is of great importance for the pediatrician to make sure that the child takes adequate quantities of fluids for at least 10 days after his return home following surgery.

Careless surgery can sometimes result in serious scarring with resultant contractures of the tonsillar fossae and soft palate.

Lung abscesses have been reported to result from aspiration of infected blood clots. Today this has been almost eliminated by operating with the patient in the Trendelenburg position and with careful suctioning of the throat.

Adenoidectomy

Immediate complications

Immediate postoperative bleeding after surgery may be the result of incomplete removal of all the adenoid tissue. Adenoid remnants may continue to bleed for hours after surgery; therefore, if there is continued bleeding from the nasopharynx postoperatively, the patient should be returned to the operating room for inspection of his nasopharynx to make sure of the complete removal of such tissue and to control any bleeding found.

Delayed complications

These usually occur 6 to 10 days postoperatively, after the child has resumed limited activities. They are caused by premature separation of the wet scab (slough) from the operative site and may result in arterial bleeding from the nasopharynx. If the bleeding persists after the child is put to bed with head elevated, the pediatrician should notify the surgeon and then take the child to the emergency area. This type of bleeding may require a trip to the operating room and/or a transfusion.

Occasionally the cartilaginous end of the eustachian tube (torus tubarius), which grows in the lateral wall of the nasopharynx, is removed by an adenoid curette or an adenotome. This may cause very little difficulty until scar tissue forms around the eustachian tube orifice. It can cause stenosis of the orifice and result in eustachian tube obstruction. The condition causes serous otitis media, barotitis media, and occasionally acute purulent otitis media. Eventually it can lead to conductive hearing loss. Reversal of this condition is very difficult and rarely accomplished.

SELECTED READING

Benson, C. D., et al. (1962): Tonsils and adenoids. In: *Pediatric Surgery, Vol. 1*. Year Book, Chicago.

Briggs, W. H., and Altenau, M. M. (1980): Acute epiglottitis in children. *Otolaryngol. Head Neck Surg.*, 88:665–669.

Brown, J. B., and Fryer, M. B. (1962): Cleft lip. In: *Pediatric Surgery*, edited by C. D. Benson et al., Year Book, Chicago.

Catlin, F. I. (1981): Pulmonary complications of tonsillectomy as described by Samuel J. Crowe. *Laryngoscope*, 91:52–62.

Dickson, R. I. (1980): Nasopharyngeal carcinoma: An evaluation of 209 patients. *Laryngoscope*, 91(3):333–354.

Everts, E. C., and Echevarria, J. (1973): Diseases of the nasopharynx. In: *Otolaryngology, Vol. 3*, edited by M. M. Paparella and D. A. Shumrick, pp. 222–224. Saunders, Philadelphia.

Everts, E. C., and Echevarria, J. (1973): Space infections of the head and neck. In: *Otolaryngology, Vol. 3*, edited by M. M. Paparella and D. A. Shumrick, pp. 318–340. Saunders, Philadelphia.

Greenfast, K. M., and Wittich, D. J. (1982): Adenotonsillar hypertrophy and upper airway obstruction in evolutionary perspective. *Laryngoscope*, 92:650–655.

Gustafson, R. O., et al. (1981): Upper aerodigestive tract manifestations of Behcet's disease. *Otolaryngol. Head Neck Surg.*, 89:409–413.

Harbild, O., and Bonding, P. (1981): Peritonsillar abscess. *Arch. Otolaryngol.*, 107:540–542.

Kuehn, D. P. (1980): Orofacial embryology, anatomy and physiology. *Ann. Otol. Rhinol. Laryngol.*, 89(Suppl. 74):138–143.

Lindsay, W. K. (1962): Cleft palate. In: *Pediatric Surgery,* edited by C. D. Benson et al., Year Book, Chicago.

Ludwig, F. W. (1939): Angina Ludovice. Translated by J. Burke, *Bull. Hist. Med.,* 7(9).

Majid, A., et al. (1979): Localization of IgE in adenoids and tonsils. *Arch. Otolaryngol.,* 105:695–697.

Muchmore, A. V. (1980): An immunologic overview of the human tonsils. *Ear Nose Throat J.,* 59:438–446.

Piersol, G. A. (1923): The visceral arches and furrows. In: *Human Anatomy.* Lippincott, Philadelphia.

Popovitch, P. (1979): Oral cysts and other developmental anomalies. *Ear Nose Throat J.,* 58:488–493.

Schaefer, W. C., and Fletcher, M. M. (1978): Diseases of the pharynx. *Surg. Rounds,* June, pp 14–19.

Schuller, D. E., et al. (1979): Childhood rhabdomyosarcomas of the head and neck. *Arch. Otolaryngol.,* 105:689–694.

Strome, M. (1981): Down's syndrome. *Laryngoscope,* 91(10):1581–1594.

Suanz, F. R. (1980): The clinical anatomy of the tonsillar (Waldeyer's) ring. *Ear Nose Throat J.,* 59:447–453.

Sweet, R. M. (1979): Lingual thyroid. *Ear Nose Throat J.,* 58(12).

Watanabe, T., et al. (1974): In vitro antibody formation by human tonsil lymphocytes. *J. Immunol.,* 113:608.

Wilds, K. J., and Hendru, W. H. (1962): Lesions of the oropharyngeal region. In: *Pediatric Surgery. Vol. 1,* edited by C. D. Benson et al. Year Book, Chicago.

Yarington, C. T. (1973): Tumors and cysts of the oral cavity. In: *Otolaryngology, Vol. 3,* edited by M. M. Paparella and D. A. Shumrick. Saunders, Philadelphia.

Chapter 6

Neck

Branchial Fistulas, Cysts, and Sinuses 383
Thyroid Problems 388
Cystic Tumors 391
Malignant Diseases Causing Neck Masses .393
Histiocytosis 396
Inflammatory Masses 397
   Pyogenic Infections 398
   Tuberculous Cervical Adenitis 398
   Brucellosis (Undulant Fever/Malta Fever) 399
   Cat Scratch Disease 399
   Rubella 400
   Syphilis 400
   Sarcoidosis 400
   Burkitt's Lymphoma 401
   Actinomycosis 401
Salivary Gland Disorders 403

BRANCHIAL FISTULAS, CYSTS, AND SINUSES

Branchial fistulas have been identified extending from the first three branchial pouches but not from the fourth or fifth (Fig. 6-1). Two types of fistulas are seen originating from the first branchial pouch. The first extends from its orifice in the neck, which presents just anterior to the sternomastoid muscle and above the hyoid bone, to the floor of the external ear. It passes through the parotid gland very near the facial nerve. A second type arises from the first branchial pouch and extends from the ear canal (Fig. 6-2) to the preauricular area (Fig. 6-3). The branchial fistula arising from the second branchial pouch passes from the lower anterior border of the sternomastoid muscle over the hypoglossal and glossopharyngeal nerves and between the external and internal carotid arteries to its internal opening just at the

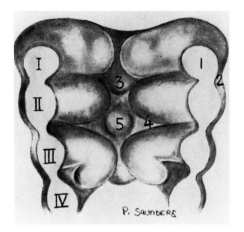

FIG. 6-1. Development of the branchial apparatus. (1) arch. (2) cleft. (3) tuberculum inpar. (4) pouch. (5) copula. (From Deweese and Saunders: *Textbook of Otolaryngology,* p. 433. Mosby, St. Louis, 1968. With permission.)

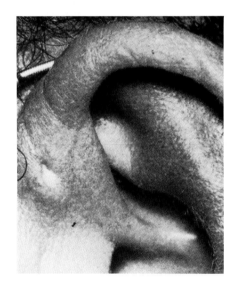

FIG. 6-2. First branchial cleft fistula in the preauricular region. Note the dimpled area. (From Deweese and Saunders: *Textbook of Otolaryngology,* p. 433. Mosby, St. Louis, 1968. With permission.)

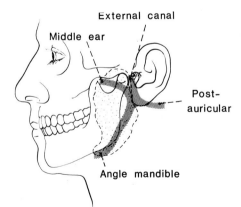

External canal

Middle ear

Post-auricular

Angle mandible

FIG. 6-3. Location of first branchial cleft anomalies. (From Olsen, K. D., et al.: First branchial cleft anomalies. *Laryngoscope,* 90(180):431, 1980. With permission.)

midpoint of the posterior border of the tonsil (Fig. 6-4). The third branchial pouch fistula passes from its opening in the neck along the lower anterior border of the sternomastoid muscle above the hypoglossal nerve and inferior to the glossopharyngeal nerve, medial to the carotid artery, and into the piriform sinus just above the superior laryngeal nerve (Fig. 6-5). Branchial pouch fistulas may form cystic dilatations almost anywhere along their courses.

Branchial cleft cysts formed from the branchial apparatus are usually identified during late childhood or middle life. Although present at birth, they are not identified until they increase in size. These cysts develop from isolated sections of a branchial fistula and are classified according to the type of lining. Those lined with columnar epithelium contain clear mucus and rarely become noticeably enlarged or cause trouble; often they are discovered by accident. The second type are lined with squamous epithelium; they usually contain pus and desquamated epithelial cells. This type expands rapidly and requires surgical removal. Such a cyst can arise from remnants of a first, second, or third branchial fistula, each of which originates from the corresponding branchial pouch (Fig. 6-6). A cyst arising from a first branchial fistula can present as a preauricular cyst, a cyst on the floor of the external canal, or it can appear in the lateral aspect of the neck, above the hyoid bone (Fig. 6-7). Those cysts related to the second pouch are the most common branchial cysts; they usually occur anterior to the anterior edge of the sternocleidomastoid muscle, or they can develop posterior to the tonsil and extend upward into the nasopharynx (Fig. 6-8). Cysts arising from a third branchial fistula present in the neck along the anterior border of the sternocleidomastoid muscle, but some develop superior to the sternomastoid muscle and lie just under the floor of the piriform sinus. Branchial cysts can expand very rapidly, accompanied by pain and fever.

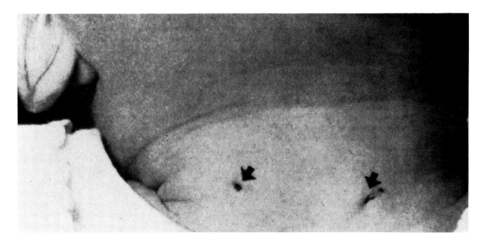

FIG. 6-4. Bilateral second branchial cleft fistulas. Exploration showed that both extended to the superior tonsillar fossa. (From Benson, C. D. et al.: *Pediatric Surgery, Vol. 1,* p. 201. Year Book, Chicago, 1962. With permission.)

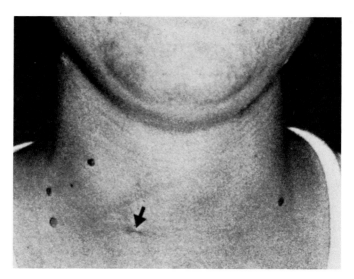

FIG. 6-5. Third branchial cleft fistula. (From May, M.: Neck masses in children, diagnosis and treatment. *Ear Nose Throat J.* 57:144, 1978. With permission.)

Branchial sinuses are incomplete fistulas that open in the same areas of the neck as fistulas. Many of them have cystic dilatations near their orifices in the neck.

Both the fistulas and sinuses normally discharge a small amount of a mucoid material, but they are extremely susceptible to infection, which produces a mucopurulent discharge. A useful method for differentiating a sinus from a fistula is to have the patient swallow; the skin around the orifice of a fistula retracts on swallowing, whereas the skin around the orifice of a sinus does not.

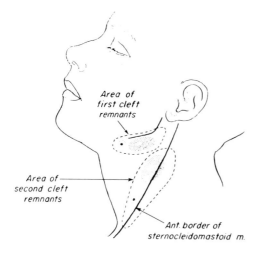

FIG. 6-6. Usual sites in the neck of first and second branchial cleft cysts and sinuses. (From Benson, C. D. et al.: *Pediatric Surgery, Vol. 1,* p. 200. Year Book, Chicago, 1962. With permission.)

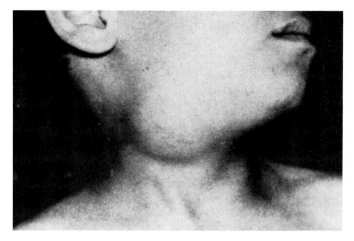

FIG. 6-7. First branchial cleft cyst in an 8-year-old boy. (From El Sarafy, S.: *Atlas of Ear, Nose and Throat Diseases,* p. 289. Ali Bin Ali, Doho, Qatar, Egypt, 1977. With permission.)

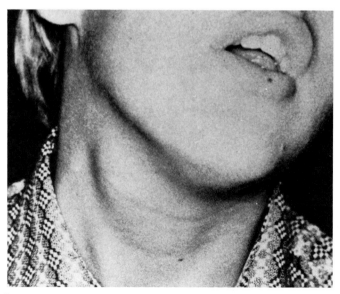

FIG. 6-8. Second branchial cleft cyst, right. (From May, M.: Neck masses in children, diagnosis and treatment. *Ear Nose Throat J.,* 57:143, 1978. With permission).

Branchial cysts, fistulas, and sinuses that are lined by squamous epithelium may contain hair follicles and remnants of sebaceous glands, and they are surrounded by lymphoid tissue that contains germinal centers.

The treatment for branchial cysts, fistulas, and sinuses is total surgical removal. In some cases, if the infection is very severe, it may be necessary to drain a cyst and place the patient on heavy antibiotic therapy before extirpation of the cyst.

THYROID PROBLEMS

Congenital goiters may be present at birth or develop during infancy as an anterior neck mass (Fig. 6-9). They are occasionally very large, firm masses that embarrass respiration and appear most frequently in European goiter areas—in Switzerland and southern Germany—the result of insufficient maternal iodine. In nongoiter areas they appear when there has been maternal consumption of thiourea for the control of hyperthyroidism. These patients recover quickly after the thiourea intake is stopped.

Juvenile goiters are the most frequently occurring goiters in areas where there is low iodine intake in the daily diet. Most of these children show marked improvement when placed on an iodine-enriched diet. However, if the mass of the tumor becomes great, it may be surgically removed to relieve respiratory embarrassment.

The goiter that appears at puberty is the most frequently occurring type in both endemic and nonendemic areas. It is smaller than the two types previously described, occurs most often in females, and improves after puberty; recovery is more rapid if desiccated thyroid is administered.

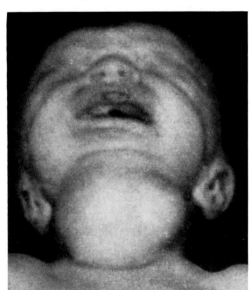

FIG. 6-9. Congenital goiter in a new-born, causing fatal respiratory difficulty. Autopsy showed it to be a teratoma of the thyroid. (From Benson, C. D. et al.: *Pediatric Surgery, Vol. 1,* p. 178. Year Book, Chicago, 1962. With permission.)

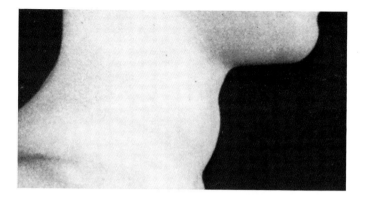

FIG. 6-10. Hasimoto's thyroiditis in an 11-year-old girl. She had a history of a neck mass without symptoms for 1 year. The PBI was elevated, the BEI was depressed, and the iodine uptake was low normal. Histologic sections showed marked lymphocytic infiltration of the gland and hyperplastic follicular epithelium. (From Benson, C. D. et al.: *Pediatric Surgery, Vol. 1*, p. 183. Year Book, Chicago, 1962. With permission.)

Hashimoto's thyroiditis is the most frequent type of thyroiditis occurring in children and is found in females much more frequently than in males. The first symptom is a slightly tender swelling of the thyroid gland accompanied by dysphagia (Fig. 6-10). The gland becomes diffusely enlarged and very firm. Many children suffering from this type of thyroiditis become hypothyroid. During the course of the disease, the child should be followed to see that the swollen gland does not cause respiratory difficulty, in which event surgery may be required to decompress the pressure on the trachea.

DeQuervain's thyroiditis and Reidel's thyroiditis occur very rarely in children.

Thyroglossal duct cyst is one of the most common cysts to present in the neck. It is a developmental anomaly that arises from the thyroglossal duct. The duct is a survivor of the diverticulum of the pharynx that elongates as the thyroid gland descends into the neck. It extends from the foramen caecum of the tongue to the pyramidal lobe of the thyroid gland, passing either anterior to or through the hyoid bone (Fig. 6-11). Cysts or fistulas may develop anywhere along the thyroglossal duct, but about 85% present below the level of the hyoid bone. They can also occur as high as the base of the tongue. Nearly all are in the midline (Fig. 6-12). They appear in the neck as nontender (unless infected), soft, fluctuant masses. When the tongue is forcibly drawn forward, this cyst moves upward in the neck (Fig. 6-13). When the cyst is just above the thyroid gland it may be confused with a thyroid cyst, and if it is very high in the neck it sometimes resembles a dermoid cyst of the floor of the mouth. Surgical removal of the cyst and the entire thyroglossal duct is necessary to cure this condition. Fistulas that normally have a small amount of mucoid discharge require total removal of the thyroglossal duct.

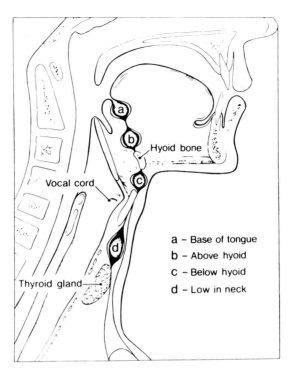

Hyoid bone

Vocal cord

Thyroid gland

a – Base of tongue
b – Above hyoid
c – Below hyoid
d – Low in neck

FIG. 6-11. Possible locations of thyroglossal duct cysts. (From Thomas, J. R.: Thyroglossal duct cysts. *Ear Nose Throat J.,* 58:511, 1979. With permission.)

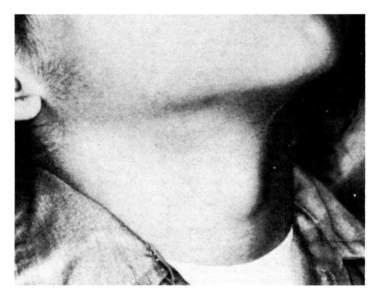

FIG. 6-12. Thyroglossal duct cyst in a young child. (From Thomas, J. R.: Thyroglossal duct cysts. *Ear Nose Throat J.,* 58:512, 1979. With permission.)

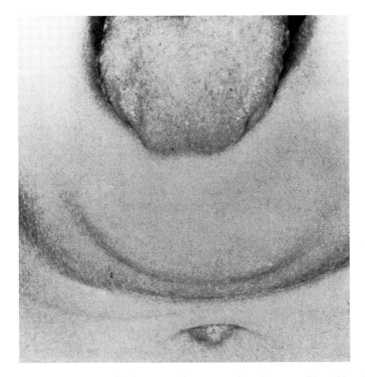

FIG. 6-13. Thyroglossal duct fistula retracted on protrusion of tongue. (From May, M.: Neck masses in children, diagnosis and treatment. *Ear Nose Throat J.* 57:145, 1978. With permission.)

CYSTIC TUMORS

Dermoids and teratomas, semicystic tumors, are classified by the difference in their lining. The dermoids are composed of layers of ectoderm and mesoderm, and teratomas include the three layers of ectoderm, mesoderm, and endoderm. The dermoid contains hair follicles, sebaceous and sweat glands, and a cheesy amorphous material. The teratomas include remnants of respiratory epithelium, cartilage, bone, smooth muscle, and blood vessels. Clinically they cannot be differentiated.

Dermoids and teratomas are relatively rare in the head and neck (7%). They most often appear in the midline, and they are usually apparent at birth and are diagnosed before the end of the first year as they slowly enlarge. They have a soft semicystic feel on palpation and are not attached to the overlying skin. When large, they may cause respiratory embarrassment. To establish a diagnosis, soft-tissue X-rays may show teeth or bone in the tumor. Aberrant thyroid tissue must be ruled out, as well as some type of lymphoma, before a definitive diagnosis can be made. Surgical removal is the treatment of choice.

Cystic hygroma was described in Chapter 5. It is a cystic mass that is usually multilocular and extremely soft and compressible on palpation. It can be transilluminated. About 80% of these tumors extend into the neck and may become a threat to the airway (Fig. 6-14). They are apparent at birth or appear shortly thereafter; expanding slowly, they become involved in the surrounding structures as they encircle the neck. They are not sensitive to X-irradiation or chemotherapy. Surgical removal of the entire tumor may be very difficult and therefore should be undertaken with some reservations; however, removal or reduction in size is necessary and can be accomplished only by surgery.

Hemangiomas are present at birth and are twice as common in females as males. The majority occur in the head and neck. They comprise a congenital anomaly of mesodermal origin; they have a characteristic bluish color and expand when the child cries. They are soft and compressible tumors that occur around the parotid gland and in the hypopharynx, orbit, and nose. On examination they may be confused with a neurofibroma; because of their soft consistency and their expansion on crying when they appear in the nose or orbit, they must be differentiated from an encephalocele. These tumors may regress as the individual grows, so they should be observed for some time before any active therapy is attempted. However, occasionally they continue to grow and may become life threatening. In such cases surgical removal is the preferred treatment.

Laryngocele acts as an air-filled mucosa-lined cyst, although it is in fact a herniation of the laryngeal ventricular appendix, which normally lies between the true and false cords. When this collapsible mass does not extend external to the larynx, it is classified as an internal laryngocele; when it appears in the neck, it is classified as an external laryngocele. The internal laryngocele is more common in children.

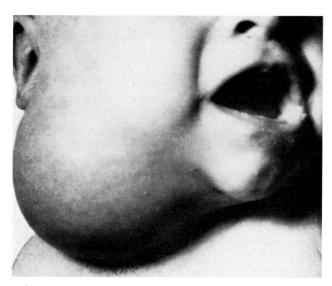

FIG. 6-14. Cystic hygroma in the anterior cervical triangle of a 3-week-old child. (From Benson, C. D. et al.: *Pediatric Surgery, Vol. 1,* p. 196. Year Book, Chicago, 1962. With permission.)

The external laryngocele passes through the thyrohyoid membrane into the lateral neck where it presents as a soft, cystic, compressible, painless mass. It expands when the child cries and then slowly disappears. The internal laryngocele causes a muffled, hoarse cry. With an external laryngocele X-ray films show an air-filled sack, and occasionally an air-fluid level is demonstrated. This cystic mass is not associated with a fistula. Such cases should be referred to a laryngologist because direct laryngoscopy is helpful in making the diagnosis of the internal or external laryngocele. The cure is surgical removal.

MALIGNANT DISEASES CAUSING NECK MASSES

Swelling of the cervical glands is frequently the initial warning of the presence of a neoplastic disease, especially when the primary site of the disease is not in the neck. Such conditions are described in the following paragraphs.

Lymphoepithelioma, the primary site of which is the nasopharynx (described in Chapter 5), metastasizes early into the posterior chain of the cervical glands. Because of the rich lymphatic communication in the nasopharynx, the spread is very often bilateral. The glands involved are swollen, firm, fixed, and nontender. They extend behind the upper portion of the ramus of the mandible, and the diagnosis can be made by biopsies obtained from the primary tumor in the nasopharynx or by removing a gland. These tumors usually originate just posterior to the eustachian tube orifice in the nasopharynx. Irradiation, sometimes combined with chemotherapy, is usually the treatment of choice, as the glands and the primary tumor are relatively sensitive to X-ray therapy. However, such treatment is not totally successful in eradicating the entire tumor, so the survival rate among these children is seldom more than 5 years.

Rhabdomyosarcoma is a solid tumor with the primary site usually in the nasopharynx or the ear. It occurs most frequently in children 5 years old or younger. Metastasis to the cervical glands may be unilateral or bilateral. The growth of the primary tumor in the nasopharynx frequently simulates hypertrophied adenoids, causing adenoid facies, noisy sleep, nasal discharge, and a mild conductive hearing loss. When the tumor arises in the ear, it causes chronic otitis media with discharge from the ear and a conductive hearing loss. Important in the differential diagnosis of this tumor with either site of origin is the steady enlargement of cervical glands and the character of the discharge, which is serosanguineous. The glands are nontender, firm, and fixed. Definitive diagnosis is made by biopsy of the primary tumor. Treatment, which has improved the prognosis over the past 10 years, is a combination of irradiation and chemotherapy (see section entitled Tumors of the Nasopharynx in Chapter 5).

Lymphosarcoma is one of the most frequently occurring malignancies in children over 5 years of age. It involves the lymphocytic mechanism and may appear alone or accompanied by leukemia (lymphocytic leukemia). It involves the glands of the groin, the mediastinum, the abdomen, and the axilla as well as those of the neck.

In adults this disease frequently runs a chronic course, but in children it is far more malignant. In the neck it occurs in the form of rapidly expanding masses that are painless and rather soft. Clinically this tumor is difficult to differentiate from Hodgkin's disease. Definitive diagnosis can be made only by biopsy. Lymphocytes of varying size with the small lymphocytes predominating invade the capsule and tissue surrounding the tumor. There are no multinucleated cells (Dorothy Reed cells) in lymphosarcomas. Blood smears and bone marrow biopsies should be done on these children to rule out lymphatic leukemia. Treatment consists of a combination of irradiation and chemotherapy.

Hodgkin's disease, which occurs more often in males, appears in older children and young adults. The presenting symptom is enlargement of the peripheral lymph nodes. The first nodes enlarged are usually in the cervical region and may be affected unilaterally or bilaterally (Fig. 6-15); this is often accompanied by glandular enlargement in the mediastinum and abdomen. The glands involved feel firm and rubbery, and when there is rapid enlargement there may be some tenderness. The microscopic picture is one of marked infiltration of the lymph nodes that progresses to granuloma formation. There is marked pleomorphism, and there are numerous multinucleated giant cells (Dorothy Reed cells). The disease may spread to the

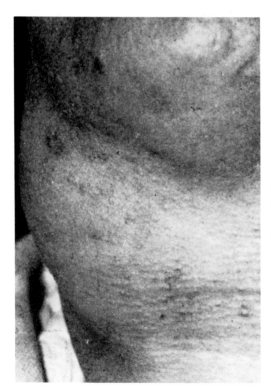

FIG. 6-15. Hodgkin's disease. The swelling was caused by matted glands in the anterior cervical triangle. (From Deweese and Saunders: *Textbook of Otolaryngology,* p. 437. Mosby, St. Louis, 1968. With permission.)

spleen and/or liver. Symptoms include fever, general malaise, and weight loss. It has been reported that in some early cases the disease is limited to a single lymph node. Differential diagnosis must eliminate lymphosarcoma, tuberculosis, and sarcoid disease. In Hodgkin's disease the lesions are not seen in extranodal areas as often as in lymphosarcoma or reticulum cell sarcoma. Biopsy sections, bone marrow studies, and tubercular tests are necessary to confirm the presence of Hodgkin's disease. Treatment, which has improved the rate of survival over the past 15 years, consists of a planned course of irradiation and chemotherapy.

Neuroblastoma is the most common solid malignant tumor (15%) seen in infants and young children, and among all childhood malignancies it is second only to leukemia in frequency. It arises from primary sympathetic neuroblasts. It is classified as a nonchromaffin tumor and almost always appears before 8 years of age. It is distributed about equally between boys and girls. Almost a third of these tumors arise in the medulla of the adrenal gland. Other sites of origin are the sympathetics of the posterior mediastinum, the cervical sympathetic chain, and the retroperitoneal area of the pelvis. A frequently presenting symptom is enlargement of cervical nodes and the development of Horner's syndrome. Increased secretion of catecholamines causes hypertension, diarrhea, and sweating in a number of children suffering from neuroblastomas. Metastasis is reported by various authors as ranging from infrequent to frequent. Invasion of the long bones can be confused with leukemic infiltration. This tumor usually grows rapidly; it is quite vascular and bleeds frequently. Regression of the tumor has been reported. There are less than 5% reported long-term survivals. Treatment has varied in different clinics. Gross et al. have reported good results with surgical removal of the tumors. They believe that removal of the primary tumor is advisable even if the tumor has spread. Surgery is followed by irradiation. Other clinicians advise chemotherapy combined with surgery when there is spread of the tumor. Bone invasion seriously worsens the prognosis in this disease.

Cervical gland enlargement is seen in children secondary to carcinoma of the nasopharynx, tonsils, tongue, oropharynx, and laryngopharynx. It may be unilateral or bilateral, and glands are enlarged, indurated, and fixed. There may be pain in the region of the primary tumor, but frequently the cervical gland enlargement is the first symptom of a malignancy. In the presence of such glands without an identified primary lesion, a thorough survey is necessary. After a careful study, if the primary site has not been located, removal of a gland for diagnostic study becomes necessary. Study of the gland may also give a clue concerning the location of the primary.

Carcinoma of the thyroid gland usually presents as an indurated mass, sometimes fixed, in the gland (Fig. 6-16). This tumor can occur at almost any age; it occurs three times as often in girls and more frequently in children who have been irradiated in the neck area. Thyroid scans should be done on these children, and a biopsy should follow. These tumors are not highly malignant, and surgical removal gives a high cure rate.

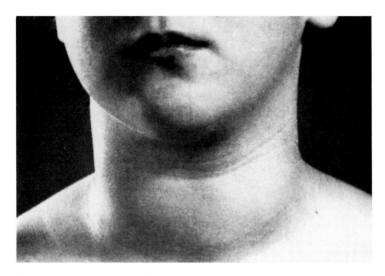

FIG. 6-16. Carcinoma of the thyroid in an 11-year-old girl. There was a 4-year history of an increasing anterior neck mass with gradually increasing respiratory difficulty. The child underwent radiation therapy to her chest for an enlarged thymus at age 3 weeks. Admission chest films showed bilateral pulmonary metastasis. (From Benson, C. D. et al.: *Pediatric Surgery, Vol. 1,* p. 186. Year Book, Chicago, 1962. With permission.)

Laryngeal carcinomas, which are extremely rare in children or young adults, may invade the glands of the neck, but the primary tumor is usually discovered before the glandular involvement because of the voice change.

HISTIOCYTOSIS

Hand–Schüller–Christian disease (histiocytosis) is an eosinophilic granuloma related to Letterer–Siwe disease. It occurs in young children, predominantly males, and is rare in black children. The lesions are disseminated, occurring in the bony skeleton, the soft tissues, and the viscera. It frequently involves the skull, mastoid bone, and maxilla. Cervical lymphadenopathy and diabetes are common, and seborrheic dermatitis and liver enlargement may also occur. Histologically, the histiocytic proliferation, the masses of eosinophils, and a few foamy histiocytes comprise the diagnostic picture. X-ray studies show a typical rounded, punched-out lesion in the bones involved (Fig. 6-17). There is usually some tenderness over such lesions. Prognosis is quite different in different individuals, but in 50% of the children, new lesions gradually stop appearing. In a few cases the disease has a rapid and fatal course. Treatment is curettage of the bony lesions and irradiation of the granulomas.

Letterer–Siwe disease begins with a greasy maculopapular skin rash that involves the face, scalp, neck, and body. There is usually marked lymphadenopathy; the

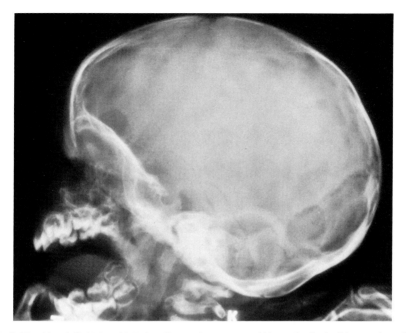

FIG. 6-17. Hand–Schüller–Christian disease in a 1-year-old boy who had a history of swelling behind the right ear and above the left eye. Note the punched-out lesion above the orbit.

liver and spleen are enlarged, and there is fever. Hemolytic anemia and jaundice frequently accompany the illness, and thrombocytopenia and leukocytosis may appear. Histiologically, the bony lesions are similar to those of Hand–Schüller–Christian disease, and there is eosinophilic granuloma formation, but the eosinophilia is less marked. Histiolytic proliferation without eosinophilic infiltration is considered to indicate a very poor prognosis. The outlook in this disease is poorer than that in Hand–Schüller–Christian disease or eosinophilic granuloma. There is no specific therapy, but steroids combined with antibiotics have been beneficial, especially during the more acute episodes.

INFLAMMATORY MASSES

The most common neck swelling is caused by enlarged cervical lymph nodes (Fig. 6-18) secondary to infections in the nasopharynx, oropharynx, laryngopharynx, tongue, gums, and scalp. When involved by such infections, the glands are swollen, tender, firm, nonindurated, movable, and warm to the touch. If the infection is severe and untreated, the glands may break down and develop abscesses, which later may progress to cervical cellulitis or a draining fistula in the neck. In most cases when the primary infection subsides, the glands return to normal.

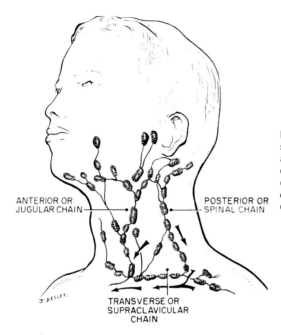

FIG. 6-18. Cervical lymphatic chains showing the positions of the anterior and posterior chains and the supraclavicular glands. (From Boies, L. R. et al.: *Fundamentals of Otolaryngology*, p. 457. W. B. Saunders, Philadelphia, 1959. With permission.)

ANTERIOR OR
JUGULAR CHAIN

POSTERIOR OR
SPINAL CHAIN

TRANSVERSE OR
SUPRACLAVICULAR
CHAIN

Pyogenic Infections

The most common infecting agents in children are pyogenic organisms: *Streptococcus, Hemophilus influenzae,* pneumococcus, and *Staphylococcus.* In children the most frequent location of the primary infection is in the lymphoid tissue of the throat and nasopharynx, and the glands involved are in the jugulodigastric triangle if the tonsils are the seat of infection and in the posterior cervical chain if the adenoids are infected. Very rarely, after the primary infection clears, a child continues to have cervical glandular enlargement, which may persist for months and be of serious concern to parents. In such cases massive antibiotic therapy is usually ineffective, and the conservative approach is to allow the child to live through at least the greater part of a summer before considering surgery. The majority of such conditions improve or clear up completely in the summer sunshine and heat, when the incidence of upper respiratory infections is low. If summer conditions fail to improve the glandular enlargement, tonsillectomy and/or adenoidectomy should be considered. However, some glandular enlargement may continue to persist in some cases after surgery.

Tuberculous Cervical Adenitis

Tuberculous infection involving a tonsil spreads into the glands of the jugulodigastric triangle. There is gradual enlargement of the glands, which rapidly increase in number and become matted together. At first they are firm and nontender, but they soon become soft and may break down completely and develop multiple draining sinuses in the neck. The drainage is serosanguineous, from which the tubercle bacillus can be cultured. The diagnosis can be established by cultures, but most often tuberculin sensitivity tests are used to make the diagnosis.

The tonsillar infection may be caused by infected milk or may be secondary to pulmonary tuberculosis. Tuberculous adenitis is frequently accompanied by a low-grade fever and weight loss. It should be considered as a generalized infection, and a complete examination with chest X-rays is indicated. The whole family should be surveyed. Treatment should be planned to combat a generalized infection, and long-term treatment and observation should be carried out. If the condition has progressed to glandular breakdown and draining sinuses, the child should be isolated until the discharge has ceased. Every effort should be made to identify the contact responsible for the child's infection.

Childhood tuberculous adenitis occurs rarely in the United States now because of the testing of dairy herds, the destruction of infected cows, and the insistence on pasteurizing milk. It still occurs in some rural areas, however, when families drink unpasteurized milk from their own cow, and it is prevalent in certain areas of Europe where pasteurization is not practiced.

Brucellosis (Undulant Fever/Malta Fever)

This disease is caused by *Bacillus abortis,* a small gram-negative rod. It is characterized by cervical adenitis and enlargement of the spleen and liver; on rare occasions it invades bone marrow. The glands contain mononuclear and epithelioid cells, and later granulomas develop. The clinical picture is one of undulating fever, sweats, anorexia, lymphadenopathy, and palpable liver and spleen. At various periods in its course it may be mistaken for infectious mononucleosis, lymphoblastoma, tuberculosis, and typhoid fever. It can be identified by specific agglutination studies.

It is contracted from infected cow's or goat's milk and is endemic in the Mediterranean basin. It has been well controlled in the United States by destruction of infected animals.

Cat Scratch Disease

This is a relatively common infection among children who play with cats. The infecting agent is thought to be rickettsial, and it can be identified by complement fixation or hemagglutination studies, which would confirm the theory that it is a virus-type infection. Cat scratch disease begins with anorexia, headache, lymphadenitis, and an elevation of temperature; in many instances it can be associated with a cat's scratch or the history of play with a cat. Glandular enlargement— which, when the scratch is around the head, includes the submandibular and/or the cervical glands—begins about 8 to 10 days after the inoculation. Glands may become fluctuant about 3 weeks later. The incubation period is 10 to 30 days, and the site of inoculation may become inflamed and swollen about 2 to 3 weeks after onset. The disease may persist for up to 3 months and has no specific therapy. Identification of infected cats has been disappointing.

Examination of sections of the infected lymph nodes shows large numbers of intra- and extracellular granule-like bodies similar to those of psittacosis. In advanced infection, the node develops multiple areas of necrosis with circumscribed areas of epithelioid and giant cells.

Rubella

This is a highly contagious viral infection in young children manifested by low fever, lymph node enlargement, skin rash, and general malaise. There is inflammation of the respiratory membranes, and in some cases there are punctate lesions on the soft palate. Rubella is included in this chapter because of the significance of the glandular enlargement. The posterior cervical, suboccipital, and postauricular glands are markedly enlarged early in the disease before the rash develops and offer an early diagnostic sign of the disease.

Syphilis

This infection occasionally manifests as a single enlarged cervical node; however, usually general glandular enlargement is seen. The definitive diagnosis can be made by serologic studies, and the treatment requires adequate penicillin therapy.

Sarcoidosis

This condition occurs widely in the United States, especially in the South. Black children in the United States are more often victims of it than white children, but it is seen rarely in the black children of Africa. The cause has not been determined, but it is thought to be closely related to tuberculosis. It is usually seen in older children and is chronic and relatively benign. The lymph nodes (peripheral and thoracic) are most often infected, and it also appears in the lungs, eyes, parotid gland, spleen, and liver. Low-grade sporadic fever, uveitis accompanied by parotid swelling and facial palsy, and uveoparotid fever are seen frequently in children suffering from sarcoidosis (Fig. 6-19). Cervical glands are discrete, rubbery, and movable and can be quite large; radiographs show mediastinal glandular masses. Biopsies demonstrate the characteristic epithelioid tubercles of the disease. There is no specific treatment, but administration of steroids is reported to decrease respiratory and renal involvement.

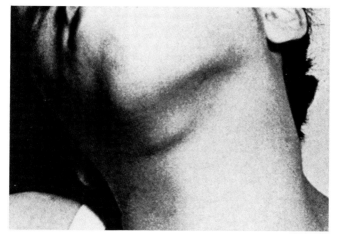

FIG. 6-19. Sarcoidosis in a black child suffering from cervical gland swelling and uveitis. (From May, M.: Neck masses in children, diagnosis and treatment. *Ear Nose Throat J.* 57:152, 1978. With permission.)

Burkitt's Lymphoma

This disease is found in children 4 to 18 years of age in Africa. Most frequently seen in black children, it can occur in children of other races living there. It invades the jaws, maxilla, salivary glands, cervical glands, and thyroid gland, causing massive swelling, fever, and weight loss; proptosis can also occur, and frequently masses can be palpated in the abdomen. Abdominal pain, nausea, and vomiting are frequently encountered in cases with visceral involvement. The disease can also involve the meninges, causing intercranial symptoms. A mass at the angle of the jaw is frequently the presenting symptom.

The lymphoma is thought to be caused by a virus, which may be mosquito-borne. Biopsies show immature lymphocytes and infiltration of histiocytes.

Treatment is by multidrug therapy. Present treatment seems to result in marked reduction of the masses, but recurrences are reported in severe cases several years after treatment and have resulted in death (see Chapter 4).

Actinomycosis

This infection usually begins in the jaw. The jaw becomes swollen and is extremely indurated and board-like on palpation. There is frequently a slight blush and some warmth over this swelling, and in a few instances multiple sinuses develop and drain a serous material containing "sulfur granules" (Fig. 6-20) (see Chapter 5).

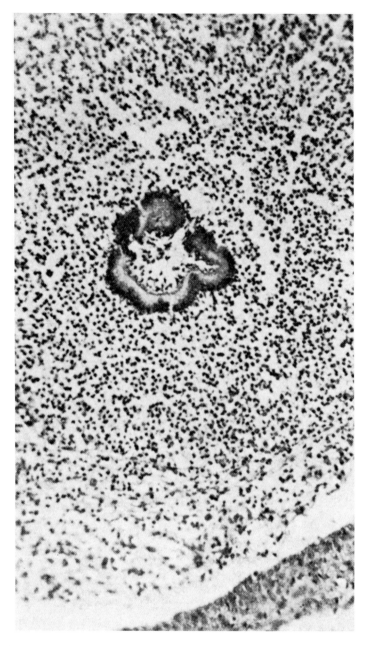

FIG. 6-20. Actinomycosis sulfur granule lying in a suppurative inflammatory reaction. (From Ash, J. E., and Raum, M.: *An Atlas of Otolaryngic Pathology.* Armed Forces Institute of Pathology, Washington, D.C., 1949. With permission.)

SALIVARY GLAND DISORDERS

Mumps in children, a frequent cause of salivary gland swelling, is a febrile disease that can affect the parotid gland on one or both sides and may also involve the submaxillary salivary glands. It is a self-limited, highly contagious disease caused by a myxovirus and may also involve other organs such as the testicles; however, in some instances the central nervous system becomes infected, resulting in encephalitis. The pathologic picture in the salivary glands is one of periductal edema and mononuclear infiltration followed by degeneration of the epithelial lining of the ducts and polymorphonuclear leukocytic infiltration. The parotid gland swelling of mumps is sometimes confused with cervical lymphadenitis, but this misdiagnosis can be avoided by careful delineation of the parotid gland. In older children suppurative bacterial infection or parotid calculi must also be considered in the diagnosis because both conditions present swollen and tender salivary glands. A history of exposure to mumps is helpful in making the diagnosis. X-ray studies can be helpful for demonstrating a calculus in the gland. The mumps virus can frequently be isolated on throat culture. There is no specific treatment, but rest in bed, analgesics, and oral hygiene are helpful. Mumps encephalitis may cause severe sensorineural deafness.

Sarcoid infiltration of the parotid gland can cause a marked painless swelling at the angle of the jaw. Biopsy may be necessary to establish a differential diagnosis between parotid infiltration and cervical adenitis associated with sarcoidosis.

Congenital cysts and hygromas (Fig. 6-21) of the salivary glands can occur during infancy. The picture is one of dilatation of the whole ductal system with multilocular

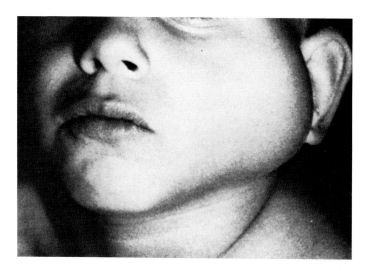

FIG. 6-21. Cystic hygroma involving the left parotid gland in a 4-year-old boy. (From Benson, C. D. et al.: *Pediatric Surgery, Vol. 1,* p. 162. Year Book, Chicago, 1962. With permission.)

cystic formation. The ducts into the cysts are patent, so that contrast media can be employed for diagnosis. Primary bacterial infection of these cysts is frequently followed by a chronic low-grade infection. This cystic formation must be differentiated from a cyst of the first branchial pouch. A solitary cyst separate from the duct system of the parotid gland can cause marked parotid gland swelling, but it does not fluctuate in size. These extraductal cysts may gradually increase in size and may cause local pain. Surgical removal of such cysts may require resection of the gland.

Chronic sialadenitis, sialectasia, and siallithiasis can lead to cyst formation and recurring acute infections; trauma around the duct can also lead to cyst formation and swelling in the upper neck. These cysts result in swelling in almost any portion of a salivary gland. When they cannot be controlled by medical measures, surgery may be required to remove them.

Although most salivary gland swelling is caused by inflammatory disease or simple ductal obstruction, some swellings of the gland may be caused by neoplasms. The mixed tumor is the most often seen benign parotid gland tumor in children, and the mucoepidermoid tumor is the most frequently encountered malignant tumor. These tumors cause solid swellings with fixation of the mass and in most instances can be differentiated only by biopsy.

The tumors of vascular origin that are found involving the parotid gland are hemangiomas, lymphangiomas, and hygromas (Fig. 6-21). On palpation these tumors compress and are soft and painless. The hemangiomas may present a bluish tint to the skin overlying them, but definitive diagnosis can be arrived at only by biopsy. Hemangiomas in children may regress.

Surgical removal of salivary tumors is the favored treatment. Frequently it is necessary to remove the involved gland. In cases in which a malignancy is involved, concurrent removal of cervical glands may be necessary. Great care must be exercised to preserve or repair the facial nerve during these operations.

SELECTED READING

Bill, A. H. (1962): Glands of the neck. In: *Pediatric Surgery, Vol. 1*, Chap. 14, edited by C. D. Benson et al. Year Book, Chicago.

Himalstein, M. R. (1980): Branchial cysts and fistulas. *Ear Nose Throat J.*, 59:23–29.

Holt, G. R., et al. (1979): Dermoids and teratomas of the head and neck. *Ear Nose Throat J.*, 58:520–531.

May, M. (1978): Neck masses in children. *Ear Nose Throat J.*, 57:136–158.

Olsen, K. D., et al. (1980): First branchial cleft anomalies. *Laryngoscope*, 90:423–436.

Ravitch, M. M., and Rush, B. F. (1962): Cystic hygroma. In: *Pediatric Surgery, Vol. 1*, Chap. 16, edited by C. D. Benson et al. Year Book, Chicago.

Chapter 7

Larynx

Embryology and Anatomy 406
Function 408
   Respiration 409
   Voice Production 409
Deformities 409
   Laryngomalacia 411
   Paraglottic Deformities 411
   Webs 411
   "Cleft" Larynx 412
   Congenital Subglottic Stenosis 412
Diseases 413
   Croup 414
   Supraglottic Laryngitis 415
Vocal Cord Paralysis 416
Papilloma and Hemangioma 417
   Papilloma 417
   Hemangioma 418
   Other Laryngeal Tumors 419
Cysts 419
Vocal Cord Nodules 420
Trauma 421
   External Trauma 421
   Intubation Injury 421
   Caustic Trauma 424
   Thermal Injury 424
Anomalies of the Great Vessels 424
Airway Problems 426
   Diagnosis 426
   Differential Diagnosis of Stridor 428
   Management 428
Corrosive Ingestion 430

EMBRYOLOGY AND ANATOMY

The entire respiratory system is an outgrowth of the primitive pharynx. At 3.5 weeks of embryonic life, the laryngotracheal sulcus develops at the ventral aspect of the foregut. By the end of the first trimester of pregnancy, the lower respiratory tract has developed, and the larynx remains at the crucial point of take-off of the respiratory tract from the primitive gut. Thus, the prime function of the larynx becomes much more obvious in that it has evolved, both on an embryologic and a comparative anatomic basis, as a switch valve that prevents inundation of the respiratory tract by the passage of material through the alimentary tract at the time of swallowing. During normal respiration, reflex adjustment of the glottic aperture assists in the regulation of gas exchange within the lungs and in maintenance of the acid–base balance. Phonation, or voice production, by vibration of the vocal cords is an incidental function of the larynx compared to the more basic respiratory and protective functions.

During fetal life, and even through infancy and childhood, the larynx continues to grow and elaborate its basic structure. In addition, its position within the organism changes throughout life: it originates essentially in the upper pharynx, progresses further into the neck throughout life, and is often found in the senescent adult within the thoracic inlet.

The upper limit of the larynx is the hyoid bone, from which the shield-shaped thyroid cartilage is suspended by the thyrohyoid membrane and its ligaments. In turn, the posterior inferior horns of the thyroid cartilage articulate with the "signet-ring"-shaped cricoid cartilage (Fig. 7-1). The cricoid, the only complete ring of cartilage in the respiratory tract, is in continuity with the trachea. Thus, the cricoid and thyroid cartilages form the basic cartilaginous skeleton of the larynx, bridging the gap between the hyoid and the first tracheal ring. (During palpation of the neonatal neck, it should be noted that the thyrohyoid membrane is so short that the body of the hyoid obscures the midline prominence of the "Adam's apple" notch of the thyroid cartilage, which is the most prominent feature of the postpubertal larynx) (Fig. 7-2).

The most obvious features of the pharyngeal aspect of the larynx (Fig. 7-3) are the epiglottis and the arytenoid eminences; the omega-shaped free margin of the epiglottis in continuity with the aryepiglottic folds bounds the laryngeal inlet. During swallowing, these structures pull together to act as the upper laryngeal sphincter. The prow-shaped vallecular aspect of the epiglottis serves primarily to divide the bolus and deflect it toward the pyriform sinuses (lateral to the arytenoids and the signet face of the cricoid). Simultaneously, the relative forward motion of the cricoid away from the cervical spine allows the bolus to pass through the relaxing crico-pharyngeal sling and enter the esophagus.

The prime sphincter function of the larynx resides in the control of the glottic aperture. The glottis is V-shaped; the point of the V is the anterior commissure formed by the attachment of the vocal ligaments to the thyroid ala. With normal

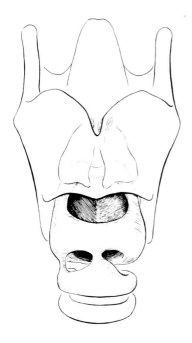

FIG. 7-1. Frontal view of the larynx. *Shaded structure* is the cricoid cartilage showing small attachments to the first tracheal ring.

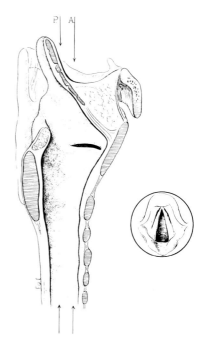

FIG. 7-2. **Left:** Midsagittal split of the larynx showing the left half of the larynx. This profile is of course often seen in the lateral X-ray film. Note the relatively large body of the hyoid bone as it rides down in front of the thyroid notch. **Right:** Endoscopic view of the larynx as it would be seen either with a laryngoscope or a laryngeal mirror. (See Figs. 7-11 and 7-12 for explanation of abbreviations.).

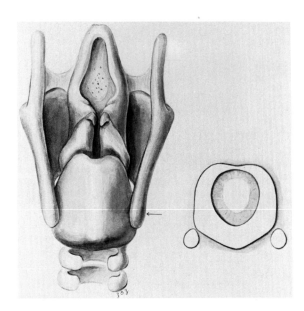

FIG. 7-3. Left: Laryngeal skeleton seen from behind showing the relationship of the thyroid cartilage to the large signet-ring posterior plate of the cricoid on which sits the arytenoid cartilages, which in turn attach to the long epiglottis. **Right:** Hortizontal section through the ring of the cricoid demonstrating the limits of the subglottic larynx. It should be noted that this is the one point at which cartilage completely encircles the airway.

inspiration, the arytenoids are held apart, and the resulting gap is the posterior commissure. If the vocal cords do not approximate closely during this swallowing act, aspiration ensues. Close approximation of the vocal cords is required to build up the "bechic blast" neccessary for effective cough; similarly, sustained expiratory approximation of the true cords is the basic requisite for phonation. To permit the inspiratory phase of breathing, the vocal cords must be actively held apart to open the glottic aperture.

FUNCTION

The prime function of the larynx lies in its ability to protect the lower respiratory tract from inundation during swallowing. The "trap door" simile taught to most elementary-school students is indeed an oversimplification. The epiglottis does serve to divide the bolus and divert it toward the pyriform fossae, and its loss via surgery (supraglottic hemilaryngectomy) or disease (tuberculosis) results in a transient tendency to aspirate that is overcome by reeducation. Failure of the laryngeal sphincter to close is a much more devastating problem and may require surgical diversion.

An essential in the coordinated act of swallowing is the lifting of the closed larynx away from the cervical spine, thus opening the relaxed cricopharyngeal sphincter. This in turn permits the bolus to be carried by the esophageal peristalitic wave to the stomach.

Respiration

The paralyzed larynx (in which the cords assume a "cadaveric" paramedian position) permits the minimal flow of air necessary for quiet inspiration. If there is need for an increase in air flow, the vocal cords must be abducted to permit the greater inflow. This synchronous opening of the larynx would normally be accomplished by the action of the cricoarytenoidius "posticus" muscles (innervated by the recurrent laryngeal nerves).

Failure of the above mechanism for any reason (interarytenoid web, cricoarytenoid joint fixation, muscular paralysis, or neurologic deficit) results in the catching of the true cord in the inspiratory air stream, producing high-pitched paradoxical inspiratory phonation (stridor). If both cords are simultaneously affected (especially in cases of posterior commissure web and in central nervous system lesions), the stridor may be heard at rest; it is increased when the patient is asleep or anesthetized and disabling on attempted exertion.

The expiratory phase of respiration forces the paralyzed cords apart and requires no active or muscular participation. The Bechic blast necessary for effective cough requires momentary closure of the larynx behind which intrathoracic pressure builds up before release of the blast of air.

Voice Production

"A rough quality of voice," or hoarseness, implies a difference in tone or impairment of normal vocal cord vibration in the act of phonation. This should be distinguished from such disorders as slurred speech, which is not true "hoarseness" but really a matter of impaired articulation—the enunciation of words and sentences; the latter is a function of the coordinated action of the tongue, lips, teeth, etc. on the sound produced by phonation. Thus, the larynx functions only as a source of sound, which is then modulated by articulatory mechanisms. The control of vocal cord tension resulting in a variety of pitches can be very elaborate. The free vibrating edges of the true cords may be impaired by inflammation, trauma, new growths, or anatomic constrictions such as webs and cysts. Spastic closure of the glottis may impair air flow just as severe subglottic or supraglottic swelling may muffle the voice.

DEFORMITIES

Most pathological processes "deform" the larynx or the airway to a recognizable extent, and they can be tabulated by the region affected (Table 7-1).

TABLE 7-1. *Deformities of the larynx*

Anatomic region	Congenital deformity	Acquired deformity
Supraglottic		
Epiglottis	Absence (rare)	
	Cleft (very rare)	Destruction
		Caustic
		Infection
Tubular		Swelling
Laryngomalacia	Epiglottic redundancy	Arytenoid dislocation during
	Aryepiglottic redundancy	intubation
	Arytenoid redundancy	
Webs between the false cords		
Paraglottic	Laryngocele	
	Laryngomucocele	Laryngomucopyocele
Glottic		
		Iatrogenic
		Papilloma therapy
		Intubation
		Intubation
	Webs, anterior and posterior	Anterior webs can be
		iatrogenic: from papilloma
		therapy, especially the laser,
		or from intubation. Posterior
		webs can also come from
		intubation
	Paralysis	Paralysis
	Unilateral	Unilateral
		Birth trauma
		PDA ligation
	Bilateral—familial?	Bilateral
Subglottic	Absence of the cricoid lumen	Subglottic stenosis
	Congenital subglottic stenosis	Postintubation
	Elliptical cricoid	
	Entrapment of the first	
	tracheal ring	
	Occult submucous cleft of	
	the posterior plate of the	
	cricoid	
	Glandular hyperplasia	
	Laryngeal cleft—TE fistula	
Tracheobronchial	Stenosis	Foreign body
	Malformation	Granuloma
	Innominate	
	Rings	
	Slings	

Laryngomalacia

The most common reason given for a "noisy baby" is laryngomalacia, which is best described as a redundancy of the supraglottic laryngeal structures (the epiglottis itself, the aryepiglottic folds, and the arytenoids). Indrawing of any or all of these supraglottic structures on inspiration tends to produce stridor. "Stress" stridor is commonly improved when the patient is prone, and it is aggravated when the patient is recumbent.

True epiglottic deformities are much more uncommon. The epiglottic edge is commonly omega-shaped in the infant and can be exaggerated to produce a "tubular" epiglottis. A true deformity such as the bifid epiglottis or congenital absence of the epiglottis is extremely unusual. Occasionally, absence of the epiglottis is acquired as a result of a caustic burn.

Paraglottic Deformities

The paraglottic larynx (those soft tissues of the larynx lateral to the glottis) contains the ventricles and saccules, the vocalis muscles, etc. The most common deformity here is a cystic deformity in which the laryngeal saccule, or "appendix," is enlarged by either retained air or mucus to produce either a true "laryngocele," a laryngomucocele (see Fig. 7-10), or, if infected, a laryngopyocoele. As a result of this ballooning of the paraglottic larynx, the airway is compromised, as is the pyriform fossa; thus, severe swelling by a laryngomucocele interferes not only with breathing but also with swallowing.

Webs

Adhesions between the anterior ends of either the false cords or the true cords are occasionally seen. False cord webs produce airway obstruction as a prime symptom. Webs of the true cords may impair the airway somewhat but also, by shortening the vibrating length of the vocal cord, make the voice more high-pitched than normal. The most common traumatic web is one secondary to intubation; a posterior interarytenoid web tends to hold the arytenoids together so that inspiratory stridor is produced. For many years, this was thought to be a "paralysis" secondary to intubation. In reality, there are probably no true "paralyses" caused by intubation. Traumatic anterior commissure webs most frequently follow overenthusiastic treatment of papillomas with forceps or the laser. Vocal cords themselves may be deformed in a number of ways to produce hoarseness. The most common deformity is the vocal nodule, or "screamer's node," which in reality is callus formation at the midportion of the membranous vocal cord. This is caused primarily by exuberance and vocal strain. Removal of such traumatically induced thickening does little unless the child changes his voice habits.

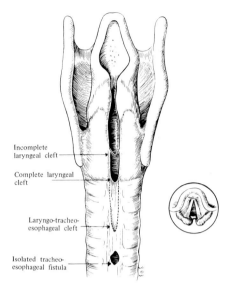

Incomplete
laryngeal cleft

Complete laryngeal
cleft

Laryngo-tracheo-
esophageal cleft

Isolated tracheo-
esophageal fistula

FIG. 7-4.   Posterior midline defects.

"Cleft" Larynx

Aerodigestive midline defects may involve part or all of the partition between the laryngotracheal (respiratory) tube and the pharyngoesophageal (alimentary) tube. Historically, the first of these to be recognized was the tracheoesophageal fistula, which was often associated with esophageal atresia and thus the obligate aspiration of all swallowed material. More subtle was the "H"-type fistula between the otherwise patent esophagus and trachea in which the bypassing of the laryngeal switch valve was only intermittent.

During the last decade a more extensive laryngotracheoesophageal cleft and its repair have been prominent in both the laryngological and pediatric surgical literature. When this defect is confined to the larynx, the symptoms are much more those of respiratory obstruction associated with a redundancy of the tissue lining the laryngeal cleft (Fig. 7-4).

An "occult" cleft associated with a slit-like cricoid has been described in which there is no fistulous connection but the spine of the cricoid is absent.

Congenital Subglottic Stenosis

Beneath the vocal cords (the glottic aperture) lies the "subglottic" larynx. To visualize this area directly from above, the vocal cords must be retracted; a bronchoscope or telescope passed between the cords also aids in evaluating the shape and caliber of the subglottic airway. Any narrowing of the subglottic airway is by definition subglottic stenosis; in practice, however, this term does not include inflammatory or tumorous distortions of the lumen. Congenital malformations may result from either a cartilaginous or a soft tissue abnormality.

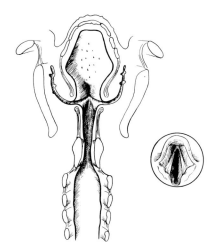

FIG. 7-5. A deformity of the cricoid in which its transverse diameter is congenitally very narrow, producing a slit-like subglottic airway. This extreme elliptical shape of the cricoid produces a situation wherein the slightest swelling will produce severe respiratory distress.

The most striking cartilaginous abnormality is that in which the cricoid is totally devoid of lumen: such an atretic cricoid produces an acute respiratory emergency in the delivery room wherein the child is seen to make respiratory attempts but to move no air whatsoever. Lesser degrees of stenosis in which there is some lumen and yet the cartilage is flattened either in an anteroposterior or a transverse (Fig. 7-5) diameter have also been described. Such hard cartilaginous stenoses do not always accept an endotracheal tube, and thus emergency tracheotomy may be required. On the other hand, lesser distortions of the cricoid may produce dyspnea that is symptomatic enough to require intubation and for which the origin is not recognized. Indeed, one of the explanations for acquired subglottic stenosis may lie in the fact that infants are intubated by visualization of the vocal cords and not of the subglottic larynx; thus, intubation of an abnormal subglottis could much more readily produce scarring and later stenosis. This is not to excuse all postintubation stenosis but may indeed explain some of the occurrence of such problems.

Children with lesser deformities of the subglottic airway may survive the neonatal period and be passed off as "noisy babies" only to become severely embarrassed when their first respiratory infection is superimposed on the distorted anatomy. Indeed, the most common time for diagnosis of congenital subglottic stenosis is between the sixth and 12th months of life, with such babies presenting as respiratory emergencies when they have been carried for the first several months as "noisy babies."

DISEASES

Inflammatory diseases of the larynx include "croup," LTB, nondiphtheric croup, pseudocroup, and acute stenotic laryngitis, all of which are examples of obstructive subglottic laryngitis. Epiglottitis may be subclassified as supraglottic laryngitis, supraglottitis, and laryngopharyngitis.

The differential diagnosis must consider laryngotracheal bronchitis, epiglottitis, and the presence of a foreign body.

Tumors that affect the larynx are papillomas, hemangiomas, rhabdomyosarcomas (rarely), and carcinoma (rarely).

External trauma that can damage the larynx may originate with intubation, caustic agents, and thermal burn.

Foreign bodies may lodge in the hypopharyngeal and esophageal areas (where they may result in retropharyngeal abscess) as well as in laryngeal, tracheal, or bronchial airways.

Croup

"Croup" is classically characterized by a resonant barking cough, hoarseness, and persistent stridor. Fearon suggested that this term is not always used with precision and preferred the term "acute obstructive subglottic laryngitis." He also acknowledged the prevalence of the terms acute laryngotracheitis and acute laryngotracheobronchitis (LTB). Senior et al., in a recent study, included "all cases with hoarseness and a barking cough—with or without inspiratory stridor" as "croup." When this term is used so variously among physicians, it is not difficult to project the degree of semantic imprecision implied when the range of persons employing this term is extended to include parents, grandparents, and others with whom the pediatrician must communicate.

If one considers the anatomy involved, it can readily be understood how swelling in the subglottic larynx can produce hoarseness, stridor, dyspnea (due to both airway obstruction and the retention of tracheobronchial secretions), and even death.

Before the study of bacteriology, "croup" probably included an exudative membranous component characteristic of diphtheria; in more recent times, the lack of bacteriologic etiology has led to the term "viral croup." Current experience suggests that many cases are caused by *Mycoplasma,* although among cases severe enough to require endoscopic intervention, *Staphylococcus* has been implicated in those patients in whom an exudative subglottic laryngitis has been observed.

The submucosa of the subglottic larynx is composed of loose areolar tissue that can swell in only one direction, at the expense of the airway. This loose tissue is surrounded by the cartilaginous cricoid and the conus elasticus, which confine the swelling on its periphery (Fig. 7-6).

This clinicopathologic process suggests an orderly progression of symptoms from the prodromal "head cold" or upper respiratory infection to hoarseness, barking cough, and stridor, which becomes dyspnea. Such symptoms are usually independent of patient position. In children under 1 year of age, one should suspect an underlying subglottic deformity (e.g., mild to moderate stenosis, hemangioma). An abrupt onset suggests the possibility of a foreign body. Dysphagia and drooling suggest either a cervical esophageal foreign body or involvement of the supraglottic larynx ("epiglottitis"), which conditions classically have a much more abrupt onset.

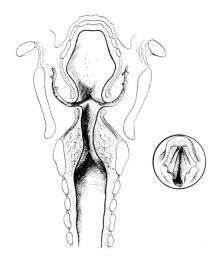

FIG. 7-6. Left: Frontal view of the larynx showing the type of swelling seen in croup. It demonstrates the bounding of this swelling by the cricoid cartilage and the conus elasticus and shows how the swelling can expand only at the expense of the airway. **Right:** Endoscopic view of this swelling, showing how it presents as a subglottic flattening of the normally concave undersurface of the vocal cords.

Treatment is therefore to reduce inflammatory subglottic swelling by the use of steroids and to provide supplementary humidification to help keep secretions fluid and encourage their migration through the narrow airway. When the airway is dangerously impaired, endoscopy may permit removal of adherent secretions from the narrowed subglottis and facilitate the aspiration of tracheobronchial secretions. Intubation may, by forcefully dilating the inflamed area, increase the airway, but only at the risk of traumatizing the inflamed subglottic tissue and promoting long-term scarring—subglottic stenosis. Tracheotomy may, of course, bypass the obstruction without further traumatizing the subglottis.

Supraglottic Laryngitis

Supraglottic laryngitis—inflammation of those parts of the larynx that intrude into the hypopharynx (epiglottis, aryepiglottic folds, arytenoids, etc.)—is manifested primarily by hypopharyngeal symptoms, dysphagia, odynophagia, and drooling. Inflammation involving the lingual surface of the epiglottis may progress rapidly with consequent curling of the epiglottis posteriorly, angulating the airway, and may lead to precipitous airway obstruction. Because of the kinking of the airway by the swollen epiglottis, intubation may be difficult if not impossible even with an open-tube bronchoscope.

Epiglottitis is the term most commonly applied to the supraglottic inflammation described above. Because of its life-threatening nature, it deserves special consideration. Possibly the organism most commonly indicted is *Hemophilus influenzae;* however, the same pathological change can be found with either thermal or chemical burns of the hypopharynx. The symptomatology is distinctly different from that of "croup" in that pharyngeal symptoms predominate. Dysphagia and even odynophagia

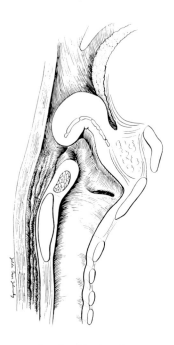

FIG. 7-7. Swelling of the lingual surface of the epiglottis, causing the epiglottis to fold on itself so that the uninvolved laryngeal surface is angulated posteriorly. In the extreme case, this can prevent endotracheal intubation and sometimes even passage of a bronchoscope.

associated with drooling are not uncommon. As the airway becomes involved, a muffled "hot potato" voice may be apparent. Because of the dysphagia and pooling of secretions in the pyriform sinuses, the patient often prefers to sit up, leaning forward and drooling. Stridor in this situation occurs immediately prior to respiratory obstruction (Fig. 7-7).

The history usually indicates a rapid course, although if shotgun antibiotic therapy has been given the course may be somewhat slower. Another consideration to bear in mind, as with other *H. -influenzae* infections, is the possibility of associated meningitis.

The management of suspected epiglottitis deserves special caution because the patient who has progressed to dyspnea or stridor may easily be completely obstructed by meddlesome use of a tongue blade or similar device. Our own practice is to take all patients who are suspected of epiglottitis to an intensive care unit where endolateral films can be obtained and emergency measures such as intubation and bronchoscopy can be carried out with the collaboration of the anesthesiology department (see Chapter 4).

VOCAL CORD PARALYSIS

Clinically, the most important paralysis is that produced by bilateral failure of the recurrent laryngeal nerves to function, i.e., bilateral recurrent nerve paralysis, also known as bilateral posticus paralysis or bilateral abductor paralysis. Such failure of the normally synchronous opening of the glottis with inspiration leaves the vocal cords in a paramedian position, which is often adequate for quiet inspiration. However, any inspiration sharp enough to cause a relative drop in tracheal subglottic air pressure results in passive inspiratory adduction of the cords. This brings the cords into median apposition, and the inspiratory airstream produces a high-pitched inspiratory phonation ("inspiratory stridor"). The relatively high pitch produced is caused by the true cords themselves vibrating.

Causes of bilateral paralysis are most commonly central (fourth ventricular pressure or lesion) or brainstem herniation via an Arnold–Chiari malformation in which the vagus nerves are compressed against the foramen magnum by herniation of the brainstem. Bilateral peripheral involvement is also seen (more commonly in the adult) with thyroid neoplasms or surgery, cervical esophageal carcinoma, or mediastinal neoplasm. Tracheoesophageal trauma or surgery may also involve one or both recurrent nerves. In unilateral paralysis, the left recurrent nerve, which has a longer course around the ligamentum arteriosum, is more often at risk than the right recurrent nerve. Patent ductus arteriosus (PDA) ligation is the most common surgical cause in infants, although either or both nerves may of course be involved in tracheoesophageal fistula surgery.

Historically, unilateral neonatal paralysis is most often associated with a birth in which the umbilical cord has been found around the neck. It has been recently suggested that cesarean section through a small uterine incision (which causes traction on the neck by the aftercoming head) may also be associated with unilateral recurrent nerve paralysis.

Paralysis resulting from contusion but not division of the nerve is usually temporary. Even with the Arnold–Chiari malformation, reduction of the herniation by relieving the increased intracranial pressure may cause the symptoms to regress. The symptoms of unilateral paralysis are usually transient; although there are those who claim that unilateral paralysis may require tracheotomy in 20% of the patients, our experience has been much less dramatic, with only the occasional unilateral paralysis requiring tracheotomy.

Bilateral paralysis commonly requires emergency intubation and subsequent tracheotomy. Conversely, it is the rare infant with bilateral paralysis who can safely avoid tracheotomy (Fig. 7-8).

PAPILLOMA AND HEMANGIOMA

Papilloma

Papilloma, a warty growth most commonly seen on the skin, may also involve any of the mucous membranes of the mouth, pharynx, larynx, or tracheobronchial tree. Those that involve the endolarynx most commonly produce hoarseness and

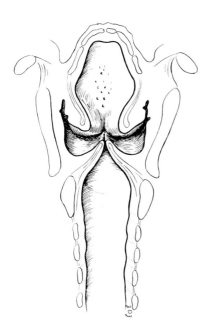

FIG. 7-8. Mechanism of inspiratory obstruction in bilateral recurrent nerve paralysis. In the absence of any abductor action, the negative inspiratory pressure in the trachea pulls the vocal cords together, producing a paradoxical inspiratory phonation that is heard as a high-pitched inspiratory stridor.

not infrequently respiratory obstruction. Recently, the correlation between infantile laryngeal papilloma and maternal vaginal wart has also been noted. Papillomas in the respiratory tract are thought to be viral in origin. They have traditionally been treated by endoscopic forceps removal; however, this has now been refined by the use of the laser, and most recently the effect of interferon on such growths is being studied. The effectiveness of any single method is extremely difficult to quantitate, as papillomas can occur and regress spontaneously. For a time it was believed that papillomas would disappear at puberty, but this has not been proved to be a statistically significant milestone.

Hemangioma

Subglottic hemangioma should always be considered in the differential diagnosis of the dyspneic infant. Characteristically, such lesions are more symptomatic during the first few months after birth than they are at the time of delivery. About half of the subglottic hemangiomas are associated with cutaneous angiomas of various sorts. Endoscopically, most angiomas are solitary lesions (Fig. 7-9). When they are seen in association with Sturge–Weber syndrome, there may be diffuse discoloration to the endolaryngeal structures. Details of the methods of handling hemangiomas vary tremendously. There is controversy over whether to biopsy. Low-voltage radiotherapy, steroids, laser, and watchful waiting have all been advocated.

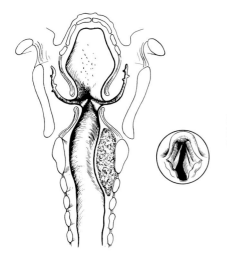

FIG. 7-9. Frontal view (**left**) showing the swelling produced by a subglottic hemangioma and the characteristic endoscopic picture (**right**).

Other Laryngeal Tumors

Rhabdomyosarcoma occasionally involves the endolarynx or the pyriform fossae. The author personally has experience with one patient, 4 years of age, who did not respond to radiotherapy but then subsequently responded nicely to laryngectomy. Carcinoma of the larynx has been reported only once or twice in children under 10 years of age. The differential diagnosis here is with the much more common papillomas. It should also be recalled in this setting that treatment of papillomas by radiotherapy has been known to induce carcinomatous change.

CYSTS

A variety of cystic lesions are found in or in close proximity to the larynx. All seem to be of glandular origin. The most superior to be noted here is a cystic mass presenting at the foramen caecum. Most of these are fluid-filled cysts that respond to simple marsupialization. However, occasionally such a mass is an undescended thyroid gland.

Simple mucosal retention cysts may originate anywhere in the hypopharynx. Those originating in the vallecula pose a special threat to the airway by depressing the epiglottis.

Cystic lesions of the laryngeal appendix or "saccule" are of particular interest because of their location deep in the superior paraglottic larynx (Fig. 7-10). They may be filled with air (laryngocele), mucus, or, if infected, pus. "Saccular" cysts usually present with respiratory distress secondary to intrusion of the paraglottic

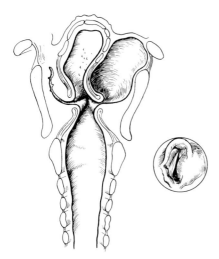

FIG. 7-10. Anterior half of the larynx in the frontal plane (**left**). The dilated structure is the laryngeal saccule or appendix. This structure is dilated to form a laryngeal mucocele or laryngeal retention cyst. This can be filled with air, pus, or mucus. The endoscopic view (**right**) shows how it compromises not only the supraglottic airway but also the swallowing passage as it impinges on the pyriform fossa.

swelling on the supraglottic airway. Endoscopically, the swelling is usually seen to involve the aryepiglottic fold and to compress the associated pyriform fossa.

Laryngoceles (more common in adults) may extend through the thyrohyoid membrane, presenting in the neck as an "external" laryngocele; these can often be inflated by the Valsalva maneuver.

Lymphangioma may involve the supraglottic laryngeal and hypopharyngeal mucosa, often in association with a "cystic hygroma" in the neck. Also seen in the laryngeal ventricle is the thin-walled oncocytoma (histologically analogous to Warthin's tumor). Ectasia of the subglottic submucosal glands has been seen to produce a form of "soft" subglottic stenosis.

VOCAL CORD NODULES

"Screamer's nodes"—paired nodules at the junction of the anterior and middle third of the membranous cords—are often found in the 2- to 4-year age group when a rival younger sibling appears on the scene. This self-inflicted trauma is also occasionally seen in more exuberant children 8 to 14 years old (Fig. 7-11). The main problem presented here lies in the differential diagnosis of hoarseness in children wherein papilloma (see above) must be excluded. As for any callus formation, treatment is best accomplished by removing the "trauma"; only rarely do very well-organized fibrotic nodules require endoscopic surgical excision. On the other hand, attempts to curb an exuberant youngster could result in suppressed emotion and subsequent bouts of greater trauma. Probably the most helpful strategy is to lessen the general level of tension if possible by reassurance of the parents.

Intubation granulomas most often occur at the junction of the membranous and cartilaginous glottis, i.e., the tip of the vocal process of the arytenoid (see below).

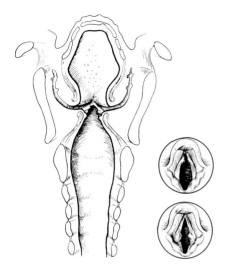

FIG. 7-11. Anterior half of the larynx cut in the plane marked *A* in Fig. 7-2. As one looks forward, one can see the anterior commissure, the cut edges of the cricoid and thyroid cartilages, and the laryngeal ventricles and saccules. **Right:** The endoscopic views show first vocal nodules of the anterior cord, which are the classic "screamer's nodes" and then nodules of the posterior cord, which are most commonly associated with the trauma of intubation. These are commonly called intubation granulomas, and they occur at the junction of the membranous and cartilaginous vocal cords.

TRAUMA

External Trauma

External trauma to the larynx itself is rare in infants and small children. However, as these children grow and ride bicycles, minibikes, and snowmobiles, the incidence of true laryngeal injury increases. The force generated by a child bicycling slowing into a clothesline may be minimal. However, as the propulsive force increases with minibikes and especially snowmobiles, the force generated can even lead to decapitation. The problem seems to lie in the fact that as higher speeds are generated, the wire or clothesline put up to discourage people from riding minibikes or snowmobiles across their property may not be visible to the rider. Such external injury, if it is less than decapitation and compatible with life, may present the physician with a child who has gross subcutaneous emphysema, hemoptysis, and respiratory distress, usually the result of a gross injury to the larynx and/or trachea that has caused discontinuity of the cervical air column. Such injury is obviously a major catastrophe and may require tracheotomy. Endoscopy for any neck injury should be approached with caution because if there has been injury to the cervical spine, hyperextension may compound the spinal cord problem and produce quadriplegia.

Intubation Injury

Intubation injuries can be classified as injuries produced during the act of intubation (e.g., arytenoid dislocation and hypopharyngeal perforation) and those produced in the larynx by the intubation tube itself. Arytenoid dislocation is best understood if it is realized that the cricoarytenoid joint is indeed a very small but true joint that is supported by small ligamentous attachments. If the square blade of an intubation laryngoscope is introduced into the cervical esophagus and then slowly withdrawn to expose the larynx, it is not difficult to postulate how such a maneuver could dislocate one or both arytenoid cartilages and tear the ligaments that attach it to the cricoid.

The far more common and definitely more serious injury is that produced within the larynx by the presence of an endotracheal tube. This can vary in intensity from simple transient vocal cord edema to ulceration and granulation at the vocal process of the arytenoid to loss of subglottic epithelium, granulation, and even chondritis and total loss of the subglottic laryngeal lumen.

As one considers intubation, one should keep in mind the fact that the glottic aperture (bounded by the true vocal cords and the posterior commissure) has approximately one-half the cross-sectional area of the human trachea. Therefore, there is no need to try to insinuate a tube that has the same diameter as the trachea itself. Indeed, the resistance implied by the reduction of the air column at the larynx may be important in the physiological prolongation of expiration. The absolute limit to the passage of an endotracheal tube is of course the diameter of the cricoid, which is the only complete ring of cartilage in the respiratory tract. However, to pass a tube that is just large enough to be forced through the lumen of the cricoid is to ignore the soft tissue that lines the lumen of the cricoid. Pressures that cause ischemia of the mucosal lining of the subglottic larynx may lead to granulation, loss of epithelium, and even chondritis of the cricoid itself. A gentler and more physiological approach is—instead of looking for the largest possible tube that will fit— to look for the smallest possible tube that will give adequate ventilation and permit a "leak" of air between the laryngeal mucosa and the tube. Such a leak would imply that there probably is no significant mucosal ischemia.

In addition to the fit of the tube itself, the state of relaxation of the patient is important. An unconscious patient or one who is therapeutically paralyzed may tolerate a relatively small tube that is changed frequently and kept clean for months without suffering laryngeal injury. On the other hand, a snugly fitting tube in a child who is restless, apprehensive, and fighting its presence may produce laryngeal injury within a period of hours. The basic concept to be appreciated here is not the time that a tube is in place but the amount of work that takes place at the interface between the patient and the tube which is causing the injury.

The long-term effects of intubation trauma may well be glottic and/or subglottic stenosis. Because of prolonged intubation, it is not uncommon to find, on inspecting the larynx a week after tracheotomy has been done, that the previously raw arytenoids and vocal cord edges are beginning to adhere to one another (Fig. 7-12). If the adhesion is deep in the posterior commissure, laryngeal "pseudoparalysis" may be produced wherein the vocal cords seem clean and indeed vibrate well on phonation but the arytenoids fail to separate on inspiration. Such a deep posterior commissure web is best diagnosed by introducing the tip of an anterior commissure laryngoscope between the cords. The distraction produced in the posterior commissure usually makes such a web stand up, where it can easily be divided with a microscissors or a laser.

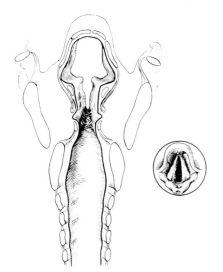

FIG. 7-12. A view of the larynx looking toward the posterior half from the plane marked *P* in Fig. 7-2. This shows scarring and webbing between the arytenoids as a result of intubation trauma. As one looks at this from above, the endoscopic view (**right**) shows that the webbing between the posterior portions of the cords tends to hold them together and prevent good opening of the larynx on inspiration.

In extreme cases in which the mucosa has been lost and there is also chondritis of the cricoid, the laryngeal lumen may be obliterated totally by the healing process (Fig. 7-13). Thus, it is not uncommon for patients who had prolonged intubation to be relatively asymptomatic for the first week or even month but to find later that they cannot tolerate even the slightest upper respiratory infection. Indeed, as the

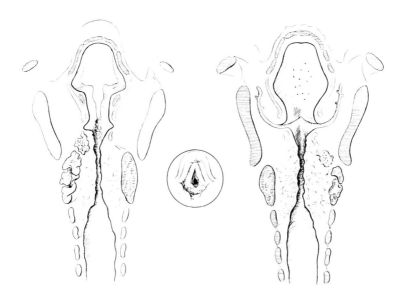

FIG. 7-13. Subglottic stenosis as a result of prolonged intubation. **Left:** Posterior view showing the scarring, swelling in the subglottic larynx, and destruction of some of the cricoid cartilage itself. **Center:** Endoscopic view with the very small residual aperture. **Right:** Frontal view of the cut larynx, showing again the tremendous scarring and compromise of the subglottic airway.

scarring progresses and the respiratory obstruction increases, tracheotomy may be required in a patient who was initially extubatable.

Caustic Trauma

Caustic injuries to the esophagus are discussed elsewhere. However, it should be noted that occasional overwhelming caustic ingestion is associated with a burn to the epiglottis and laryngeal inlet and produces a true chemical epiglottitis, which is an extreme respiratory emergency.

Thermal Injury

Thermal injury can be caused by steam, hot water, flame, or entrapment in a burning building. This can vary from hot water injury similar to the caustic injury wherein the epiglottis is swollen and edematous to a hot gas injury wherein the larynx may even be bypassed and the trachea and bronchi burned by inhaled substances. The treatment in these situations may vary from simply steroid administration or humidification to intubation or even tracheotomy to bypass an upper respiratory obstruction and permit ready evacuation of lower respiratory tract secretions.

ANOMALIES OF THE GREAT VESSELS

A "double" aortic arch is the abnormal persistence of the posterior limb of the vascular "ring" that leads to encirclement of both the trachea and esophagus (Fig. 7-14). Such encirclement causes esophageal compression, which is readily diagnosed by esophagram. More subtle are the primarily respiratory compressions produced by an aberrant innominate artery (Fig. 7-15) and the pulmonary sling (Fig. 7-16). The aberrant innominate artery bears no relationship to the esophagus. A left pulmonary artery arising from the right and "slinging" between the trachea or left bronchus and the esophagus is occasionally suggested by the esophagram. Of significance here are the variety of bronchial malformations often seen in association with this vascular anomaly. Indeed, the bronchial malformations are often less amenable to surgical correction than the anomalous origin of the left pulmonary artery.

Needless to say, neither of the above is ruled out by a "normal" esophagram. The aberrant innominate artery is probably more readily diagnosed by endoscopy with monitoring of the right brachial, radial, and/or temporal pulses. When suspected, the pulmonary sling is most expeditiously demonstrated by pulmonary arteriogram; however, this does not quantitate the bronchial malformation often associated with the "pulmonary sling."

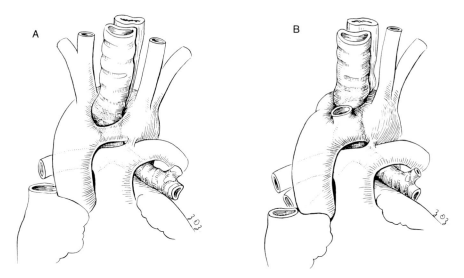

FIG. 7-14. Vascular ring, double aortic arch. **A:** Right arch predominating. **B:** Left arch predominating. In both cases, symptoms are predominantly expiratory stridor with some dysphagia. The diagnosis is readily made by the characteristic indentation demonstrable on esophagram.

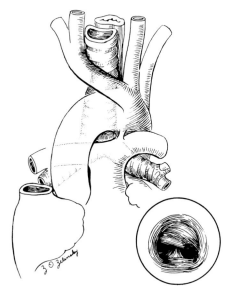

FIG. 7-15. "Aberrant" innominate artery in which the artery makes an oblique compression of the trachea, presenting a characteristic endoscopic profile (see **inset**). Endoscopic compression of this possible flattening should diminish palpable pulses peripheral to the point of compression. Symptomatically, such a compression may be the site of an expiratory wheeze; it may be associated with "dying spells" or reflex (nonobstructive) apnea.

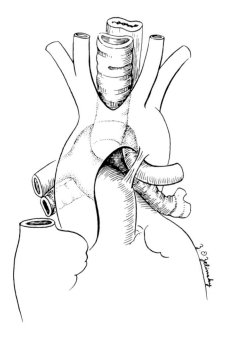

FIG. 7-16. Pulmonary sling in which the left pulmonary artery is derived from the right pulmonary artery (instead of the auricles); the path of this anomalous vessel often produces slit-like compression of the left bronchus. Also affecting pulmonary aeration may be a variety of associated bronchial anomalies.

AIRWAY PROBLEMS

Diagnosis

The term "airway problem" implies that the patient is having difficulty moving air through his major air passages. During the first 6 weeks of life, before the neonate has learned to breathe through his mouth, nasal or nasopharyngeal obstruction may be life threatening. Beyond this period, air hunger is usually manifested by mouth breathing associated with stridor.

If the patient is capable of moving sufficient air to produce sound, one may readily infer that the patient who is breathing easily and quietly gives little cause for concern. As one listens carefully to noisy respiration, one should try to characterize such noise by its pitch, the phase(s) of respiration during which the noise is produced, and the work performed by the patient in producing effective respiratory exchange. The loudness of the sound is indicative of the degree of obstruction only when taken in the context of adequate ventilation, since, as an extreme example, the patient who is totally obstructed and is thus moving no air is silent.

If one considers the mechanics of respiration, the logic of those sounds produced by the redundant soft tissues of the pharynx and supraglottic larynx are most apt to be heard on the negative-pressure or inspiratory phase of respiration. The site of production of sound best heard on expiration is lower, i.e., the main bronchi and trachea. An obstruction in the relatively fixed areas of the subglottic larynx and/or extrathoracic trachea is most apt to produce a biphasic sound that is heard well in both phases of respiration.

Observation of the soft tissues of the neck and chest may give an insight into the work involved as well as the site of the obstruction. Synchronous indrawing of the supraclavicular, suprasternal, and substernal soft tissues indicates a relatively high point of obstruction. Similarly, on radiographic examination the hypopharynx and pyriform sinuses may be seen to balloon on inspiration above a laryngeal obstruction. Effortless indrawing of the lower sternum with quiet easy respiration may be diagnostic of the anomalous attachment of the lower sternum to the diaphram known as primary pectus excavatum.

Asymmetric filling or emptying of the chest may imply partial obstruction of one of the main bronchi by a foreign body or the deformity associated with the "pulmonary sling" or other vascular anomalies. The absence of such asymmetry on physical or radiographic examination does not rule out the more dangerous situations in which the obstruction may be in the lower trachea or even caused by separate foreign bodies in each main bronchus. Hoarseness implies interference with vocal cord vibration and may have a variety of causes: inflammation, neoplasm such as papilloma, a foreign body, or asymmetry of muscle tone.

A weak cry may result from shortening of the vibrating edge of the cord by a web or neural or muscular failure of approximation. The cry may be muffled by supraglottic obstruction as seen in epiglottitis or a lingual thyroid or thyroglossal cyst.

Foreign bodies in or impinging on the airway are probably the most frequently missed cause of airway obstruction. Fewer than half of the patients with foreign bodies removed present with a history of choking or aspiration.

Sudden complete obstruction of the supraglottic larynx is usually fatal unless the child is treated successfully by first aid, as with the Heimlich maneuver. A laryngotracheal foreign body (small enough to transgress the glottis but too large to enter a main bronchus) usually causes severe respiratory obstruction unless its shape is unusual (Fig. 7-17). A watermelon seed may cause coughing. (An audible slap is often heard when the foreign body strikes the subglottis.) Such a tracheal obstruction does not cause an inequality of pulmonary aeration; there may, however, be bilateral pulmonary air trapping on expiration. Inversion of such a patient may prove fatal if a foreign body that permits air to pass the carina (which is larger than the glottis) impacts in the subglottis. Similarly, if there are simultaneous foreign bodies in both main bronchi (e.g., two peanuts), there may be wheezing, dyspnea, and bilateral hyperinflation but no radiologic localization.

Only when there is unequal aeration can the diagnosis be confirmed radiographically. Partial obstruction of a bronchus may permit air to enter as the bronchus opens on inspiration; on expiration, however, the ipsilateral partially obstructed lumen will be the first occluded, trapping air during the expiratory phase, while the contralateral bronchus continues to empty (obstructive emphysema). Such a shift of the mediastinum may be misinterpreted as early atelectasis. With atelectasis,

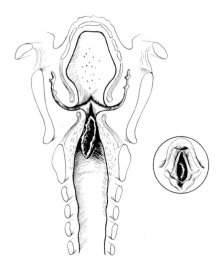

FIG. 7-17. A fragment of peanut husk has lodged in the subglottic larynx. The clinical picture here is often very similar to that of croup, as is the compromise of the airway.

of course, the air is absorbed distal to a complete obstruction, causing collapse of the unaerated segment, lobe, or lung.

With time and ensuing bronchial reaction to the foreign body, it is not uncommon to have a scenario in which the initial aspiration causes a cough that subsides as the bronchus accommodates to the presence of the foreign object. After a "silent" interval of hours or even days, early bronchial reaction to the foreign body may produce obstructive emphysema that progresses to atelectasis as the bronchial obstruction becomes complete. If such a case is misdiagnosed as "pneumonia" or "asthma," the bronchial reaction may subside with antibiotic and/or steroid treatment, thus improving the aeration and X-ray only to have the symptoms recur when therapy is withdrawn. Indeed, localized bronchial obstruction (often by foreign body) is the leading cause of "recurrent pneumonia," especially if the same lobe or segment is recurrently involved by emphysema or atelectasis.

Differential Diagnosis of Stridor

The differential diagnosis of stridor is outlined in Table 7-2. Of course, total obstruction is silent. Therefore, a patient whose noisy respirations become less noisy may have a progressive obstruction that is almost total.

Management

The physician responsible for a child in whom a mechanical airway obstruction is suspected should not hesitate to seek consultative assistance. Radiologic consultation is occasionally diagnostic (as with a radiopaque foreign body, vascular ring, pulmonary sling, and choanal atresia). Conversely, "negative" X-rays exclude

LE 7-2. *Differential diagnosis of stridor*

ulbar) paralysis
  syndrome

ıle

ıtal and/or acquired)
Expiratory stridor
  Vascular compression (ring, sling, or innominate)
  Esophageal pathology including foreign body
  Tracheal papilloma
  Laryngotracheal foreign body
  Tracheobronchial anomaly
Apnea
  Reflex, associated with aberrant innominate artery
  Gastroesophageal reflux
  Central nervous system origin
  Choanal atresia
Stridor associated with subcutaneous emphysema
  Asthma
  Foreign body
  Trauma
    Minibike
    Laryngotracheal perforation

relatively few causes of obstruction in an absolute sense; that is, a radiograph that does not demonstrate a foreign body does not rule out such a diagnosis. The child in whom epiglottitis is suspected is certainly safer in an intensive care unit or an operating room, where such an obstruction can be aggressively managed, than he might be on an X-ray table far from the equipment and expertise necessary for his very survival.

Intubation, which may be life saving for an infant with vocal cord paralysis or respiratory distress because of cardiopulmonary disease, may produce serious trauma to an inflamed or deformed larynx. In cases of a laryngotracheal foreign body, intubation has in some cases been directly responsible for the death of the patient.

An endoscopist should work with instruments that permit not only visualization of the mechanical obstruction but also such operative procedures as the aspiration of cysts, division of webs, and the removal of foreign objects, granulomas, papillomas, etc. Needless to say, such an endoscopist must be ready and able to perform a tracheotomy should the need arise. To perform an endoscopic examination with the idea of "just taking a peek at the problem" is as dangerous and meddlesome as presuming to make the diagnosis of epiglottitis with a tongue depressor and being unequipped to manage the total respiratory obstruction that may be precipitated by such a maneuver.

Tracheotomy may be employed to achieve one or more goals in airway management: It may be used to:

1. Relieve obstruction: (a) neonatal nasal and/or nasopharyngeal obstruction at an age when the infant cannot relieve such obstruction by mouth breathing; and (b) pharyngeal, laryngeal, or tracheal obstruction by trauma, inflammation, tumor, cyst, or deformity.

2. Provide long-term ventilatory support when it is believed that prolonged intubation would injure the larynx.

3. Provide long-term access for the removal of tracheobronchial secretions.

CORROSIVE INGESTION

We can safely assume that toddlers do not set out to poison themselves, nor have they learned to sip or taste carefully an unknown substance. They have learned that a whitish crystalline substance is sweet and that good things come from plastic cups, Coca-Cola bottles, baby food jars, etc. We are loath to admit that child abuse plays a significant part, but it is extreme carelessness (even without malice) when grandfather leaves his dentures to soak in a caustic cleanser in a plastic cup or drinking glass, especially if the dentures are removed and the cleanser is left sitting on the sink. A child's mother will wear rubber gloves to paint the oven cleaner paste on the inside of an oven and then return the jar (the size and color of a junior food container) filled with a lye and flour mixture (not unlike the flour and fruit mix the child expects) to an unprotected place under the kitchen sink. "Child-proof" containers have helped to limit the number of caustic poisonings as well as to raise the level of awareness of the problem. However, the protection of such a top is lost once the material is transferred to a drinking glass, plastic cup, or the ever seductive Coca-Cola bottle. The most compulsive parent may have a perfectly safe home only to have her child poisoned at the babysitter's house or in grandmother's kitchen.

The most significant indication for management is a history suggestive of ingestion. Dysphagia, pain, drooling, and in severe cases respiratory distress are significant symptoms. The presence of burns around the lips, mouth, and oropharynx may indicate that the substance was tasted, found unpleasant, and spit out. The absence of such findings may indicate that the child drank greedily and stopped only when he felt pain in his esophagus and/or stomach. *Thus the absence of oral burns cannot safely be assumed to preclude an esophageal or even a gastric burn.* This is especially true of the "heavy" (high specific gravity) drain cleaners such as Liquid Plumber® and Plunge®, which may pass so rapidly to the stomach that esophageal burns are thought to be produced primarily by regurgitation. The worst pharyngoesophageal burns seem to be produced by slowly dissolving solids (lye, Draino®) and thick pastes such as Easy-Off® oven cleaner.

It has been suggested that the ingestion of bleach, Clorox®, ammonia, etc., seldom produces a serious burn; some authors suggest that if the patient has no obvious burn and no dysphagia, it may be safe to simply follow up with a barium X-ray study within 6 weeks or so. Following this routine may rule out a long-standing stenosis, but if one is found, it suggests that the patient would have been better treated prophylactically with steroids until the mucosa had been found to be intact endoscopically.

When a more damaging caustic agent is suspected, the patient should be started on prophylactic steroid therapy until the mucosa can be demonstrated to be intact. Once the patient has been started on this regimen, his dysphagia may regress sufficiently to permit at least a liquid diet. This also allows time for a more deliberate medical evaluation, esophagram, and assurance that the patient is a good candidate for endoscopy under general anesthesia.

If the burn is sufficiently ulcerative to be demonstrated radiographically, or if there are signs of respiratory distress or peritoneal irritation, steroids may be withheld. This is especially true when the "heavy" agents are suspected or in adult suicide attempts wherein the caustic has been gulped down with determination, a situation that is likely to produce gastric burn and even peritonitis. Steroids are contraindicated here because of the possibility that the signs and symptoms of peritonitis could be masked by the suppression of the inflammatory response. If an overwhelming burn is suspected, the airway is under control, and the presence of a burn is certain, one might proceed to elective exploratory gastrotomy.

SUGGESTED READING

Benjamin, B. (1981): *Atlas of Paediatric Endoscopy: Upper Respiratory Tract and Oesophagus.* Oxford University Press, New York.

Healy, G. B., and McGill, T. J. I., editors (1979): *Laryngo-Tracheal Problems in the Pediatric Patient.* Charles C Thomas, Springfield, IL.

Tucker, G. F. (1980): Laryngeal development and congenital lesions. *Ann. Otol. Rhinol. Laryngol.,* 89:142–145.

Tucker, J. A. and O'Rahilly, R. (1972): Observations on the embryology of the human larynx. *Ann. Otol. Rhinol. Laryngol.,* 81:520–523.

Subject Index

Abscess
  alveolar, 332–333
  aural, 357
  brain, 300–301
  cervical, 397
  epidural, 300
  extradural, 91
  orbital, 294
  parapharyngeal, 357,361–363
  peritonsillar, 357,360
  pharyngomaxillary, 361–363,364
  pulmonary, following tonsillectomy, 380
  retropharyngeal, 322,357,361,362,363
  submaxillary, 363–366
  submental, 360
Acoustic reflexes, measurement of, 167–169
Acoustic trauma, 140–143
Actinomyces, 60
Actinomycosis, 401,402
  of the jaw, 342
Adenitis
  cervical glands, 393–402
  tuberculous cervical, 399
Adenoidectomy
  cleft palate and, 85
  complications of, 381
  indications for, 368,379,380
  middle ear effusions and, 73
  otitis media and, 381
  velopharyngeal incompetence masked by, 205
Adenoiditis
  acute, 355–356
  causative organisms, 356
  cervical glands in, 357
  chronic, 356
  complications of, 357
  eustachian tube obstruction and, 70
  hearing loss and, 356
  pneumococcal, 357
  streptococcal, 356–357
  viral, 356
Adenoids, 323
  atrophy of, age of onset, 352,368
  hypertrophy of, 368–369
    facial development and, 368
    hearing loss and, 369
    nasal disorders and, 258
    obstructive sleep apnea and, 368–369
    sinusitis and, 369
  immune function, 352–353
  infection of, see Adenoiditis
Adenoma, chromophobe, 374

Adenovirus, 356
  hearing loss and, 126
Agammaglobulinemia, Bruton's type, 353
Agranulocytosis, 350
Airway obstruction, 426–429
Albright's syndrome, 281
Alcohol, ototoxicity, 123
Alexander's aplasia, 101,111
Allergic reactions
  to antibiotics, 61
  middle ear effusions and, 82
  otitis media and, 70
Alport's syndrome, 107,114
  hearing loss and, 101
Alveolar process, formation of, 319
Alveoli, epithelial lining of, 2
γ-Aminobutyric acid, 38
Aminoglycosides, ototoxicity, 123–125
Amphotericin
  in mucormycosis, 270
  in oral candidiasis, 348
  in otomycosis, 61
Ampicillin
  bacterial resistance to, 81
  in epiglottitis, 377
Analine dyes, ototoxicity, 123
Angiofibroma, 285
  epistaxis and, 285
  nasal obstruction in, 285
  nasopharyngeal, 285,371,372,373
Anosmia, 8
Anotia, 24
Anoxia, hearing loss and, 99,122–123
Anterior faucial pillar, formation of, 320
Antibiotics
  allergic reaction to, 61
  in otitis media, 76,81
    suppurative, 72
Antihistamines, in nonsuppurative otitis media, 82
Apgar score, hearing loss and, 99,122–123
Arnold-Chiari malformation, vocal cord paralysis
  and, 417
Arsenic, ototoxicity, 123
Aspartate, 38
Aspergillus, 60
Atopy, external otitis and, 62
Atropine, ciliary action and, 18
Atticoantrostomy, 94
Audiogram, interpretation of, 156–157
Audiometry; see also Auditory brainstem response
  behavioral observation, 151–153
  conditioned play, 152,153–154

Audiometry (*contd.*)
  tangible reinforcement operant conditioning, 152,154
  visual reinforcement, 152,153
Auditory brainstem response, 100,151
  in child with normal hearing, 162
  in intensive care nursery, 162–163
  limitations, 164
  in postmeningitic children, 163–164
  technique of, 161
Auditory discrimination, 155
Auditory neurons, neurotransmitters in, 38
Auditory pathways, CNS, 36–37
Autonomic dysfunction, 9
Autosomal dominant disorders, 112–116
Avitaminosis, effect on mucous membranes, 9

Barany chair, 176
Barotitis, 45
Barotitis media, adenoidectomy and, 381
Barotrauma, eustachian tube and, 70
Behcet's disease, oral ulceration in, 348–349
Blood dyscrasias, epistaxis and, 260
Brain abscess, 300–301
Branchial fistula, 383,388; *see also* Cysts, branchial cleft; Sinuses, branchial
  differentiation from branchial sinus, 386
Brucellosis, 399
Bullous myringitis, 63, 101
Burkitt's lymphoma, 276–277,401
  differential diagnosis, 277
Burns, mouth, 345–346

Calcium deficiency, mucous membranes in, 9
Caloric testing, vestibular assessment via, 183–184
Candidiasis, oral, 348
Carbon monoxide, ototoxicity, 123
Carcinoma; *see also* Malignancy; Tumors
  laryngeal, 419
  tonsillar, 367
Cat scratch disease, 399–400
Cauliflower ear, 25,53
Cauterization, in nasal hemangioma, 285
Cellulitis
  cervical, 397
  as a complication of acute sinusitis, 293
  orbital, 289,290,293
Cerebrospinal fluid, rhinorrhea, 309
Cerumen
  composition of, 55
  curettage of, 55,57
  function of, 25
  impactation, 56
Cervical glands, swelling of
  as indicator of malignancy, 393,394,395
  secondary to infection, 397–402

Cheyne-Stokes respiration, 92
Chickenpox
  hearing loss and, 101
  mucous membranes in, 12
  tonsil hypertrophy after, 353
Chloramphenicol
  in epiglottitis, 377
  ototoxicity, 123
Chloroquine, ototoxicity, 125
Cholera, thrombotic desquamation of mucous membranes and, 9
Cholesteatoma, 45,88–89,93
  in acute necrotizing otitis media, 78
  attic retraction, 86
  with chronic mastoiditis, 90,94
  congenital, 95,96
  diagnosis, 78
  extirpation of, 89
  hearing loss and, 101
  tympanic membrane perforation and, 87,88
Cholesterol granuloma, 87
Chondroma, nasal, 275
Chondrosarcoma, 275,276,277
Chordoma, in nasopharynx, 374
Cilia, activation of, 5
Ciliary streaming, 7
  autonomic dysfunction and, 9
Cleft palate, 337–339
  adenoidectomy and, 85
  congenital heart defects and, 338
  hypertelorism and, 338
  middle ear effusion and, 70
  otitis media and, 339
  repair, 339
  speech production and, 205–207
Cochlear, 31–33
Collagen diseases, eustachian tube and, 70
Common cold, 291
Communication, functions necessary for effective, 211–212
Computer tomography
  in acute petrositis, 89–90
  in diagnosis of
    in acoustic neuroma, 77
    brain abscess, 92
    extradural abscess, 91
  in evaluation of hearing loss, 107
  of frontal sinus fracture, 309
  of internal auditory canal, 77
  nasal sinuses, 246
  of temporal bone fractures, 145–146
Computerized rotational testing, 63
Congenital disorders, 247,249,377; *see also* Congenital malformations
  cholesteatoma, 95,96
  goiters, 388
  macroglossia, 343
Congenital malformation, 24,48–53,101,108,111,417

cardiac, cleft palate and, 338
laryngeal, 410–413
mouth, 336–341
Corrosives, ingestion of, 430–431
Cortilymph, 32
Cortisone, in treatment of nasal polyps, 256,257
Corymebacterium, 59
Coryza, 356
Coxsackie virus, associated with
pharyngotonsillitis, 348
Craniopharyngioma, in nasopharynx, 374
m-Cresyl acetate, in otomycosis, 61
Crib death, obstructive sleep apnea and, 368
Cribriform plate, 2
Cricoid cartillage, 406,407,413,414–415
Cyclophosphamide, in Burkitt's lymphoma,
277
Cysts
benign bone, 288
branchial cleft, 383,385,387,388
congenital, 377
dental, 333
dentigenous, 333,335
dermoid, 287
in nasopharynx, 374
in hypopharynx, 377–378
laryngeal, 419–420
median maxillary, 342
mucous retention, 286,377,419
nasal, 286–288
nasopalatine, 341
oral, 351
radicular, 333
saccular, 419
salivary gland, 404
thyroglossal duct, 389,390
thyroid, 389
on the tonsil, 367
Cytomegalovirus infection
congenital infection, 127–128
hearing loss and, 101

Decibel, defined, 156
Decongestants, 82
DeQuervain's thyroiditis, 389
Dermatitis, seborrheic, external otitis and, 62
Diabetes mellitus, mucormycosis associated with,
13
Digital examination, of pharynx, 332
Dihydrostreptomycin, ototoxicity, 123
Diphtheria
nasal, 253
pharyngeal, 253
pseudomembranous-type tonsillitis in, 358
treatment, 253
Dopamine, 38
Duane's retraction syndrome, 118

Dysentery, nasal perforations and, 260
Dyspnea, subglottic hemangioma and, 418

Ear; *see also* External ear; Inner ear; Middle ear
anatomy and physiology of, 25–39
cauliflower, 25,53
clinical examination of, 40–46
congenital malformations of, 24,48–53,101
diseases and disorders, 47–148
embryology of, 20–24
wax, *see* Cerumen
Eardrum, *see* Tympanic membrane
Ecchymosis, nasal fractures and, 257,307
Education, for hearing-impaired child,
158,159,171,172
Eighth nerve, tumors, 96
Electric cauterization, mucous membrane injury
and, 18
Electric coagulation, mucous membrane injury
and, 18
Electrocochleography, 160,161
Electronystagmography, 175,176
Encephalitis, mumps, 403
Encephalocele, 283
nasopharyngeal, 373–374
Endolymph, volume of, 32
Endolymphatic duct, formation of, 20
Enophthalmos, following "blow-out" fractures,
308
Enterobacter aerogenes, 60
Epidural abscess, otomastoiditis and, 29
Epiglottis, 377,406,415–416
studor, 416
subclassification 413
Epistaxis, 258–265
angiofibroma and, 285
blood dyscrasias and, 260
control of, 261–264,265
environmental conditions in etiology of, 260
etiology, 259–261
Foley catheters in control of, 264
in granuloma, 260
hemangioma and, 260,284
in hemophilia, 260–261
hypertension associated with, 259
as indication of malignancy, 260
leukemia and, 260
nasal septum perforation and, 260
nasal septum ulceration and, 260
in Osler-Weber-Rendu disease, 261
papilloma and, 260, 273
phenylephrine in, 262
purpura and, 260
rheumatic fever and, 261
site of bleeding, 259
trauma and, 259–260
tumor-induced, 273

Epstein-Barr virus
  in etiology of Burkitt's lymphoma, 277
  hearing loss and, 126
Erysipelas, 251,252,253
  in external otitis, 61
Erythromycin
  in combined therapy for otitis media, 81
  in congenital syphilis, 133
Escherichia coli, 60
Ethacrynic acid, ototoxicity, 123,126
Ethmoid bone, 233
Ethmoid cells, osteosarcoma of, 278
Ethmoid complex
  carcinoma of, 270
  drainage, 236
  hemangioma, 285
  mucormycosis of, 270
  osteomyelitis in, 294
Eustachian tube
  anatomy and physiology, 68–69
  congenital deformities, 69
  function, 69
  "lock", 70
  obstruction of, 69–70
  surgical measures for restoring function of, 85
"Expanded rubella syndrome," 129
External auditory canal, 23
  anatomy of, 54
  atresia of, 24,48,51,64,101
  dermatoses, 26
  examination landmarks, 42
  fibrous dysplasia, 63
  foreign bodies in, 57–58,59
  irrigation, 56
  kertinizing squamous epithelium in, 55
  microflora of, 59
  osteoma, 63
External ear
  disorders of, 47–48
  rhabdomyosarcoma, 64
  tumors, 63–64
External otitis, 59–63
  antibiotic treatment in, 61
  chronic, 62
  diffuse, 59–61
  eczematous, 62
  localized, 62
  "malignant", 62–63
  mycotic, 60
  neurodermatitis and, 62
  tubercular, 62
Eye movement examination, in vestibular
    assessment, 84

Facial nerve palsy, 90
Fibroma
  of the nasopharynx, 371
  ossifying, 63–64,280,341,342

Fibrosarcoma
  of the jaw, 341
  nasal obstruction in, 278
Fibrous dysplasia, 281–282
  of the jaw, 341
Fistula
  branchial, 383–388
  thyroglossal duct, 389,391
Foley catheter, in epistaxis, 264
Fracture
  blow-out, 308
  CSF rhinorrhea as indicator of, 309
  facial, 303–314
  frontal sinus, 309–310
  mandible, 314
  maxillary sinus, 310
  nasal, 304–307
Frontal sinus, 233,235
  carcinoma of, 270
  drainage, 236
  fracture, 309–310
  hemangioma, 285
  mucoceles in, 302
  osteoma in, 279
  transillumination, 246,247
  venous drainage, 238
Fungal infections, 270,271
Furosemide, ototoxicity, 123
Furuncle, 62
Furunculosis
  carvernous sinus thrombosis secondary to, 299
  nasal, 251,252

Genetics, role in hearing loss, 108–122
Gentamicin, ototoxicity, 123,124
Gentian violet, 61
Glioma, frontonasal, 283
Glutamate, 38
Goblet cells, 1
Goiters, 388
Gold, ototoxicity, 123
Goldenhar's syndrome, 119
Gradenigo's syndrome, 89
Granuloma
  cholesterol, 45,66
  epistaxis in, 260
  intubation, 420
  lethal midline, 267
  nasal, 265–269
  nasal obstruction due to, 265–269
  tuberculous, 265–266
Griseofulvin, in mucormycosis, 271
Growth retardation, hearing loss and, 99,135
Guarnieri's bodies, 12,14

Hair cells, 34
Hairy tongue, 345

Hand-Schueller-Christian disease, 396–397
Hard palate, formation of, 319
Harelip, 332
  repair of, 337
Hashimoto's thyroiditis, 389
Hearing
  as essential factor in effective communication, 212
  loss of, *see* Hearing loss
  measurement of, 149–173
Hearing aid, selection of, 169–170
Hearing loss
  adenoid hypertrophy and, 369
  adenoiditis and, 356
  age of onset, 213,218
  age at time of identification, 150
  Alport's syndrome and, 101,114
  anoxia and, 99,122–123
  Apgar score and, 99,122–123
  autosomal disorders and, 112–120
  categorization of, 156,157
  chickenpox and, 101
  cholesteatoma and, 101
  conductive, 213,218
  cytomegalovirus infection and, 101
  drug-induced, 99,101,123–126
  Duane's retraction syndrome and, 119
  early detection of, 98–100
  education for child with, 158,159,171,172
  etiology, 101,108–148
  evaluation of, 102,223–224
  genetic evaluation in, 120–122
  Goldenhar's syndrome and, 119
  growth retardation and, 99
  hereditary, 99,108–122
  identification of, 150,219–220
  indicator of, 99
  influenza and, 101
  Jervell and Lange-Nielsen syndrome and, 117
  Klippel-Feil malformation and, 118
  language development and, 207–209
  measles and, 101
  Melnick-Fraser syndrome and, 113–114
  meningitis and, 163–164
  mental retardation and, 99
  metabolic disorders and, 101
  middle ear effusions and, 73,74
  mumps and, 101
  neurofibromatosis and, 114–115
  noise-induced, 140–143
  Norrie's disease and, 118
  otitis media and, 101,157,213
  otopalatodigital syndrome and, 118
  otosclerosis and, 115–116
  Pendred's syndrome and, 117
  physical examination of child with, 222
  questionnaire for evaluating for, 103
  risk factors, 99
  sensorineural, 213,218
  sickle cell anemia and, 101
  speech development and, 219
  sudden, 136–140
  syphilis and, 101
  toxoplasmosis and, 101
  from trauma, 101
  Treacher Collins syndrome and, 114
  Turner's syndrome and, 120
  tympanic membrane perforation and, 101
  tympanosclerosis and, 101
  types of, 213,218–219
  Usher's syndrome and, 116–117
  Waardenburg's syndrome and, 101,112–113
  Wildervaank's syndrome and, 118
Heart defects, congenital, cleft palate and, 338
Hemangioma, 284–285
  epistaxis and, 260,284
  of frontal sinus, 285
  head and neck, 392
  parotid gland, 404
  subglottic, 418,419
  tonsil, 367
Hematoma, as complication of cerumen curettage, 55
Hemophilia, epistaxia in, 260–261
Hemophilus influenza, 356
  in acute otitis media, 79,81
  in epiglottitis, 377
Herpes, mucous membranes and, 12
Herpes hominis virus, in oral cavity, 348
Herpes simplex, in external otitis, 61
Histamine phosphate, in sudden hearing loss, 139
Histiocytosis, 396–397
Hoarseness, 409
Hodgkin's disease, 394–395
Horner's syndrome, in neuroblastoma, 395
Hygroma, 351
  cystic, 391–392
  parotid gland, 404
Hyperemia, otitis media and, 75
Hypertelorism, associated with cleft palate, 338
Hypertension, epistaxis associated with, 259
Hypogammaglobulinemia, otitis media and, 80
Hypopharynx
  carcinoma of the, 395
  cysts in, 377–378,419
  disorders and, diseases of, 376–378
  examination of, 331–332
Hypothyroidism, eustachian tube and, 70

Immunoglobulin electrophoresis, in otitis media, 80
Incus, 27
  lenticular process, 29
  necrosis, 87
Infections; *see also* Abscess
  of adenoids, 354–358
  bacterial, 356

Infections (*contd.*)
  congenital, 127–128
  dental, 332–333
  ear, *see* External otitis; Otitis media
  involving pharyngeal spaces, 359–366
  nasopharyngeal, 361
  of the oral cavity, 346–350
  streptococcal, 356
  of tonsils, 354–359
  viral, 356
Infectious mononucleosis, differential diagnosis,
    359
Influenza
  destruction of ciliated membranes in the trachea
    from, 10
  hearing loss and, 101
Inner ear
  embryologic development, 21
  structural malformation, 111
Innominate artery, laryngeal function and aberrant,
    424,425
Internal auditory canal, size, 78
Intubation
  complications of, 429
  otitis media and, 78
Iodine, in otomycosis, 61

Jaw, tumors of, 341–342,343–344
Jendrassik position, 188,190
Jervell and Lange-Nielsen syndrome, 107
  hearing loss and, 117

Kanamycin, ototoxicity, 123,125,142
Kernicterus, 134
Klebsiella pneumoniae, 60
Klebsiella rhinoscleromatis, 269
Klippel-Feil malformation, 118
Koplik's spots, 12–13

Labyrinth
  membranous, 20,22
    fluids surrounding, 32–33
  periotic, 20
Labyrinthitis
  nonsuppurative, 90–91
  rubella and, 126
  suppurative, 90
  temporal bone fracture and, 92
  viral infections and, 126
Language
  communication and, 212,213
  early development of, 212–213
  problems, criteria for referral for evaluation of,
    200
  skills
    development of, 194,195–197,207–209

Laryngitis, supraglottic, 413,415–416
Laryngocele, 410,411,419,420
  external, 393
  internal, 392
Laryngomalacia, 411
Laryngomucocele, 410,411
Laryngopharyngitis, 413
Laryngopharynx, *see* Hypopharynx
Laryngotracheitis, mucous membranes and, 10
Larynx, 2
  carcinoma of, 396,419
  caustic trauma to, 424
  "cleft", 412
  congenital subglottic stenosis, 412–413
  deformities, 409–413
    congenital, 410
  disorders and diseases of, 210,413–420
  embryonic development of, 406
  external trauma to, 421
  function, 408–409
    anomalies of great vessels and, 424,425
    assessment of, 202
    speech and, 202
  inflammatory diseases of, 413–416
  intubation injury, 421–424
  obstruction of, 426–430
  respiratory function, 406,408,409
  sphincter function, 406
  thermal injury of, 424
  webs, 411
  voice production and the, 406,409
Lateral nasal wall, 231–232
Lead
  toxicity, 333
    ototoxicity, 123
Learning disability, maternal and fetal factors
    contributing to, 198
Leprosy
  external otitis associated with, 62
  nasal obstruction in, 269
Letterer-Siwe disease, 396–397
Leukemia
  epistaxis and, 260
  oral ulceration in, 350
Ludwig's angina, 363–366
Lues, external otitis associated with, 62
Lupus erythematosus, systemic, 62
Lymph node
  cervical, 398
    infected, 400; *see also* Cervical glands,
      swelling of
Lymphangioma, 420; *see also* Adenitis
  macroglossia from, 345
  parotid gland, 404
Lymphoepithelioma
  metastasis into cervical glands, 393
  nasopharyngeal, 375
  tonsillar, 367

Lymphoma
  Burkitt's, 276–277
  malignant, 275–276
Lymphosarcoma, 393
  differentiated from Hodgkin's disease, 394
  nasal, 275
  tonsillar, 367
Lysozyme, bacteriostatic activity, 241

Macroglossia, 338
  congenital, 343
  from lymphoangioma, 345
Malignancy, epistaxis an indicator of, 260; *see also* Carcinoma; Tumors
Malleus, as a diagnostic landmark in otoscopy, 27
Malocclusion, 333
Mandible, osteomyelitis in, 334
Mandibular process, 318,319
Mandibulofacial dysostosis, 340–341
  micrognathia in, 340
Mastoidectomy
  cholesteatoma extirpation via, 89
  radical indications for, 95
Mastoiditis
  cholesteatoma and, 90
  chronic, 90
  coalescent, 92
Maxilla, osteomyelitis in the, 333
Maxillary process, 319
Maxillary sinus, 232
  air capacity, 233
  carcinoma of, 270
  dental infection and health of, 233
  drainage, 236
  fracture, 310
  ossifying fibroma, 280
  transillumination, 246,247
Measles; *see also* Rubella
  acute necrotizing otitis media and, 78
  hearing loss and, 101
  mucous membranes and, 13
Meckel's cartilage, 23
Melanoma, nasal, 270
Melnick-Fraser syndrome, 113–114
Meningioma, 283–284
  temporal bone, 96
Meningismus, otitis media and, 75
Meningitis
  following pneumococcal tonsillitis or adenoiditis, 357
  hearing loss and, 135–136
  otitis media and, 78
  otogenic, 92
  otomastoiditis and, 29
  recurrent, 301
  sinusitis and, 300
  temporal bone fracture and otogenic, 92

Mental retardation, hearing loss and, 99
Mercury, ototoxicity, 123
Metabolic disorders, hearing loss and, 101
Michael's aplasia, 101,111,136
Microglossia, 338
Micrognathia, 338
  in mandibulofacial dysostis, 340
Microtia, 49
Middle ear
  effusions, 44–46,67,68,70,72,73,82,83; *see also* Otitis media
  exteriorization of, 64
  function, measurement of, 150,164–169
  hyperemia, 43,75
  mucosa membranes, destruction of, 13
Mikulicz cell, in rhinoscleroma, 268
Mondini's aplasia, 101,111
Monilia, hairy tongue and, 345
Mononucleosis, infectious, 359
Mouth
  agranulocytosis and ulceration of, 350
  burns of, 345–346
  congenital deformities, 336–341
  diseases and disorders of, 332–359
  examination of, 328
  floor, potential spaces in, 321
  stratified epithelium, 2
  tubercular lesions in, 350
Mow response, 151
Mucocele, following sinusitis, 301–302
Mucormycosis
  mucous membranes and, 13
  nasal, 270,271
Mucous membranes
  arteritis of, 13
  avitaminosis and, 9
  calcium deficiency and, 9
  dehydration and, 8
  in digestive tract, 1
  drugs and ciliary action of, 18
  electric cauterization and injury to, 18
  electric coagulation and, 18
  epithelial cells of, 1
  functions, 2–8,242
  goblet cells of, 1
  injury due to infections, 9–18
    cholera, 9
    herpes, 12
    influenza, 10,11,12,13
    laryngotracheitis, 10
    measles, 13
    mucormycosis, 13
    pemphigus, 13
    smallpox, 12
    tuberculosis, 16
    typhoid fever, 9
  keratinization of, 9
  middle ear, 13

Mucous membranes (*contd.*)
olfactory, 4,8,236,242,243
premalignant lesions in, 16
in respiratory tract, 1,2
silver nitrate-induced scarring of, 18
thrombotic desquamation of, 9
thrombotic infarction of, 13
trichloroacetic acid-induced scarring of,
18
Mucous retention cyst, 377,419
Mucus
bacteriostatic effect, 5
function of, 5
lysozyme in, 241
streaming of. 6–7
Multilocular cyst, 23,24
Mumps, 403
differentiated from cervical lymphadenitis,
403
hearing loss and, 101,126
sudden, 137
Mycobacterium leprae, 269
Myoclonus, palatal, eustachian tube and, 70
Myringitis, bullous, 63,101
Myringoplasty, repair of tympanic membrane
perforations with, 94
Myringotomy
in otitis media, 79–80
technique, 83,84
Myxomas, 285–286

Nasal disorders, 247–289
adenoids and, 258
allergic rhinitis, 253–254
bacterial infections and, 250–253
congenital, 247,249
fractures, 257; *see also* Nasal fractures
infection-induced, 249–253
polyps, 254–257
in syphilis, congenital, 249
vasomotor rhinitis, 254
viral infections and, 249–250
Nasal endotracheal tube, mucous membrane injury
from, 18
Nasal fractures, 257,304–307
ecchymosis associated with, 257,307
Nasal obstruction
angiofibroma and, 285
conditions resulting in, 265–289
in fibrosarcoma, 278–279
from granuloma, 265–269
in leprosy, 269
in rhinoscleroma, 269
in rhinosporidosis, 273
in sarcoidosis, 265
Nasal passage, atresia of, 247,248,249

Nasal septum, 231,232
abscess, 250,251
blood supply, 237,259
chondrosarcoma of, 275,277
common deflections of, 233
fetal, 319
hemangioma of, 284
melanoma of, 270
nerve supply, 240
perforation, 9–10
chondrosoma-induced, 277
dysentery and, 260
epistaxis and, 260
typhoid fever and, 260
ulceration, epistaxis and, 260
in Wegener's granulomatosis, 266
Nasal sinuses; *see also* specific sinuses, i.e.,
Frontal sinus
accessory
anatomy, 232–235,289
fractures involving, 307
function of, 243
infection of, 289–303
osteomyelitis of, 294–299
bacterial infections of, 250,254
computer tomography scan, 246
examination of, 246,247
infection of, *see* Sinusitis
lymphosarcoma of, 275
myxoma in, 285–286
papilloma of, 274
polytomography scan, 246
Nasal turbinates, 236
blood supply, 237
hypertrophied, 257
Nasal vestibule, 2
Nasofrontal process, 319
Nasopharyngeal bursa, 329
Nasopharyngitis, eustachian tube obstruction
and, 70
Nasopharyngoscope, 331
Nasopharyngoscopy, 46,246,255
in diagnosis of middle ear effusion, 74
Nasopharynx, 367–376
angiofibroma of the, 371,372,373
carcinoma of, 395
ciliated columnar epithelium of, 2
crangiopharyngioma of, 374
dermoid cysts in, 374
encephalocele in, 373–374
examination of, 329–331,332
fibroma of, 371
foreign bodies in, 369,370
function of, 367
infections of, 361
lymphoepithelioma in, 375
plasmacytoma in, 375–376
rhabdomyosarcoma in, 375

teratoma in, 374
tumors of, 369,371,372,374,375
Neck
    abscess, 397
    diseases and disorders, 383–404; *see also*
        Cervical glands, swelling of
    malignancies, 393–396
Neomycin
    allergic response to, 61
    ototoxicity, 123
Neurilemmoma, 284
Neuroblastoma
    Horner's syndrome in, 395
    nasal, 282
Neurodermatitis, external otitis and, 62
Neurofibroma, 284
Neurofibromatosis, 96,114–115
Neuroma, computer tomography in, 77
Newborn
    auditory brainstem response in, 162–163
    otitis media and, 78
Nicotinic acid, in sudden hearing loss, 139
Nisseria catarrhalis, in acute otitis media, 79
Nitrogen mustard
    in Burkitt's lymphoma, 277
    ototoxicity, 123
Noise exposure, risk criteria, 141
Noma, 346,347
Norepinephrine, 38
Norrie's disease, 118
Nose; *see also* Nasal terms
    bleeding of, 258–365; *see also* Epistaxis
    blood supply, 237–238,239,258
    cilia of, 5
    deformity, 257
    disorders of, *see* Nasal disorders
    examination, 243–246
    expiratory current, 241
    fetal development, 229–232
    filtering of inspired air by vibrissae of, 5
    foreign bodies in, 258
    fractures, 257,304–307; *see also* Nasal fractures
    functions of, 241–243
    inspiratory current, 241
    mucous blanket in, function of, 241
    mucous membranes, function of, 5
    mucus in, 241
        direction and rate of flow, 242
    nerve supply, 239–241
Nose drops, vasoconstrictors in, 254
Nystatin
    oral candidiasis, 348
    in otomycosis, 61

Obstructive sleep apnea, adenoid hypertrophy and, 368–369

Ocular motor system, 177
Oil of chenopodium, ototoxicity, 123
Olfaction, 8
Optokinetic testing, 186
Optokinetics, 178–179
Oral cavity, embryologic development, 318–319
Organ of Corti
    innervation of, 37
    receptor hair cells of, 31
Oropharynx
    carcinoma of, 395
    examination of, 328–329
Osler-Weber-Rendu disease, 261
Ossicular osteolyses, 87
Osteoma, 279
Osteomyelitis
    as a complication of sinusitis, 294–299
    in ethmoid complex, 294
    in the mandible, 334
    of the maxilla, 333
Osteosarcoma, 278
Otitis
    adhesive, 87
    barotrauma, 81
Otitis externa, *see* External otitis
Otitis media
    acute necrotizing, 78
    adenoidectomy and, 381
    allergy and, 70
    antibiotics in, 76,81
    brain abscess from, 91–92
    cleft palate and, 339
    diagnosis, 73–76
    differential diagnosis, 75
    follow-up of patients with, 76
    gram-negative pathogens in neonatal, 78
    hearing loss and, 101,157,213
    immunoglobulin electrophoresis in, 80
    incidence among children, 68
    intubation and, 78
    meningismus and, 75
    meningitis and, 78
    myringotomy in, 79–80
    neonatal, 78
    nonsuppurative, 66,67
        signs and symptoms, 73–74
        treatment, 81–85
    persistence of effective following acute, 67
    recurrent,
        hearing loss and, 135
        hypogammaglobulinemia in, 80
    septicemia and, 78
    serous, 45
    sulfonamides in, 81
    suppurative, 66,67
        acute, 75–76,79
        antibodies in, 72
        treatment, 81,82

Otitis media (*contd.*)
  treatment of, 76,81–85
  tympanic membrane perforation in, 76
Otomastoid system, radiologic examination, 76,78
Otomastoiditis, 76
  acute, 90
  acute petrositis and, 89
  chronic suppurative, 94
  complications of, 29
  facial nerve palsy in acute, 90
Otomycosis, 61
Otopalatodigital syndrome, 118
Otosclerosis, 46,115–116
Otoscope, surgical, 41
Ototoxicity, drug-induced,
  alcohol-induced, 123–126
Oxygen, exchange in alveoli, 4
Ozena, 288–289

Palatoglossus, 320
Palatopharyngeus, 320
Papilloma
  differential diagnosis, 274
  epistaxis and, 260,273
  of the larynx, 417–418
  malignant degeneration in, 274
  microcysts in, 274
  on the tongue, 352
  on the tonsil, 336
Parainfluenza virus, hearing loss and, 126
Parapharyngeal space, 323
  infection, 361–363,364
Paresis, eustachian tube and, 70
Parotid gland
  anatomy of, 321–322
  calculi, 403
  cystic hygroma involving, 403
  hemangioma, 404
  sarcoid infiltration, 403
  tumors, of vascular origin, 404
Patent ductus arteriosus ligation, 417
Pediatrician
  in rehabilitation of hearing-impaired child,
    224–227
  role in identification of hearing loss, 219–224
Pendred's syndrome, 107,117
Pendular eye tracking, 184–185
Penicillin
  in congenital syphilis, 133,249
  in Trench mouth, 347
Penicillium, 60
Periarteritis, Wegener's granulomatosis and,
    266,267
Perichondritis, 53, 54
Perilymph, volume, 32
Perilymphatic duct, 22
Peritonsillar space infection, 360–361
Petrositis, acute, 89–90

Pertussis, 10
Pharmacetin, ototoxicity, 123
Pharyngotonsillitis, 348
Pharynx
  anatomy, 322
  blood supply, 325
  lymphatic drainage, 326
  muscles of, 325
  nerve supply, 325
  primitive, 318
  stratified squamous epithelium of, 2
Phenylephrine, in epistaxis, 262
Phycomycetes, 60
Pierre-Robin syndrome, 206,339–340
Pinna, 53
  anatomy, 25
  formation of, 23,24,48
Plasmacytoma, in nasopharynx, 375–376
Plaut Vincent's infection, 347–348,354,355
Pneumootoscopy, 45
Politzerization, 83
Polybrene, ototoxicity, 123
Polymorphic reticulosis, 267
Polyp(s), 371
  nasal, 265
  verrucous, 274
Polypectomy, 257
  cavernous sinus thrombosis following, 299
Polytomography, nasal sinuses, 246
Positional tests, for vestibular assessment, 186
Pott's puffy tumor, 295
Pregnancy, vasomotor rhinitis and, 254
Prematurity, hearing loss and, 134
Proptosis, in orbital cellutitis, 293
Proteus, 60
  in acute otitis media, 79
Pseudomonas, 59,60
Pseudomonas aeruginosa, in acute otitis media,
    79
Psoriasis, external otitis and, 62
Purpura
  epistaxis associated with, 260
  hereditary, 261
Pyocele, 301–302

Queckenstedt test, 91
Quinine, ototoxicity, 123,125

Radiation therapy, carcinomatous change induced
    by, 419
Ramsey Hunt syndrome, 61
Ranula, 351
Reading
  disability, 199
  oral language comprehension and, 194
von Recklinghausen disease, 96,284

Reichert's cartilage, 22
Reidel's thyroiditis, 389
Reissner's membrane, 33
Resorcin, 61
Respiration, role of nose in, 241–242
Retropharyngeal space infections, 361,362,363
Rhabdomyosarcoma, 95
  external ear, 64
  of the larynx, 419
  in nasopharynx, 375
Rheumatic fever, epistaxis and, 261
Rhinitis
  allergic, 253–254
  atrophic, 254,288–289
  vasomotor, 254
Rhinitis medicamentosa, associated with topical
  decongestants, 82
Rhinoscleroma, nasal obstruction in, 268,269
Rhinoscopy, 246
  in diagnosing of middle ear effusion, 74
Rhinosinusitis, eustachian tube obstruction and, 70
Rhinosporidium seeberi, 270,272
Rhinosporidioris, nasal, 270,273
Rhinotomy, in frontonasal glioma, 283
Rhizopus, 60
Ristocetin, ototoxicity, 123
Rotational tests
  computerized, 188,189
  vestibular assessment via, 186–190
Rubella; *see also* Measles
  congenital, 127,128–131,132
  expanded syndrome, 129
  hearing loss associated with, 127,128–131,
    132
  lymph node enlargement in, 400
Rubeola, hearing loss and, 126
Russell body, in rhinoscleroma, 268

Saccades, 178
Saddle nose, 257
Salicylates, ototoxicity, 123,125–126
Salivary glands, 321–322
  disorders, 403
Sarcoidosis
  cervical gland swelling in, 400,401
  external otitis associated with, 62
  nasal obstruction in, 265
  uveitis in, 400,401
Sarcoma, of the jaw, 342,344
Saucerization, of nasal cysts, 286
Scarlatina rash, as complication of adenoiditis or
  tonsillitis, 357
Scarlet fever
  acute necrotizing otitis media and, 78
  tonsil hypertrophy following, 353
Scheibe's aplasia, 111
Schwannoma, 284

Sclerosing agents, mucous membrane scarring
  and, 18
Scopolamine, ciliary action of mucous membranes
  and, 18
Screamer's nodes, 420
Septicemia
  as complication of streptococcal tonsillitis or
    adenoiditis, 357
  epiglottitis and, 377
  otitis media and, 78
Sialadenitis, 404
Sialectasia, 404
Siallithiasis, 404
Sickle cell anemia, hearing loss and, 101
Sigmoid sinus, thrombophlebitis of, 91
Silver nitrate, mucous membrane scarring by, 18
Sinuses, branchial, 386,388; *see also* Nasal
  sinuses
Sinusitis, 289–303
  acute, 289–290,292
  adenoid hypertrophy and, 369
  chronic, 291–293
  common cold and, 249
  complications of, 293–303
  etiology, 290
  meningitis following, 300
  mucocele after, 301–302
  osteoma and, 279
  osteomyelitis secondary to, 294–299
  prevention of, 291
Soft palate, development of, 320
Somatostatin, 38
Speech
  communication and, 212
  development of, hearing loss and, 219
  disorders, 201–202,202–205
  laryngeal function and, 202
  normal development, 194–197
  potential risk factors for delayed, 199
  production of, 195
    cleft palate and, 205–207
    disorders of, 202
Sphenoid sinus, 235
  carcinoma of, 270
  mucocele in, 302
Staphylococcus, in furunculosis, 251,252
Staphylococcus aureus, 59,60
  in acute otitis media, 79
Staphylococcus epidermis, 59,60
Stenson's duct, 321–322
Steroid therapy, associated with, oral candidiasis,
  348
Stickler's syndrome, 206
Streptococcus, 60,356
  beta hemolytic, in acute otitis media, 79
  in erysipelas, 251
Streptococcus pneumoniae, in acute otitis media,
  79,81

Streptococcus viridans, 59
Streptomycin, ototoxicity, 123,124
Stridor
    differential diagnosis, 428
    in epiglottitis, 416
Sturge-Weber syndrome, hemangioma in, 418
Stuttering, 203–205
Submaxillary gland, 322
Submental space infection, 360,363–366
Sulfonamides, in combined therapy for otitis
        media, 81
Superior turbinate, 2
Supraglottitis, 413
Syphilis
    cervical gland swelling in, 400
    congenital
        hearing loss in, 101,133–134
        nasal disorders in, 249
        saddle nose and, 257
    hearing loss and, 101,133–134

Tandem Romberg testing, 188,190
Tangier disease, 359
Teeth
    development of, 326,327
    milk, eruption of, 327
Temporal bone, 29
    fractures, 144–147
        CSF otorrhea in, 146
        otogenic meningitis and, 92
    meningioma, 96
    neuroanatomy, 30–31
Temporal lobe abscess, otomastoiditis and, 29
Teratoma
    head and neck, 391
    in nasopharynx, 374
Tetracycline, in congenital syphilis, 133
Thalidomide, ototoxicity, 123
Thornwaldt's disease, 356
    nasopharyngeal bursa, 329
Thrombophlebitis, sigmoid sinus, 91
Thrombosis
    cavernous sinus, 299
    lateral sinus, otomastoiditis and, 29
    vascular, 357
Thyroglossal duct
    cysts of, 389,390
    fistula, 389,391
Thyroid gland, carcinoma of, 395,396
Thyroiditis, types of, 389
Tobacco, ototoxicity, 123
Tobramycin, ototoxicity, 124
Tomography, 52,246
Tongue
    abnormalities of, 343,345
    anatomy of, 320–321
    carcinoma of, 395
    hairy, 345
    stratified squamous epithelium of, 2

Tonsils, 323
    abscess of the, 357,360
    vs adenoids, 324
    anatomy of, 324
    antibody production and, 353
    as an antigen trap, 353
    atrophy of, age of onset, 352
    carcinoma of the, 367,395
    cysts on the, 367
    faucial, 323
    hemangioma in the, 367
    hypertrophy, 353–354
        viral infections and, 353
    immune function, 352–353
    infections of the, *see* Tonsillitis
    lingual, 323,324
    lymphocytes in, 353
    papilloma on the, 366
    tuberculous infections of the, 398–399
    tumors of the, 366–367
Tonsillectomy
    complications of, 380
    contraindications to, 379
    hemangioma diagnosis during, 367
    indications for, 354,379
    pulmonary complications following, 380
Tonsillitis
    acute, 354,357
    causative organisms, 356
    cervical glands in, 357
    chronic, 355
    complications of, 357
    diphtheria, 253
    exudative, 354
    follicular, 354,355
    inflammatory, 354
    lingual, 358
    membranous, 354
    middle ear effusions and chronic, 85
    pneumococcal, 356,357
    pseudomembranous, 354,358
    streptococcal, 356–357
    symptoms of, 354
    ulcerative, 354
    viral, 356
Tonsilloliths, 358–359
Torus mandibularis, 341
Torus palatinus, 340,341
Toxoplasmosis
    congenital, 132–133
    hearing loss and, 101,132–133
Transillumination, nasal sinuses, 246,247
Trauma
    acoustic, 140–143
    epistaxis and, 259–260
Treacher Collins syndrome, 49,50,114,340–341
Trench mouth, 347–348
Trichloroacetic acid, mucous membrane scarring
        by, 18

Triethanolamine, ciliary action of mucous
  membranes and, 18
Trimethoprim-sulfamethoxazole, in otitis media,
  81
Tubal inflation, in nonsuppurtive otitis media, 83
Tuberculosis
  external otitis associated with, 62
  mucous membranes and, 16
Tuberculous infection
  adenitis from cervical, 399
  nasal obstruction in, 265–266
  of the oral cavity, 350
  retropharyngeal abscess from, 322
Tunica propria, 1
Turbinates, as regulators of tissue fluids, 5
Turner's syndrome, 120,206
Tumors
  angiofibroma, 285
  Burkitt's lymphoma, 276–277,401
  chondroma, 275
  chrondrosarcoma, 275,276,277
  chordoma, 374
  connective tissue, 275–279
  cystic, 286–288,391–393
  eighth nerve, 96
  encephalocele, 283
  epithelial, 270–274
  Ewing's sarcoma, 277
  fibroma, 63–64,280,341,342,371
  fibromyxoma, 286
  fibrosarcoma, 278–279,341
  glioma, 283
  granuloma, 45,66,260,420
  head and neck, 391–397
  hemangioma, 260,284–285,367,
    392,404,418,419
  hygroma, 351,391–392
  of the jaw, 341–342,343,344
  lymphangioma, 345,404,420
  lymphoepithelioma, 367,375,393
  lymphoma, 275–277
  lymphosarcoma, 275–276,393,394
  melanoma, 270
  meningioma, 96,283–284
  mesodermal, 285–286
  mixed, of salivary origin, 352
  of the mouth, 351–352
  myxoma, 285
  nasal, 265–288
  nasopharyngeal, 369,371,376
  neurilemmoma, 284
  neuroblastoma, 282,395
  neurofibroma, 284
  neurogenic, 282
  neuroma, 77
  nonepithelial, 270
  osseous, 279
  osteoma, 279
  osteosarcoma, 278

  papilloma, 260,273–274,336,352,417–418
  sarcoma, 342,344
  schwannoma, 284
  of the tonsils, 366–367
  vascular, 284–285
Tympanic membrane, 23
  atrophy, 46,86
  bulging, 45
  bullous myringitis of the, 63
  calcific plagues in, 43
  complex with ossicular chain, disarticulation of,
    29
  conical apex, 28
  evaluation of, 42–43
  examination landmarks, 43
  hypermobility, 44
  hypervascularity, 75
  in middle ear effusions, 74
  necrosis, in acute otitis media, 78
  pars flaccids of, 27
  pars tensa of, 27
  perforation, 87–93
    hearing loss and, 101
    in otitis media, 76
    traumatic, 143–144
  physiology of, 28
  retraction of, 44
    middle ear effusions and, 83
  site of, 25
Tympanometry, 165–167
  in acute suppurative otitis media, 75
  in diagnosis of middle ear effusion, 74
Tympanoplasty, 93
Tympanosclerosis, 43,46,85,93
  hearing loss and, 101
Typhoid fever
  nasal perforations and, 260
  thrombotic desquamation of mucous membranes
    and, 9

Ultrasonography, in assessment of laryngeal
  function, 202
Usher's syndrome, 116–117
Uveitis, in sarcoidosis, 400,401

Vancomycin, ototoxicity, 123
Varicella-zoster virus, hearing loss and, 126
Vascular thrombosis, as complication of
  adenoiditis or tonsillitis, 357
Vasoconstrictors, in nose drops, 254
Velocardiofacial syndrome, 206
Vestibular dysfunction, postmeningitic deafness
  and, 136
Vestibular function, 175–176
  assessment of, 179–190
  computerized rotational testing for, 63
Vestibulo-ocular reflex, 178

Viomycin, ototoxicity, 123
Viral infections, 249–250
   pertussis associated with, 10
   tonsil hypertrophy and, 353
Vision loss, craniopharyngioma and, 374
Visual pursuit, 177,184–185
Voice disorders, 201
Vocal cord
   nodules, 420
   paralysis, 416–417
      Arnold-Chiari malformation and, 417
      neonatal, 417
      patent ductus arteriosus ligation and, 417

Waardenburg's syndrome, 112–113
   hearing loss and, 101

Waldeyer's ring, 323,352
Wax, ear, *see* Cerumen
Wegener's granulomatosis, 266–267
Wharton's duct, 322
Wildervaank's syndrome, 118

X-ray
   of nasal sinuses, 246
   otomastoid d system, 76,78

Yaws, external otitis associated with, 62

Zygoma, fracture of, 307